Handbook of Reoperative General Surgery

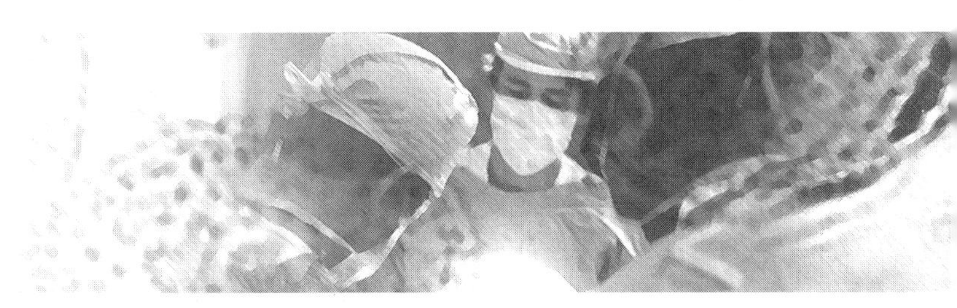

Brief Contents

Handbook of Reoperative General Surgery

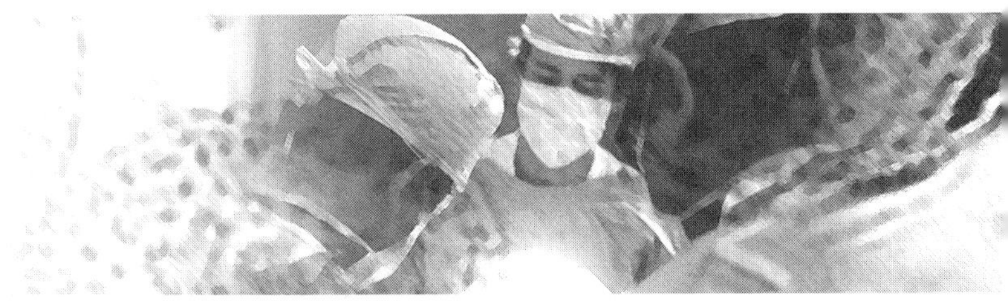

Mark P. Callery, MD, FACS

Chief, Division of General Surgery

Beth Israel Deaconess Medical Center

Associate Professor of Surgery

Harvard Medical School

Boston, Massachusetts

Foreword by Josef E. Fischer, MD, FACS

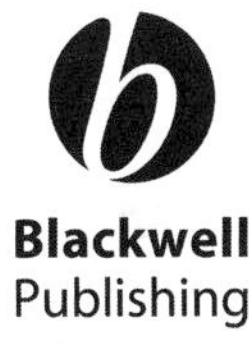

Blackwell
Publishing

Blackwell Publishing, Inc., 350 Main Street, Malden, Massachusetts 02148-5018, USA
Blackwell Publishing Ltd, 9600 Garsington Road, Oxford OX4 2DQ, UK
Blackwell Publishing Asia Pty Ltd, 550 Swanston Street, Carlton, Victoria 3053, Australia

05 06 07 08 5 4 3 2 1

ISBN-13: 978-1-4051-0473-9
ISBN-10: 1-4051-0473-2

Library of Congress Cataloging-in-Publication Data

Handbook of reoperative general surgery/edited by Mark P. Callery;
foreword by Josef E. Fischer.
p. ; cm.
Includes index.
ISBN-13: 978-1-4051-0473-9 (pbk. : alk. paper)
ISBN-10: 1-4051-0473-2 (pbk. : alk. paper)
1. Reoperation—Handbooks, manuals, etc. I. Callery, Mark P.
[DNLM: 1. Reoperation. WO 500 H236 2005]
RD33.65.H36 2005
617'.91—dc22

2005010291

A catalogue record for this title is available from the British Library

Acquisitions: Nancy Anastasi Duffy
Development: William Deluise
Production: Jennifer Kowalewski
Cover and Interior design: Leslie Haimes
Typesetter: International Typesetting and Composition in India
Printed and bound by Sheridan Books in Ann Arbor, MI

For further information on Blackwell Publishing, visit our website:
www.blackwellmedicine.com

Notice: The indications and dosages of all drugs in this book have been recommended in the medical literature and conform to the practices of the general community. The medications described do not necessarily have specific approval by the Food and Drug Administration for use in the diseases and dosages for which they are recommended. The package insert for each drug should be consulted for use and dosage as approved by the FDA. Because standards for usage change, it is advisable to keep abreast of revised recommendations, particularly those concerning new drugs.

The publisher's policy is to use permanent paper from mills that operate a sustainable forestry policy, and which has been manufactured from pulp processed using acid-free and elementary chlorine-free practices. Furthermore, the publisher ensures that the text paper and cover board used have met acceptable environmental accreditation standards.

With love and gratitude to Angela and our daughters,
Leah, Jacqueline and Brooke.

Table of Contents

Contributors

Christopher D. Anderson, MD
Division of Hepatobiliary Surgery and Liver Transplantation
Department of Surgery
Vanderbilt University Medical Center
Nashville, Tennessee

Mercedeh Baghai, MD
Emory Endosurgery Unit, Department of Surgery
Emory University School of Medicine
Atlanta, Georgia

Michel A. Bartoli, MD
Research Fellow in Vascular Surgery
Washington University School of Medicine
St. Louis, Missouri

George Blackburn, MD, PhD, FACS
Associate Professor of Surgery & Nutrition
Harvard Medical School
Director, Center for the Study of Nutrition Medicine
Beth Israel Deaconess Medical Center
Boston, Massachusetts

Mai N. Brooks, MD
Department of Surgery, Division of Surgical Oncology
UCLA David Geffen School of Medicine
Los Angeles, California

Darren R. Carpizo, MD, PhD
Department of Surgery, Division of Surgical Oncology
UCLA David Geffen School of Medicine
Los Angeles, California

Helena Chang, MD, PhD
Professor of Surgery
David Geffen School of Medicine at UCLA
Director of the Revlon/UCLA Breast Center
UCLA Medical Center
Los Angeles, California

Ravi S. Chari, MD
Chief, Division of Hepatobiliary Surgery and Liver Transplantation
Vanderbilt University Medical Center
Associate Professor of Surgery and Cancer Biology
Vanderbilt University School of Medicine
Nashville, Tennessee

Herbert Chen, MD, FACS
Chief of Endocrine Surgery
Department of Surgery
University of Wisconsin
Madison, Wisconsin

Eric J. DeMaria, MD, FACS
Director, Center for Minimally Invasive Surgery
Chair, Division of General & Endoscopic Surgery
Medical College of Virginia
Professor of Surgery
Chair, Division of General Surgery
Virginia Commonwealth University
Richmond, Virginia

David R. Fischer, MD
Assistant Professor of Surgery
University of Cincinnati
Attending Surgeon, Surgery
University of Cincinnati Surgeons, Inc.
Cincinnati, Ohio

Josef E. Fischer, MD
Chairman, Department of Surgery
Beth Israel Deaconess Medical Center
Mallinckrodt Professor of Surgery
Harvard Medical School
Boston, Massachusetts

Daniel B. Jones, MD, FACS
Chief, Section of Minimally Invasive Surgery
Beth Israel Deaconess Medical Center
Associate Professor of Surgery
Harvard Medical School
Boston, Massachusetts

Scott F. Gallagher, MD
Assistant Professor of Surgery
University of South Florida Health Sciences Center
Tampa, Florida

Kathrin Mayer, MD
Assistant Professor of Surgery
University of California, Davis School of Medicine
Attending Surgeon
University of California, Davis Medical Center
Sacramento, California

Michel M. Murr, MD, FACS
Director of Bariatric Surgery
Associate Professor of Surgery
University of South Florida Health Sciences Center
Tampa, Florida

Michael Nussbaum, MD, FACS
Associate Professor of Surgery
Vice Chairman, Clinical Affairs
Chief of Staff, The University Hospital
University of Cincinnati
Cincinnati, Ohio

Ram Nirula, MD
Assistant Professor of Surgery
Medical College of Wisconsin
Attending Surgeon, Division of Trauma/Critical Care
Froedtert Hospital
Milwaukee, Wisconsin

David A. Provost MD, FACS
Director, Center for the Surgical Management of Obesity
Associate Professor of Surgery
University of Texas Southwestern
Dallas, Texas

Sharona Ross, MD
Department of Surgery
University of South Florida Health Sciences Center
Tampa, Florida

Vivian M. Sanchez, MD
Instructor of Surgery
Section of Minimally Invasive Surgery
Beth Israel Deaconess Medical Center
Harvard Medical School
Boston, Massachusetts

Charles R. Scoggins, MD
Assistant Professor, Surgical Oncology
University of Louisville
Attending Surgeon
University and Norton Hospital
Louisville, Kentucky

Shimul A. Shah, MD
Fellow in Hepatobiliary Surgery
University of Toronto
Toronto, ONT, Canada

Rebecca S. Sippel, MD
Chief Resident in General Surgery
University of Wisconsin Hospitals and Clinics
Madison, Wisconsin

C. Daniel Smith, MD
Chief, General and Gastrointestinal Surgery
Emory University Hospital
Professor of Surgery
Emory University School of Medicine
Atlanta, Georgia

Nicholas E. Tawa, Jr., MD, PhD
Assistant Professor of Surgery
Harvard Medical School
Attending Surgical Oncologist
Beth Israel Deaconess Medical Center
Boston, Massachusetts

Robert W. Thompson, MD
Professor of Surgery, Cell Biology and Physiology
Washington University School of Medicine
Attending Surgeon
Barnes-Jewish Hospital
St. Louis, Missouri

Kent R. VanSickle, MD
Associate of Surgery
Emory University School of Medicine
Fellow, Department of Surgery
Emory University Hospital
Atlanta, Georgia

Charles M. Vollmer, Jr., MD
Visiting Assistant Professor of Surgery
Harvard Medical School
Department of Surgery
Beth Israel Deaconess Medical Center
Boston, Massachusetts

Mark L. Welton, MD
Associate Professor of Surgery
Stanford University School of Medicine
Stanford, California

Tonia Young-Fadok, MD, MS, FACS, FASCRS
Associate Professor of Surgery
Mayo Clinic College of Medicine
Consultant, Division of Colon and Rectal Surgery
Mayo Clinic
Scottsdale, Arizona

Foreword

I am delighted to write a foreword for Dr. Mark Callery's book on reoperative surgery. Dr. Callery was the first person that I recruited into the building of the Department of Surgery at Beth Israel Deaconess Medical Center. He has done spectacularly well at establishing a superb Division of General Surgery, several members of which are represented in this book, namely Dr. Nick Tawa, Dr. Daniel Jones, and Dr. Charles Vollmer. I'm also glad to see Dr. Michael Nussbaum's name as author of the chapter, "Reoperative Surgery for Intestinal Fistula," as he and I were very closely associated in the University of Cincinnati for many years. Most, if not all, of the individuals in this book are associated with tertiary quaternary centers. They deal, by nature, with problems that community hospitals, even the large ones, often do not relish to undertake largely because of absence of resident staff and other infrastructure.

The first component for caring for patients who need reoperative surgery is the nature of institution and the surgical residency. The surgical residency is the heart of every department of surgery, and its quality determines the quality of patient care that the department of surgery renders. However, there must be other components, including the ready availability of imaging and what I call "heavy radiology" which means CT scans, MRI, and angiography, the last of which now can be carried out by divisions of vascular surgery. In the study of results, it has become increasingly clear that the association of better outcomes with higher volume institutions is not just the result of the resources and abilities to care for complications, including ICUs, critical care, "heavy radiology," and other diagnostic or therapeutic techniques, but with surgeon volume and expertise as well. Dr. John Birkmeyer's recent article in the *New England Journal of Medicine* clearly suggests that in high volume hospitals, there are differences between high volume surgeons whose expertise apparently brings about better outcomes and those surgeons with less experience in difficult areas.[1] There is probably no truer situation where this applies than in reoperative surgery in which the cases are difficult to diagnose and evaluate; the patients must have pre-operative evaluations by skilled clinicians as well as consultants; and the surgeon must have the ability to test certain physiological parameters that determine what kind of reoperative surgery will take place. I found it interesting when Dr. Birkmeyer, in our mutual discussions, told me that he had expected, when undertaking the study, that it would be hospital volume that would be predominant in the outcomes and not surgical volume. This most recent paper in the *New England Journal of Medicine* reaffirms what all of us intrinsically know. At least partially, it is the skill of the individual surgeon, his or her judgment, and the surgeon's ability to prepare for a difficult operation that in large measure determines the outcome.

[1] Birkmeyer, John D., M.D. et al. "Surgeon Volume and Operative Mortality in the United States." *New England Journal of Medicine*. Volume 349:2117–2127, No. 22. Novermber 27, 2003.

In addition to operative skill, the successful reoperative surgeon must have developed a system of dealing with the complex reoperative surgery on the basis of not only experience, but also an underlying knowledge of the anatomy and physiology that enables safe approaches in difficult anatomic situations. There is also a necessity for some reality testing. To those of us who have dealt with reoperative surgery all of our careers, we know that, at least in abdominal surgery and the surgery of gastrointestinal fistulas, that the mortality varies directly with the state of the adhesions. While these may be modified somewhat by Separafilm, which in my own personal experience has proved useful in patients on whom I knew I was going to reoperate, in general, operations are most favorable when performed within 10 days after the prior operation and after 120 days when the adhesions have matured and become more filmy and less fleshy with a tendency to bleed and provoke enterotomies. This practice is something that is intrinsically known by surgeons and has been documented as being associated with the mortality of 20 percent when reoperative surgery has been performed between 10 and 120 days and only 10 percent when surgery is performed before 10 days and after 120 days. When I carry out reoperative surgery or operate on patients with fistulas, I always try to perform the operation more than 120 days after the last operation. This is possible when one is dealing with a large referral practice in which patients are referred often after unsuccessful attempts to close the fistula with failure, and the fistula has been present for some time.

There are certain characteristics that are essential to the successful reoperative surgeon. I've already pointed out the importance of familiarity with anatomy and pathophysiology and excellent judgment. Moreover, the surgeon must also have confidence in his or her ability to do the operation. The surgeon must use adequate exposure and help. Most importantly, he or she must set aside time for the performance of the operation. For example, it does little good to attempt to undertake an operation on a patient with a gastrointestinal fistula, an area with which I am intimately familiar, and think that the surgeon is going to complete it in three to four hours. The technically brilliant surgeon may accomplish this some of the time, but there will be times when the going is just so difficult that an indefinite amount of time should be allowed. One cannot do one's best job in reoperative surgery when one has their mind on an office full of patients waiting to see the surgeon.

Of the characteristics of the surgeon who does successful reoperative surgery, meticulous technique ranks high on the list. When there are two ways to do an operation, one of which in the surgeon's mind yields the best results, then that is the technique that should be followed. There should be adequate drainage of areas that are potentially infected or where the surgeon has to undertake preventative measures, for example, when one has to take bowel off the pancreas in which a pancreatic leak may be possibly expected.

Before the operation, the patient must be adequately prepared nutritionally and immunologically. If the patient's short turnover proteins are inadequate, and one has time to plan the operation, then the serum transferrin should be restored to normal (greater than 220 μg/dL) prior to the procedure. In patients with gastrointestinal fistulas, particularly those that are associated with mesh, inflammatory bowel disease, and colorectal disease, the ability to allow enough time for what is undoubtedly going to be a very difficult procedure is essential. Judgment as to what is acceptable, the ability to persevere when fatigued, and knowing that when one is fatigued one should not take on an entirely new area are attributes of a surgeon who will get a successful result with a low morbidity and mortality.

During the operation, one should enter the abdomen, if abdominal surgery is what is being discussed, or other areas, in a way that one can gain entrance to the operative area with less chance of doing any damage. In the case of the abdomen, one may choose to make a transverse incision when the original incisions may be vertical. If one has decided on a vertical incision, it may be that the original incisions may be short, in which case one can enter the abdomen cephalad or caudad. One must explore the entire abdomen, free up the entire bowel from the ligament of Treitz to the rectum, and get a clear idea of what the anatomy is.

In dissection, I have always used the technique of "taking what the abdomen will give me." In other words, if I am not making progress in one area, I have usually placed laparotomy sponges soaked in antibiotic solution on the bowel elsewhere so that when progress is at a standstill, I can go to a different area in a similar fashion where there is slight edema and one can see between the loops. Then, I dissect in that area.

Post-operatively, provisions should be made for post-operative nutrition, and I usually use a feeding jejunostomy of 14-Fr latex whistle-tip catheter, which may be above several of the anastomoses. I've always used hypo- or iso-osmolar enteral solutions. Bowel that is compromised in a vascular or an immunological sense cannot tolerate hyper-osmolar solutions. One should try and provide adequate post-operative nutrition either enterally, or, if caloric or protein parity cannot be achieved with enteral solutions alone, TPN should be utilized early. I always start with a hypo-osmolar solution, and in tube feeding, never try to stress a small bowel with significant solutions greater than an osmolality of 310 or 320. One can thus avoid pneumatosis and bowel necrosis in this fashion. Remember that manufacturers' labels are intended to sell more of the product, not to accurately describe the pathophysiology of tube feeding.

In the various chapters, there are different characteristics which should characterize each approach to reoperative surgery. In the case of gastric surgery and post-gastrectomy syndromes, it is wise to point out to the patient that they will not be 100 percent after the operation. They may get back to 60 or 70 percent of their pre-morbid state, but their eating mechanism will never resemble what was there previously. If they do, one has good fortune rather than surgical skill working in their direction. It is absolutely essential that the surgeon does his or her own endoscopy in patients with a post-gastrectomy syndrome to make certain that stenosis of the anastomosis, a scenario that is particularly applicable to stapled gastric anastomoses, be revised. Remember, few gastrointerologists, no matter how skillful, ever come into the operating room to feel an anastomosis and correlate it with its endoscopic appearance.

To be a reoperative gastric surgeon, it is critical that one is familiar with the post-gastrectomy literature and the various combination and permutations including Henle's loops, the length of bowel, and the size of the loop bowel, which can be reversed, for example, in post-vagotomy diarrhea (an operation which I never do as currently described). If one reads the original literature, one can see that a reversed 10 cm loop in post-gastrectomy and vagotomy diarrhea is almost certain, as it has been in my experience, to result in long-term intestinal obstruction.

Whether reoperative bariatric surgery should continue to be done laparoscopically really depends on the skill of the laparoscopist, and Dr. Jones is a superb laparoscopist. However, one suspects that, under these circumstances, it is probably extraordinarily difficult to do everything laproscopically, and an open approach may be necessary.

Reoperations on hernias are done for a number of reasons, including recurrence, but an increasing number of reoperations are attributed to the entrapment of nerves following a mesh repair, an unfortunate area in which I have ample experience. I see many individuals with this problem, and sometimes tincture of time or injections with steroids into the area of the trigger point or neuroma is appropriate. In many instances, it is required to take out whatever mesh one can and do an inguinal neurectomy of both nerves by tracing them laterally until they are relatively clean and free of adhesions then transecting them, tying them, and placing them under the muscle. In most patients, this would result in the ability to go on living their lives without excruciating pain.

With melanoma, Dr. Tawa will tell you that an adequate margin, especially in areas where the initial margin was inadequate, as well as taking fascia where available is essential if one is to salvage these patients. Nonetheless, the old adage that the best shot one has of curing a melanoma is the initial one is well taken. And no matter how skilled the surgeon is, there are a certain number patients who will be lost to melanoma even with the best of hands carrying out reoperative surgery.

Dr. Callery is a superb hepatobiliary surgeon technically, but he also excels because he has a comprehensive knowledge of the pathophysiology and anatomy of the field, which is essential if one is to save some of these patients, many of whom are reoperated on for malignant disease. In benign disease, such as chronic pancreatitis, the operation is difficult enough the first time, but the second and third time, one must have an extraordinary technique, as well as good appreciation for what is possible and what will work. Operations for relieving pain either by the identification of the splanchnic nerves within the abdomen, coeliac blocks, or transthoracic thoracoscopic splanchnic neurectomy, may be useful as an adjunct to this area.

Physiological evaluation as well as the knowledge of what tests to use is essential in gastroesophageal, gastric, and colorectal reoperation. Physiological testing of sphincter tone, gastroesophageal motility and reflux, the ability to differentiate spasm versus esophageal obstruction, the ability to do endoscopy and dilatation, and the use of non-operative approaches including medication and the knowledge of such medication cannot be overstated for the individual treating these disease areas. Sometimes, as the court for last resort, for example, in gastroesophageal surgery and particularly inflammatory bowel disease, the surgeon does the patient a great favor by rendering an opinion which states that operation is inappropriate and a judicious use of medication may be more efficacious for that particular patient.

In short, I am pleased to see this book on reoperative surgery. One would hope that since reoperative surgery is not an area that is well represented in the surgical literature, perhaps this book would be a basis of a larger work of reoperative surgery. While there have been some in the past, there is paucity of good textbooks in reoperative surgery. I salute the authors, and especially Dr. Callery, for their efforts and skill in caring for their patients with difficult surgical problems.

Josef E. Fischer, MD, FACS
Mallinckrodt Professor and Chairman
Department of Surgery
Beth Israel Deaconess Medical Center
June 2005

Preface

Why offer a new *Handbook of Reoperative General Surgery*? After all, reoperations have become more and more common as our field continues to grow, and as we care for patients living longer. Just about everyone gets experience, or thinks they do, in many types of reoperation during their training. Once on one's own, however, the real stakes become clear. Patients rarely present as straightforward and therefore require precise decision-making and tenacious management. The safety and predictability normal anatomy offers is gone. Unusual complications occur. Basic surgical principles may help, but innovation and insight are usually required to achieve the best operative and perioperative care. Will you be ready? Will your care reflect logic, knowledge, and confidence? Will you know key principles to help you succeed? Do you have the resources you need?

The guiding objective of this new *Handbook* is to help you succeed. At the concept level, this book was received enthusiastically by nearly all medical students, surgical residents, and faculty that I surveyed. They confirmed that very few published resources for reoperative general surgery are available. Those that are, while helpful, require updating, given the recent changes across our field. What follows is a current analysis of the elements of general surgery which most commonly require reoperation. I have invited, as senior chapter authors, some of America's most admired and talented young surgeons, all accepting with enthusiasm. For you, they have delivered what you need to know to succeed, developing each element along traditional principles of pathophysiology, anatomy, and diagnosis, while revealing the non-traditional challenges reoperation will create. Each chapter provides the key literature citations, both older and new, that you'll need.

Who better to provide your invited foreword than Josef E. Fischer, MD, FACS, whose clinical legacy is reoperative general surgery? With over 35 years' experience and countless lessons learned, Dr. Fischer continues to embark on clinical journeys from which most rightfully recoil. Indeed he has what it takes, but more importantly, he now lays it out for you in clear language. He emphasizes preparation, and recommends leaving no stone unturned in your workup. To proper nutritional care he weds meticulous operative technique. His foreword will make you think, but it may also instill a new confidence in you as a clinician.

Because highlighting each chapter will only delay your entry into this *Handbook,* I will not. Instead, I welcome you to consider what formidable opponents the liver, biliary tract, and pancreas are during reoperation. Consider how critical diagnosis and operative strategy are for breast cancer. Learn the principles and realities of getting the multiply injured patient through repeated operations safely. Galvanize your approach to dealing with reoperations on all areas of the gastrointestinal tract, including the fistulas it can haunt you with. Learn how to reassure and help the patient with yet another hernia recurrence and pain. Enjoy the only précis on reoperative bariatric surgery I know of.

With this *Handbook,* you can be ready, and you can succeed. You'll learn basic principles for reoperation that will carry you forward. You'll hear from experience which will help you understand how to benefit from your own. You'll learn to understand why and when you yourself or your resources have reached the limit. We hope that both you and your patients will benefit from this *Handbook*. Best wishes for success!

Mark P. Callery, MD, FACS
June 2005

Acknowledgements

In addition to my co-contributors, I thank William Deluise and Jennifer Kowalewski of Blackwell Publishing for their professionalism, talents, and tenacity in bringing *Handbook of Reoperative General Surgery* to press. My administrative assistants Ailicet Montilla and Amy Hayward also helped ease the process along. I thank my many teachers and colleagues in Surgery from medical school through today. A few warrant special mention and gratitude for their extraordinary mentorship including Martin McKneally, Samuel Wells Jr, Wayne Flye, Nathaniel Soper, Sir David Carter, O. James Garden, Steven Strasberg, William Meyers, and Josef Fischer. Finally, I thank my patients and their families.

CHAPTER 1

Reoperative Hepatobiliary Surgery

Christopher D. Anderson, MD; Charles R. Scoggins, MD; Ravi S. Chari, MD

Précis

Reoperative hepatic and biliary surgery are common strategies aimed at increasing the resectability of primary hepatobiliary and metastatic hepatic tumors. This chapter discusses the most common indications for reoperative hepatobiliary surgery, alternatives to reoperation, and important perioperative considerations.

Reoperative Hepatic Surgery

RECURRENT METASTATIC COLORECTAL CANCER

Nearly 150,000 cases of colorectal carcinoma (CRC) will be diagnosed in the United States in 2003.[1] Over one-half of patients will metastasize, most commonly to regional lymph nodes and the liver.[2,3] Hepatectomy has become the treatment of choice for metastatic colorectal cancer to the liver.[3–5] Modern surgical techniques and perioperative care have allowed for an ever-increasing number of hepatic resections to be performed with a minimum of complications. Unfortunately, recurrent liver disease occurs in up to 60% to 70% of resected patients, thus necessitating retreatment in a number of patients.[5–7]

Numerous studies have shown efficacy of hepatectomy for the treatment of metastatic colorectal cancer.[2,8–13] Low rates of morbidity and mortality for liver resection, along with 5-year survival rates of over 35%, have led to widespread acceptance of liver resection for this disease.[9,12,14] As more patients are treated with liver resection, the number of patients experiencing recurrent disease has increased.

Studies attempting to preoperatively predict those patients at greater risk of failure following hepatectomy for metastatic CRC have been conducted. In a study by Fong et al with 1001 patients from the Memorial Sloan-Kettering Cancer Center,

Table 1-1 Survival Data for Second Hepatectomy for Metastatic CRC

Author	Recurrence (n)	Morbidity (%)	Mortality (%)	Survival
Nordlinger 1994[16]	130	24.7	0.9	3-year 33%
Pinson 1996[19]	10	ND	0	2-year 88%
Adam 1997[17]	64	20	0	5-year 41%
Tuttle 1997[23]	23	22	0	5-year 32%
Chiappa 1999[15]	26	20	0	4-year 44%
Suzuki 2001[22]	26	27	0	5-year 32%
Yamada 2001[21]	11	ND	0	5-year 45%
Petrowsky 2002[18]	126	28	1.6	5-year 34%

ND, not defined.

several clinical factors were found to be predictors of recurrence following metastasectomy.[13] These clinical predictors were margin positivity, the presence of extrahepatic disease, number of tumor nodules greater than 1, carcinoembryonic antigen (CEA) above 200 ng/mL, tumor size greater than 5 cm, node-positive primary lesions, and disease-free interval of less than 12 months. When combined into a clinical score, the predictive power of failure was felt to be significant, with no patients with a score of 5 being a long-term survivor.[13]

Patients who recur following liver resection pose a therapeutic dilemma. Those with failure confined to the liver may be considered for reresection. The morbidity rate associated with reoperative liver resection in this setting has been reported between 20% and 25%—this is no different than that seen with primary hepatectomy.[15–19] Survival data following second hepatectomy for metastatic CRC has demonstrated acceptable results (Table 1-1). There is a survival benefit to repeat hepatectomy when compared to patients with unresectable recurrence.[23] Long-term survival rates approaching 40% have been reported.[15,17,18,21] Factors associated with poor survival after repeat hepatectomy include extensive disease, short time interval (less than 12 months) between hepatectomies, and positive surgical margins.[17,18,20–22]

RECURRENT HEPATOCELLULAR CARCINOMA

Hepatocellular carcinoma (HCC) is a relatively uncommon disease in the United States; however, in Asian countries it is one of the most common causes of cancer-related death.[1] For patients with early HCC and decompensated cirrhosis, liver transplantation is considered the treatment of choice.[24,25] The overall 5-year survival for patients undergoing transplantation is greater than 50%.[26,27] Surgical resection remains one of the best treatment modalities in patients without concomitant cirrhosis, but because of recurrence in 40% of patients, resection may only be used as a "bridge" to transplantation in selected patients.[28,29] Repeat hepatectomy, when possible, has been demonstrated as the best treatment modality for recurrent disease.[28,29]

Multicentricity of disease and early portal venous invasion have been postulated as causes of the high recurrence rate following hepatectomy for HCC.[29,30]

Table 1-2 Survival Data for Repeat Hepatectomy for Recurrent HCC

Author	Reference	Recurrence (n)	Morbidity (%)	Mortality (%)	Survival
Nakajima 1993[35]	34	14	ND	ND	5-year 92%
Matsuda 1993[28]	27	22	9	0	5-year 51.2%
Lee 1995[29]	28	13	46	0	3-year 44.8%
Hu 1996[30]	29	59	15	3	3-year 44%
Poon 1999[34]	33	11	ND	ND	5-year 69.3%

ND, not defined.

Surgical factors relating to hepatectomy that have been shown to negatively affect outcome with respect to recurrence are positive margins of resection, very high AFP level, venous invasion, and large tumor size.[31–33] While the disease-free survival following repeat hepatectomy is shorter than that for primary resection, the 5-year survival following repeat hepatectomy for recurrent HCC is as high as 92% (Table 1-2).[28–30,33–35]

Repeat hepatic resection for recurrent HCC has also been shown to be superior to chemoembolization and ethanol injection.[34,35] In a study from Hong Kong, Poon et al demonstrated the 5-year survival rate for recurrent patients treated with percutaneous ethanol injection to be 0%, as compared to 20.9% following chemoembolization, and 69.3% for patients undergoing repeat hepatectomy.[34]

ALTERNATIVES TO REPEAT RESECTION

Radiofrequency ablation (RFA) is an evolving technology that is gaining popularity for the treatment of patients with unresectable primary and metastatic liver tumors.[34] This technique is becoming an important alternative and a complementary modality in the treatment of unresectable HCC and liver metastatic colorectal carcinoma.[36] It can be performed percutaneously, laparoscopically, or during laparotomy with a complication rate of 5% to 13% in most series.[37–41] Efficacy, however, is not as clear; most published reports have short follow-up periods, thus there is poor data regarding recurrence and disease-free survival following RFA. The largest of the clinical series report local recurrence rates of up to 39%, but this modality may be a viable option for recurrent, unresectable liver tumors.[42–50]

INTRAOPERATIVE CONSIDERATIONS IN REPEAT HEPATIC SURGERY

For both initial and repeat hepatic surgery, safe hepatic resection and biliary surgery are dependent on control of hemorrhage. Dissection of adhesions between the hepatic remnant and adjacent viscera must be careful and deliberate and should be conducted with electrocautery. An important consideration for repeat hepatic resection are the hepatic veins, which can be very close to the surface of the previous resection. Care should be taken, especially when mobilizing the liver off the diaphragm, as small tears in the liver capsule can result in significant lacerations during retraction and manipulation of the liver and give rise to significant blood loss. To prevent this hemorrhage, maintaining a low CVP from the onset of these cases is important. Hemorrhage from the low-pressure veins can be controlled with digital pressure or parenchymal compression. Another maneuver that can minimize hemorrhage is circumferential access to the hepatoduodenal ligament. When recurrent tumor mandates mobilization of the liver off the vena cava, and previous mobilization of the liver off the vena cava has occurred, careful exposure of the vena cava above and below the liver should be performed as an initial maneuver, in the event that total vascular exclusion of the liver is necessary to control vena caval bleeding.

Intraoperative ultrasound is critical to clarify distorted anatomy that may be encountered in repeat hepatic surgery. Because previous liver resection induces an asymmetric regenerative response, normal anatomic relations often vary. Preoperative CT and MRI can be used to create a three-dimensional picture in the surgeon's mind, but final clarification is often left to the operating room. Intraoperative U/S will help clarify the relation between hepatic vascular structures (with the aid of color-flow Doppler), biliary structures, and viscera. Bile duct injury is a significant potential source of major morbidity, and mandates absolute identification before ligation of any major branches. If ductal anatomy is unclear, identification by way of interoperative U/S or cholangiogram may be useful. Alternatively, deferring ductal ligation until parenchymal transection may also eliminate the risk of ductal injury.

Following mobilization of the liver, hepatic parenchymal transection can be conducted much the same as it is in a primary operation. The techniques available are many and are beyond the scope of this chapter. The choice of anatomic versus subsegmental/wedge resection should be made on the basis of margin, quality of liver, and anticipated remnant following the second operative intervention.

Reoperative Biliary Surgery

Postoperative biliary strictures are the most common indication for reoperation on the biliary tract. The majority (80%) of benign biliary strictures result from bile duct injury during laparoscopic cholecystectomy. Most large series report the incidence of ductal injury following laparoscopic cholecystectomy to be 0.3% to 0.85%.[51] Other, less common benign postoperative biliary strictures occur following bile duct reconstruction, tumor resection, or liver transplantation. More rare indications for reoperative biliary surgery include retained or recurrent choledocholithiasis and nonstricture complications of hepatobiliary surgery.

The clinical presentation of patients with benign postoperative biliary strictures following a bile duct injury varies with the type of injury and the time after injury. Historically, following open cholecystectomy, 10% of patients presented within the first week, 70% within 6 months, and 80% within 1 year.[52] In a recent study of 156 patients referred for management of biliary strictures resulting from bile duct injuries, 9.3% of injuries were recognized during laparoscopic versus 0% during open cholecystectomy.[53] In this series of 156 patients with postoperative biliary strictures, 49 (31.4%) presented with leaks, 42 (26.9%) presented with jaundice, and 50 (32.1%) presented with cholangitis.[53] In general, patients with a bile leak will present early, whereas patients with postoperative biliary strictures alone often present with jaundice or cholangitis months to years following the initial injury.

Inappropriate management of biliary strictures may result in significant morbidity and mortality secondary to complications such as biliary cirrhosis or cholangitis. In a 12-year review of 130 patients with postoperative biliary strictures, the causes of mortality were all related to the presence of liver parenchymal disease with portal hypertension. Of these patients, 23 (17.7%) had evidence of portal hypertension at the time of referral.[54]

DIAGNOSIS

Abdominal imaging with U/S or CT should be performed in patients with signs of peritonitis, sepsis, or any other clinical suspicion of biloma. Such patients must be stabilized with immediate parenteral antibiotics and image-guided percutaneous drainage of any fluid collections. Patients with signs and symptoms of cholangitis should undergo urgent cholangiogram with biliary drainage. In patients with a biliary stricture following resection of a biliary tumor, triple-phase contrasted CT, and possibly a positron emission tomography (PET), will help distinguish a benign stricture from a tumor recurrence.[55]

Cholangiography should be performed to establish the presence of ductal stricture, identify the level of the stricture, and identify the nature of the injury when necessary. In one study of 88 patients with bile duct injuries from laparoscopic cholecystectomy, attempts at repair were unsuccessful in 27 (96%) of 28 when preoperative cholangiograms were not performed, and 28 of 41 (69%) were unsuccessful when data from cholangiograms were incomplete.[56] It is important that the method of cholangiography provide detail of the intrahepatic ductal system and the bile duct confluence. Although percutaneous transhepatic cholangiography (PTC) is the imaging method of choice for most postoperative biliary strictures, expertise with this method is not available at all centers. Endoscopic retrograde cholangiopancreatography (ERCP) may be easier to obtain in a patient with a biliary stricture and cholangitis who requires urgent cholangiography and biliary decompression. However, this is only useful in patients with bile duct continuity. If the biliary stricture is too tight to pass with ERCP, PTC may be performed for proximal biliary decompression. A number of centers employing similar algorithms have demonstrated successful outcomes.[57–59] In patients who have had a previous biliary resection with biliary enteric bypass, cholangiography is usually best achieved with PTC.

Arteriography should be considered in the preoperative evaluation of patients with benign biliary strictures. Unrecognized injury to the hepatic artery or a portal vein branch occurs with a frequency of 12% to 47% concomitant with a bile duct injury.[54,60–62] Certainly, if significant bleeding required urgent control at the time of the original operation, a vascular injury should be considered. However, the clinical consequences of hepatic artery injury are not fully known, but at least one study suggests that the presence of a right hepatic artery disruption should not affect the surgical repair of a bile duct injury.[62] In patients presenting with late strictures and evidence of liver dysfunction, an arteriogram should be performed to evaluate for evidence of portal hypertension.

INTRAOPERATIVE CONSIDERATIONS IN REPEAT BILIARY SURGERY

The management of postoperative biliary strictures following ductal injury depends on the degree of injury, the presence of stricture-induced complications, and the operative risk of the patient. A multidisciplinary team consisting of experienced interventional radiologists, endoscopists, and surgeons is essential to the success of these challenging complications.[57,59,61,63,64] After recognition of a bile duct injury or stricture, this team, coordinated by an experienced hepatobiliary surgeon should plan the following specific goals: (1) control of infection (abscess or cholangitis), (2) drainage of biloma, (3) complete cholangiography, and (4) definitive therapy with controlled reconstruction or stenting.[65]

These goals do not mandate elaborate workup and delayed repair in all cases. Some data suggest that immediate repair of bile duct injury from cholecystectomy can give good results with low morbidity when performed properly;[66] more recent data, however, suggest that inexperience with the repairs leads to recurrent stricture, failure of the repair, and potentially secondary liver parenchymal damage from unrelieved obstruction.[67–69] One recent study has suggested that the independent predictors of stricture recurrence following an initial operative repair include cholangitis before the initial repair, incomplete cholangiography, and primary repair within 3 weeks of the bile duct injury.[69] When a bile duct injury is recognized at the time of cholecystectomy (or other operation) conditions should be optimized before repair. If immediate repair is to be attempted, consultation with more experienced surgeons should be made. If expertise is not available at the time of a recognized injury, or if difficult circumstances preclude elaborate reconstructive attempts, external biliary drains will allow the patient to recover before being transferred to a center of excellence.

Successful repair of biliary strictures following appropriate preoperative management requires adherence to specific surgical principles: (1) the use of proximal bile duct with minimal inflammation, (2) the creation of a tension-free anastomosis with the use of a Roux-en-Y jejunal limb, and (3) a direct mucosa-to-mucosa anastomosis. Historically, an end-to-end bile duct anastomosis was encouraged, because it preserved the normal anatomy and theoretically reduced the possibility of cholangitis. However, multiple reports suggest that primary repair of the bile duct is associated with a 40% to 50% long-term failure rate.[70,71] Direct operative biliary-enteric bypass is the gold standard procedure for the long-term treatment of biliary strictures. These procedures have low operative mortality and acceptable morbidity.[53,54,64,72,73]

An adequate incision permitting full visualization is necessary for a good biliary enteric anastomosis. A right subcostal incision extended to either the midline or the left (chevron incision) is usually necessary. The liver should be completely freed from the diaphragm, and adhesions from previous operations should be taken down to facilitate creation of a Roux-en-Y jejunal limb if necessary. Patients who have had previous biliary tract operations will inevitably require an extensive adhesiolysis to separate the duodenum and colon from the hilum and gallbladder fossa. Great care should be used to avoid colotomy or enterotomy. In reoperative biliary surgery, the need for extensive liver mobilization is less than in reoperative hepatic surgery. Because reoperative surgery often requires hilar dissection, however, the risk of bleeding is still high. Often, the plane around the vascular structures (i.e., hepatic artery and portal vein) has not been accessed in previous surgery. By following the tissue planes around the major vessels, not only is their safety ensured, but dissection is facilitated. In most cases, the biliary system is anterior to both the hepatic artery and portal vein, and by mobilizing the structures anterior to the portal vein and hepatic artery, the bile duct is defined. Additionally, the hilar plate is frequently intact from previous surgery. The hilar plate can be raised with minimal risk to enable broad access to the biliary tree.

The Hepp-Couinaud approach to bile duct reconstruction is the best option in most circumstances.[74] This technique requires dissection of the hilar plate to expose the left hepatic duct and allow for a side-to-side anastomosis of the left hepatic duct to the Roux-en-Y jejunal limb.[75-78] The technical aspects of this and other biliary-enteric anastomosis have been well reviewed by Blumgart.[73,76-78] In general, care should be taken not to devascularize any portion of the proximal bile ducts to prevent the occurrence of a late ischemic stricture. A widely patent mucosa-to-mucosa anastomosis is essential, and creation of an "access loop" from the proximal portion of the Roux-en-Y limb for future interventional radiologic access is useful.[76,79]

INTERVENTIONAL RADIOLOGIC AND ENDOSCOPIC TECHNIQUES

Interventional radiologic techniques are useful in patients with bile duct injuries, leaks, or postoperative strictures. These techniques allow percutaneous drainage of abdominal fluid collections, preoperative identification of the ductal anatomy via PTC, and stricture dilation with or without placement of palliative stents for bile drainage in the patient whose overall physiologic status precludes a major operation. Percutaneous transhepatic dilatation can be used in patients with intrahepatic ductal disease or those in whom ERCP is not possible. It is often used as an adjunct to operative repair to assist with identification of the proximal biliary tree for reconstruction and for the dilation of anastomotic strictures.

The success rate of percutaneous transhepatic dilation is reported between 50% and 70%.[80,81] Patients with anastomotic strictures (including biliary-enteric anastomotic strictures) have the highest success rates.[79] A study of 89 patients treated for major bile duct injuries following laparoscopic cholecystectomy showed that percutaneous dilation yielded only a 64% success rate at 27 months in patients with ischemic strictures versus 92% at 33.4 months in patients with biliary-enteric anastomotic strictures.[82] In addition, while mortality following percutaneous dilation is low, the complication rates are reported as high as 35%, and consist mainly of hemobilia, cholangitis, and bile leaks.[83] These procedures often require multiple sessions of dilation to achieve long-term success rates.

When reported from large-volume centers, endoscopic and percutaneous methods of dilation have equivalent efficacy.[84,85] Endoscopic dilation of benign extrahepatic biliary strictures is also a useful adjunctive option in patents with a dominant extrahepatic stricture causing clinical symptoms. In general, treatment of biliary strictures with this technique, as with interventional radiologic methods, requires multiple sessions of dilations, and nonischemic strictures (i.e., anastomotic strictures) respond best. Endoscopic dilation also has a low mortality, but it has a significant morbidity rate. The more common complications following endoscopic biliary interventions include hemobilia, bile leak, pancreatitis, and cholangitis. In one early study of 25 patients with biliary strictures treated with endoscopic dilation, clinical improvement was noted in 22 (88%), with only an 8% complication rate.[86] In another study of 101 patients with benign biliary strictures, 66 patients were treated endoscopically with a reported restricture rate of 12 (18%) at 3 months and a complication rate of 35%.[87] While endoscopic and interventional radiologic procedures are not ideal long term treatments for biliary strictures, endoscopic stenting and drainage is a very successful treatment option for cystic duct leak or small common bile duct leaks following laparoscopic cholecystectomy.[88,89]

Careful long-term follow-up of patients with biliary strictures treated with percutaneous or endoscopic dilation methods is required, because ischemic biliary strictures will not respond permanently to dilation. Early retreatment (via repeat dilation or biliary-enteric reconstruction) of postdilation recurrent strictures is essential to prevent secondary biliary cirrhosis. The risk of additive morbidity from the required repeat sessions and of late stricture recurrence should be discussed with patients when treatment options for benign biliary strictures are being considered.

Percutaneous and endoscopic methods of dilation and stent placement are good methods for palliative care in patients with unresectable or recurrent biliary tract tumors. A discussion on this topic is beyond the scope of this chapter, but has been recently reviewed.[90]

CHOLEDOCHOLITHIASIS FOLLOWING BILIARY SURGERY

Approximately 1% to 2% of patients undergoing cholecystectomy will have stones left in the common bile duct that will require further intervention.[91] While there is debate over the ideal treatment for stones discovered by intraoperative cholangiogram, retained or recurrent bile duct stones can usually be managed with nonoperative methods. Traditionally, mechanical extraction of stones via a T tube fistula tract was the treatment of choice, but in the era of laparoscopic cholecystectomy, the use of a T tube is essentially obsolete. The preferred initial procedure for the extraction of recurrent or retained bile duct stones is ERCP with sphincterotomy.[92] This method has a reported success rate of more than 85%.[93–97] If this method fails or is technically impossible because of previous biliary enterostomy, percutaneous methods may be attempted. If these methods fail, operative re-exploration is necessary. Reoperation for retained or recurrent stones can be performed by experienced surgeons with an operative morbidity and mortality identical to endoscopic sphincterotomy.[97–100] The operation for patients with retained or recurrent stones must clear the common duct of stones and ensure free distal ductal drainage. Simple common bile duct exploration has reported failure rates of up to 33%.[101–103] Transduodenal sphincteroplasty can allow clearance of common bile duct stones and dependable long-term biliary drainage when there is no proximal biliary stricture and the common bile duct is less than 1.5 cm in diameter.[104] In settings of stone formation secondary to stricture or inflammation of the bile ducts, choledochoduodenostomy, Roux-en-Y choledochojejunostomy, or Roux-en-Y hepatojejunostomy are the procedures of choice.[97]

BILIARY REOPERATIONS FOLLOWING LIVER TRANSPLANTATION

Biliary complications occur frequently (4% to 29%) following liver transplantation.[71,105–107] These complications represent a major source of morbidity following transplantation. The majority of these complications have historically been attributed the use of T tubes for the biliary reconstruction.[108–112] Despite the decreased use of T tubes in the transplant biliary reconstruction, the overall rate of anastomotic stricture remains significant.[107] The initial management of extrahepatic posttransplantation strictures is via percutaneous or endoscopic techniques. Overall success of stricture dilation in this setting is between 45% and 80%.[83,84,112,113] Intrahepatic biliary strictures occurring after liver transplantation are much more difficult to manage, and up to 50% of these patients may require liver resection with segmental bypass procedures or retransplantation.[107,114,115]

Biliary stones occurring posttransplantation can usually be managed with endoscopic or operative techniques similar to those for retained stones in nontransplant patients.

REFERENCES

1. Jemal A, Murray T, Samuels A, et al. Cancer statistics, 2003. CA Cancer J Clin 2003;53:5–26.
2. Steele G, Jr., Ravikumar TS. Resection of hepatic metastases from colorectal cancer. Biologic perspective. Ann Surg 1989;210:127–138.
3. Scheele J. Hepatectomy for liver metastases. Br J Surg 1993;80:274–276.
4. Scheele J, Stangl R, Altendorf-Hofmann A, Gall FP. Indicators of prognosis after hepatic resection for colorectal secondaries. Surgery 1991;110:13–29.
5. Fortner JG. Recurrence of colorectal cancer after hepatic resection. Am J Surg 1988;155:378–382.
6. Holm A, Bradley E, Aldrete JS. Hepatic resection of metastasis from colorectal carcinoma. Morbidity, mortality, and pattern of recurrence. Ann Surg 1989;209:428–434.

7. Hughes KS, Simon R, Songhorabodi S, et al. Resection of the liver for colorectal carcinoma metastases: a multi-institutional study of patterns of recurrence. Surgery 1986;100:278–284.

8. D'Angelica M, Brennan MF, Fortner JG, et al. Ninety-six five-year survivors after liver resection for metastatic colorectal cancer. J Am Coll Surg 1997;185: 554–559.

9. Hughes KS, Rosenstein RB, Songhorabodi S, et al. Resection of the liver for colorectal carcinoma metastases. A multi-institutional study of long-term survivors. Dis Colon Rectum 1988;31:1–4.

10. Jarnagin WR, Gonen M, Fong Y, et al. Improvement in perioperative outcome after hepatic resection: analysis of 1,803 consecutive cases over the past decade. Ann Surg 2002;236:397–406.

11. Scheele J, Stangl R, Altendorf-Hofmann A. Hepatic metastases from colorectal carcinoma: impact of surgical resection on the natural history. Br J Surg 1990;77: 1241–1246.

12. Scheele J, Stang R, Altendorf-Hofmann A, Paul M. Resection of colorectal liver metastases. World J Surg 1995;19:59–71.

13. Fong Y, Fortner J, Sun RL, et al. Clinical score for predicting recurrence after hepatic resection for metastatic colorectal cancer: analysis of 1001 consecutive cases. Ann Surg 1999;230:309–318.

14. Nordlinger B, Quilichini MA, Parc R, et al. Hepatic resection for colorectal liver metastases. Influence on survival of preoperative factors and surgery for recurrences in 80 patients. Ann Surg 1987;205:256–263.

15. Chiappa A, Zbar AP, Biella F, Staudacher C. Survival after repeat hepatic resection for recurrent colorectal metastases. Hepatogastroenterology 1999;46:1065–1070.

16. Nordlinger B, Vaillant JC, Guiguet M, et al. Survival benefit of repeat liver resections for recurrent colorectal metastases: 143 cases. Association Francaise de Chirurgie. J Clin Oncol 1994;12:1491–1496.

17. Adam R, Bismuth H, Castaing D, et al. Repeat hepatectomy for colorectal liver metastases. Ann Surg 1997;225:51–60.

18. Petrowsky H, Gonen M, Jarnagin W, et al. Second liver resections are safe and effective treatment for recurrent hepatic metastases from colorectal cancer: a bi-institutional analysis. Ann Surg 2002;235:863–871.

19. Pinson CW, Wright JK, Chapman WC, et al. Repeat hepatic surgery for colorectal cancer metastasis to the liver. Ann Surg 1996;223:765–773.

20. Nakamura S, Sakaguchi S, Nishiyama R, et al. Aggressive repeat liver resection for hepatic metastases of colorectal carcinoma. Surg Today 1992;22:260–264.

21. Yamada H, Katoh H, Kondo S, et al. Repeat hepatectomy for recurrent hepatic metastases from colorectal cancer. Hepatogastroenterology 2001;48:828–830.

22. Suzuki S, Sakaguchi T, Yokoi Y, et al. Impact of repeat hepatectomy on recurrent colorectal liver metastases. Surgery 2001;129:421–428.

23. Tuttle TM, Curley SA, Roh MS. Repeat hepatic resection as effective treatment of recurrent colorectal liver metastases. Ann Surg Oncol 1997;4:125–130.

24. Helton WS, Di Bisceglie A, Chari R, et al. Treatment strategies for hepatocellular carcinoma in cirrhosis. J Gastrointest Surg 2003;7:401–411.

25. Bruix J, Llovet JM. Prognostic prediction and treatment strategy in hepatocellular carcinoma. Hepatology 2002;35:519–524.

26. Klintmalm GB. Liver transplantation for hepatocellular carcinoma: a registry report of the impact of tumor characteristics on outcome. Ann Surg 1998;228: 479–490.

27. Figueras J, Jaurrieta E, Valls C, et al. Survival after liver transplantation in cirrhotic patients with and without hepatocellular carcinoma: a comparative study. Hepatology 1997;25:1485–1489.

28. Matsuda Y, Ito T, Oguchi Y, et al. Rationale of surgical management for recurrent hepatocellular carcinoma. Ann Surg 1993;217:28–34.

29. Lee PH, Lin WJ, Tsang YM, et al. Clinical management of recurrent hepatocellular carcinoma. Ann Surg 1995;222:670–676.

30. Hu RH, Lee PH, Yu SC, et al. Surgical resection for recurrent hepatocellular carcinoma: prognosis and analysis of risk factors. Surgery 1996;120:23–29.

31. Ikeda K, Saitoh S, Tsubota A, et al. Risk factors for tumor recurrence and prognosis after curative resection of hepatocellular carcinoma. Cancer 1993;71: 19–25.

32. Kimura H, Yabushita K, Konishi K, et al. Prognostic factors in resected hepatocellular carcinomas and therapeutic value of transcatheter arterial embolization for recurrences. Int Surg 1998;83:146–149.

33. Shimada M, Takenaka K, Taguchi K, et al. Prognostic factors after repeat hepatectomy for recurrent hepatocellular carcinoma. Ann Surg 1998;227:80–85.

34. Poon RT, Fan ST, Lo CM, et al. Intrahepatic recurrence after curative resection of hepatocellular carcinoma: long-term results of treatment and prognostic factors. Ann Surg 1999;229:216–222.

35. Nakajima Y, Ohmura T, Kimura J, et al. Role of surgical treatment for recurrent hepatocellular carcinoma after hepatic resection. World J Surg 1993;17:792–795.

36. Parikh AA, Curley SA, Fornage BD, Ellis LM. Radiofrequency ablation of hepatic metastases. Semin Oncol 2002;29:168–182.

37. Poon RT, Fan ST, Tsang FH, Wong J. Locoregional therapies for hepatocellular carcinoma: a critical review from the surgeon's perspective. Ann Surg 2002;235: 466–486.

38. Bilchik AJ, Wood TF, Allegra DP. Radiofrequency ablation of unresectable hepatic malignancies: lessons learned. Oncologist 2001;6:24–33.

39. Curley SA, Izzo F, Ellis LM, et al. Radiofrequency ablation of hepatocellular cancer in 110 patients with cirrhosis. Ann Surg 2000;232:381–391.

40. Wong SL, Edwards MJ, Chao C, et al. Radiofrequency ablation for unresectable hepatic tumors. Am J Surg 2001;182:552–557.

41. Livraghi T, Solbiati L, Meloni MF, et al. Treatment of focal liver tumors with percutaneous radio-frequency ablation:complications encountered in a multicenter study. Radiology 2003;226:441–451.

42. Bilchik AJ, Rose DM, Allegra DP, et al. Radiofrequency ablation: a minimally invasive technique with multiple applications. Cancer J Sci Am 1999;5:356–361.

43. Curley SA, Izzo F, Delrio P, et al. Radiofrequency ablation of unresectable primary and metastatic hepatic malignancies: results in 123 patients. Ann Surg 1999;230:1–8.

44. de Baere T, Elias D, Dromain C, et al. Radiofrequency ablation of 100 hepatic metastases with a mean follow-up of more than 1 year. AJR Am J Roentgenol 2000;175:1619–1625.

45. Machi J. Radiofrequency ablation for multiple hepatic metastases. Ann Surg Oncol 2001;8:379–380.

46. Siperstein A, Garland A, Engle K, et al. Local recurrence after laparoscopic radiofrequency thermal ablation of hepatic tumors. Ann Surg Oncol 2000;7: 106–113.

47. Wood TF, Rose DM, Chung M, et al. Radiofrequency ablation of 231 unresectable hepatic tumors: indications, limitations, and complications. Ann Surg Oncol 2000;7:593–600.

48. Solbiati L, Ierance T, Tonolini M, et al. Radiofrequency thermal ablation of hepatic metastases. Eur J Ultrasound 2001;13:149–159.

49. Solbiati L, Livraghi T, Goldberg SN, et al. Percutaneous radio-frequency ablation of hepatic metastases from colorectal cancer: long-term results in 117 patients. Radiology 2001;221:159–166.

50. Berber E, Flesher N, Siperstein AE. Laparoscopic radiofrequency ablation of neuroendocrine liver metastases. World J Surg 2002;26:985–990.

51. Adamsen S, Hansen OH, Funch-Jensen P, et al. Bile duct injury during laparoscopic cholecystectomy: a prospective nationwide series. J Am Coll Surg 1997; 184:571–578.

52. Pitt HA, Miyamoto T, Parapatis SK, et al. Factors influencing outcome in patients with postoperative biliary strictures. Am J Surg 1982;144:14–21.

53. Lillemoe KD, Melton GB, Cameron JL, et al. Postoperative bile duct strictures: management and outcome in the 1990s. Ann Surg 2000;232:430–441.

54. Chapman WC, Halevy A, Blumgart LH, Benjamin IS. Postcholecystectomy bile duct strictures. Management and outcome in 130 patients. Arch Surg 1995;130: 597–602.

55. Anderson CD, Rice M, Pinson CW, et al. Fluorodeoxyglucose PET imaging in the evaluation of gallbladder carcinoma and cholangiocarcinoma. J Gastrointest Surg 2004;8:90–97.

56. Stewart L, Way LW. Bile duct injuries during laparoscopic cholecystectomy. Factors that influence the results of treatment. Arch Surg 1995;130:1123–1128.

57. Asbun HJ, Rossi RL, Lowell JA, Munson JL. Bile duct injury during laparoscopic cholecystectomy: mechanism of injury, prevention, and management. World J Surg 1993;17:547–551.

58. Cates JA, Tompkins RK, Zinner MJ, et al. Biliary complications of laparoscopic cholecystectomy. Am Surg 1993;59:243–247.

59. Soper NJ, Flye MW, Brunt LM, et al. Diagnosis and management of biliary complications of laparoscopic cholecystectomy. Am J Surg 1993;165:663–669.

60. Wudel LJ, Jr., Wright JK, Pinson CW, et al. Bile duct injury following laparoscopic cholecystectomy: a cause for continued concern. Am Surg 2001;67:557–563.

61. Davidoff AM, Pappas TN, Murray EA, et al. Mechanisms of major biliary injury during laparoscopic cholecystectomy. Ann Surg 1992;215:196–202.

62. Alves A, Farges O, Nicolet J, et al. Incidence and consequence of an hepatic artery injury in patients with postcholecystectomy bile duct strictures. Ann Surg 2003;238:93–96.

63. Branum G, Schmitt C, Baillie J, et al. Management of major biliary complications after laparoscopic cholecystectomy. Ann Surg 1993;217:532–540.

64. Jarnagin WR, Burke E, Powers C, et al. Intrahepatic biliary enteric bypass provides effective palliation in selected patients with malignant obstruction at the hepatic duct confluence. Am J Surg 1998;175:453–460.

65. Anderson CD, Kim R, Chari R. Biliary strictures. In: Pappas TN, Eubanks S, Tyler DS, Purcell GP, eds. Unbound Surgery. http://www.unboundmedicine.com/unboundsurgery.htm. Salt Lake City, UT: Unbound Medicine, Inc., 2002.

66. Browder W, Dowling JB, Koontz KK, Kitwin MS. Early management of operative injuries to the extrahepatic biliary tree. Ann Surg 1987;205:649–658.

67. Jarnagin WR, Krygier A, Fong Y, Blumgart LH. Immediate repair of cholecystectomy injuries: more harm than good. Gastroenterology 1997;112(supp):A1451.

68. Lillemoe KD, Martin SA, Cameron JL, et al. Major bile duct injuries during laparoscopic cholecystectomy. Ann Surg 1997;25:459–471.

69. Chaudhary A, Chandra A, Negi SS, Sachdev A. Reoperative surgery for postcholecystectomy bile duct injuries. Dig Surg 2002;19:22–27.

70. Rossi RL, Tsao J. Biliary Reconstruction. Surg Clin North Am 1994;74: 825–841.

71. Colonna JO, Shaked A, Gomes AS, et al. Biliary strictures complicating liver transplantation. Incidence, pathogenesis, management, and outcome. Ann Surg 1992;216:344–350.

72. Moraca RJ, Lee FT, Ryan JA, Jr., Traverso LW. Long-term biliary function after reconstruction of major bile duct injuries with hepaticoduodenostomy or hepaticojejunostomy. Arch Surg 2002;137:889–893.

73. Blumgart LH, Jarnagin WR. Biliary-enteric anastamosis. In: Blumgart LH, Fong Y, eds. Surgery of the Liver and Biliary Tract. New York: WB Saunders, 2002:595–614.

74. Hepp J, Couinaud C. [Approach to and use of the left hepatic duct in reparation of the common bile duct]. Presse Med 1956;64:947–948.

75. Murr MM, Gigot JF, Nagorney DM, et al. Long-term results of biliary reconstruction after laparoscopic bile duct injuries. Arch Surg 1999;134:604–609.

76. Blumgart LH. Hilar and intrahepatic biliary enteric anastomosis. Surg Clin North Am 1994;74:845–863.
77. Blumgart LH, Kelley CJ. Hepaticojejunostomy in benign and malignant high bile duct stricture: approaches to the left hepatic ducts. Br J Surg 1984; 71:257–261.
78. Voyles CR, Blumgart LH. A technique for the construction of high biliary-enteric anastomoses. Surg Gynecol Obstet 1982;154:885–887.
79. Barker EM, Winkler M. Permanent-access hepatojejunostomy. Br J Surg 1985;71:188–191.
80. Dawson SL, Mueller PR. Interventional radiology in the management of bile duct injuries. Surg Clin North Am 1994;74:865–874.
81. Mueller PR, vanSonnenberg E, Ferrucci JTJ. Biliary stricture dilation: a multi-center review of clinical management in 73 patients. Radiology 1986;160:17.
82. Lillemoe KD, Martin SA, Cameron JL, et al. Major bile duct injuries during laparoscopic cholecystectomy. Followup after combined surgical and radiologic management. Ann Surg 1997;225:459–471.
83. Pitt HA, Kaufman SL, Coleman J. Benign postoperative biliary strictures. Operate or dilate? Ann Surg 1989;210:417.
84. Sherman S, Jamidar P, Shaked A, et al. Biliary tract complications after orthotopic liver transplantation: endoscopic approach to diagnosis and therapy. Transplantation 1995;60:467.
85. Kuo PC, Lewis WD, Stokes K, et al. A comparison of operation, endoscopic retrograde cholangiopancreatography, and percutaneous transhepatic cholangiography in biliary complications after hepatic transplantation. J Am Coll Surg 1994;179:177–181.
86. Geenen DJ, Geenen JE, Hogan WJ, et al. Endoscopic therapy for benign bile duct strictures. Gastrointest Endosc 1989;35:367.
87. Davids PH, Tanka AK, Rauws EA, et al. Benign biliary strictures. Surgery or endoscopy? Ann Surg 1993;217:237.
88. Bergman JJ, van den Brink GR, Rauws EA, et al. Treatment of bile duct lesions after laparoscopic cholecystectomy. Gut 1996;38:141.
89. Kozarek RA. Endoscopic techniques in management of biliary tract injuries. Surg Clin North Am 1994;74:883–893.
90. Anderson CD, Pinson CW, Berlin J, Chari RS. Diagnosis and treatment of cholangiocarcinoma. Oncologist 2004;9:43–57.
91. Roslyn JL. Calculous biliary disease. In: Greenfield LJ, ed. Surgery: Scientific Principles and Practice. Philadelphia: JB Lippincott, 1993:936–953.
92. Himal HS. Common bile duct stones: the role of preoperative, intraoperative, and postoperative ERCP. Semin Laparosc Surg 2000;7:237–245.
93. Cotton PB. Endoscopic methods for relief of malignant obstructive jaundice. World J Surg 1984; 8:854–861.
94. Lambert ME, Betts CD, Hill J, et al. Endoscopic sphincterotomy: the whole truth. Br J Surg 1991;78:473–476.

95. Vlavianos P, Chopra K, Mandalia S, et al. Endoscopic balloon dilatation versus endoscopic sphincterotomy for the removal of bile duct stones: a prospective randomised trial. Gut 2003;52:1165–1169.

96. Schreurs WH, Juttmann JR, Stuifbergen WN, et al. Management of common bile duct stones: selective endoscopic retrograde cholangiography and endoscopic sphincterotomy: short- and long-term results. Surg Endosc 2002;16: 1068–1072.

97. Girard RM. Stones in the common bile duct-surgical approaches. In: Blumgart LH, Fong Y, eds Surgery of the Liver and Biliary Tract. New York: WB Saunders, 2002:725–748.

98. Cameron JL. Retained and recurrent bile duct stones: operative management. Am J Surg 1989;158:218–221.

99. Girard RM, Legros G. Retained and recurrent bile duct stones. Surgical or nonsurgical removal? Ann Surg 1981;193:150–154.

100. Miller BM, Kozarek RA, Ryan JA, Jr., et al. Surgical versus endoscopic management of common bile duct stones. Ann Surg 1988;207:135–141.

101. Way LW. Retained common bile duct stones. Surg Clin North Am 1974;53:1139–1147.

102. Allen B, Shapiro H, Way LW. Management of recurrent and residual common duct stones. Am J Surg 1981;142:41–47.

103. Braasch JW, Fender HR, Bonneval MM. Refractory primary common bile duct stone disease. Am J Surg 1980;139:526–530.

104. Ribotta G, Procacciante F. Transduodenal sphincteroplasty and exploration of the common bile duct. In: Blumgart LH, Fong Y, eds. Surgery of the Liver and Biliary Tract. New York: WB Saunders, 2002:841–850.

105. Egawa H, Uemoto S, Inomata Y, et al. Biliary complications in pediatric living related liver transplantation. Surgery 1998;124:901–910.

106. Lopez RR, Benner KG, Ivancev K, et al. Management of biliary complications after liver transplantation. Am J Surg 1992;163:519–524.

107. Sawyer RG, Punch JD. Incidence and management of biliary complications after 291 liver transplants following the introduction of transcystic stenting. Transplantation 1998;66:1201–1207.

108. Iwatsuki S, Shaw BW, Starzl TE. Biliary tract complications in liver transplantation under cyclosporine-steroid therapy. Transplant Proc 1983;15:1288.

109. Lerut J, Gordon RD, Iwatsuki S, et al. Biliary complications in human orthotopic liver transplantation. Transplantation 1987;43:47.

110. Ramirez P, Parrilla P, Bueno FS, et al. Reoperation for biliary tract complications following orthotopic liver transplantation. Br J Surg 1993;80:1426.

111. Ferraz-Neto BH, Mirza DF, Gunson BK, et al. Bile duct splintage in liver transplantation: is it necessary? Transpl Int 1996;9(suppl):185.

112. Randall HB, Wachs ME, Somberg KA, et al. The use of T tube after orthotopic liver transplantation. Transplantation 1996;61:258.

113. O'Conner TP, Lewis WD, Jenkins RL. Biliary tract complications after liver transplantation. Arch Surg 1995;130:312.

114. Campbell WL, Sheng R, Zajko AB, et al. Intrahepatic biliary strictures after liver transplantation. Radiology 1994;191:735.

115. Li S, Stratta RJ, Langnas AN, et al. Diffuse biliary tract injury after liver transplantation. Am J Surg 1992;164:536.

CHAPTER 2

Reoperative Surgery in Trauma

Ram Nirula, MD

Précis

The operative approach to the polytrauma patient has evolved over the past three decades from a complete repair of all injuries at the initial surgery to a damage control approach in the metabolically deranged individual. Many patients with severe injuries could not withstand the prolonged time, hypothermia, coagulopathy, and acidosis associated with definitive operation. This has given rise to rapid stabilization of lethal injuries and a planned delayed repair of less-threatening injuries after resuscitation in the intensive care unit (ICU). Mortality from this approach has been significantly reduced, and this has led to the application of damage control techniques in other surgical subspecialties.

Introduction

The concept of reoperative surgery in trauma evolved from the damage control approach to the critically injured patient with abdominal hemorrhage. Traditionally, surgeons repaired all injuries at the initial operation regardless of the patient's physiologic state. Those patients afflicted with the triad of hypothermia, acidosis, and coagulopathy undergoing major reparative surgery of all injuries were subjected to continued traumatic insult in the face of severe metabolic derangements, often resulting in death. Perhaps the earliest reports of planned reoperative surgery for trauma can be found in Pringle's description of hepatic packing of liver injuries.[1] Since then, abdominal packing for hemorrhage was discouraged after the military experience in World War II and Vietnam.[2] In the late 1970s and early 1980s, the practice of damage-control laparotomy regained popularity with several reports of improved mortality for patients with injuries that were previously deemed nonsurvivable.[3–6] The widespread acceptance of deliberate abbreviated laparotomy with a planned reoperative strategy has now become the standard of care for major trauma centers managing the metabolically challenged, injured patient.

Given the frequent presence of associated injuries requiring the surgical expertise of other specialties, the principles of damage control have spread across surgical disciplines to include thoracic,[7–9] urologic,[10] orthopedic,[11–14] and vascular surgery.[15–19] The surgeon managing the critically injured must be aware of these techniques as well as their indications and complications to improve patient outcomes.

Pathophysiology of Severe Injury

To recognize the need for damage control techniques and to identify a patient's possible progression toward irreversible shock, one must understand the mechanisms leading to metabolic compromise. The lethal triad of hypothermia, acidosis, and coagulopathy is now the well-recognized foe of the trauma surgeon, and so must be avoided or minimized during the resuscitative and damage control phases of care.

HYPOTHERMIA

Heat loss begins at the time of injury and may be worsened by prolonged exposure, severity of shock, injury severity, and extremes of age. Hypothermia may then be potentiated by the infusion of crystalloids, exposure in the emergency room, cold trauma bays, and operating rooms, and prolonged operative times. The association between hypothermia and death is well established. Slotman et al. identified a 40% mortality rate for prolonged hypothermic patients admitted to the ICU.[20] Similarly, Jurkovich et al. noted that patients with a core temperature at or below 89.6°F (32°C) carried a 60% increased mortality over those with temperatures of 93.2°F (34°C) or greater. More convincingly, in 1997 Gentilello et al. published the results of the first randomized, prospective trial to assess the effect of rapid active rewarming versus standard rewarming methods on hypothermic trauma patient outcome. Patients undergoing active rewarming required less fluid resuscitation and had lower mortality compared to those randomized to the standard warming protocol.[21] These studies indicate that hypothermia is an independent predictor of mortality, and rapid reversal is associated with a significant reduction in mortality. Efforts to minimize heat loss through use of warmed fluids, minimizing exposure and operative times, and restoring adequate circulating volume are paramount to a successful outcome in a damage-control patient.

Acidosis

As tissue hypoperfusion increases secondary to hypovolemic shock, a shift from aerobic to anaerobic metabolism leads to lactate acidosis, thereby exacerbating the coagulopathic state.[22] The rate of improvement in acidosis is linked to survival in several series.[23–28] More specifically, persistent acidosis at the conclusion of damage control ($pH < 7.2$) is strongly associated with death.[29] Recognition of severe acidosis using the base deficit from the admission arterial blood gas (ABG) or intraoperative ABGs indicates the presence of significant metabolic compromise and

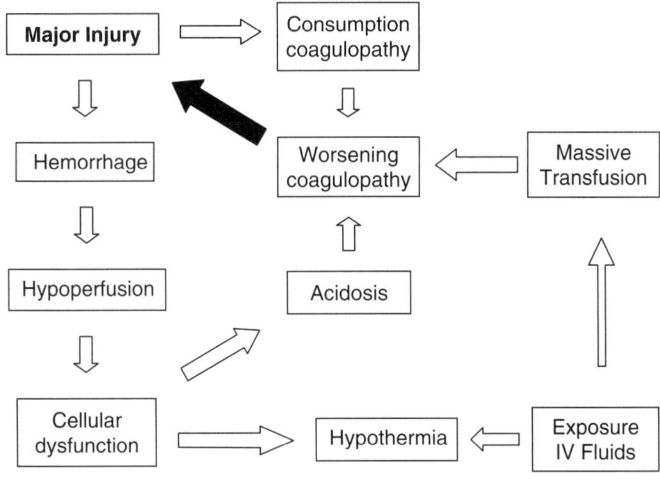

Figure 2-1 The triad of hypothermia, acidosis and coagulopathy following injury combine to worsen hemorrhage and physiologic demands on the severely injured patient.

should prompt the surgeon toward an abbreviated laparotomy before the onset of irreversible shock and coagulopathy.

COAGULOPATHY

As hemorrhagic shock progresses, coagulopathy intensifies and is exacerbated by acidosis and hypothermia. The body's utilization of coagulation factors secondary to ongoing bleeding leads to a consumption coagulopathy. This is worsened by resuscitation, which produces a dilutional coagulopathy. Furthermore, hypothermia leads to a reduction in clotting cascade enzyme function as well as platelet dysfunction and aggregation abnormalities.[22,30,31] To make matters worse, many laboratories perform partial thromboplastin time (PTT) and prothombin time (PT) studies at normal body temperature, which is typically higher than the temperature of the patient. As a result, the degree of coagulopathy is often underestimated, since these tests do not take into account the effect of hypothermia on the clotting cascade. It is clear that the pathway to coagulopathy is intimately related to the physiologic insult imposed by hemorrhage and, therefore, must be anticipated in hypothermic, acidotic patients indicating the need for damage control (Figure 2-1).

Indications for Damage Control Celiotomy

Damage-control laparotomy is actually only one step in the resuscitation of the polytrauma patient. It begins with the following four steps: (1) recognizing the patient's metabolic compromise, (2) performing an abbreviated laparotomy, (3) resuscitation in the ICU setting, and (4) reoperation for reconstruction once the resuscitation is adequate. The key to successful management is early recognition of the "maximal injury subset"[22] of patients (approximately 10% of celiotomies for trauma) requiring this approach.[5,32] Ideally, the decision should be made within the first few minutes of the operation, or even beforehand, on the basis of the patient's physiology and constellation of injuries. Injury patterns that have frequently benefited from the bail-out approach include combined major vascular injury with hollow or solid organ injury, destruction of the pancreaticoduodenal complex, high-grade liver injury, and multiregional injuries with competing priorities.[33] Furthermore, the resuscitation itself may mandate a planned reoperation simply because the degree of visceral edema precludes closure of the abdomen without the development of abdominal compartment syndrome (ACS).

Several investigations have identified physiologic data regarding the degree of hypothermia, acidosis, and coagulopathy to provide objective evidence indicating the need for a damage control approach. Krishna et al. determined, after reviewing 40 patients with severe injury (ISS over 35) undergoing complete initial reparative laparotomy instead of damage control, that mortality was strongly associated with severe hypothermia (below 91.4°F [33°C]), severe acidosis (base deficit > 12 mEq/L), or a combination of moderate hypothermia and acidosis (below 92°F [33.5°C] and base deficit over 5 mEq/L).[34] Another retrospective review of 58 patients requiring more than 10 units of packed cells in the first 24 hours identified ISS, hypothermia, acidosis, and hypotension as significant risk factors for the development of life-threatening coagulopathy. In fact, the risk of severe coagulopathy according to their prediction model was 98% when the pH was less than 7.10, systolic blood pressure (SBP) was below 70 mm Hg, temperature was below 93.2°F (34°C) and ISS was over 25.[35,36] More recently, the value of partial pressure arterial CO_2 ($PaCO_2$) less the end-tidal CO_2 ($ETCO_2$) may be useful intraoperatively as a marker for cellular metabolic derangement in the face of reduced cardiac output. Since CO_2 is an end-product of aerobic metabolism, lower $ETCO_2$ levels suggest reduced tissue perfusion and increased anaerobic metabolism. In fact, during cardiopulmonary resuscitation (CPR), often the first sign of return in spontaneous circulation is an increase in $ETCO_2$.[37] Using this strategy, Tyburski et al. reviewed 501 patients undergoing emergent laparotomy for trauma. The authors found a strong association between mortality and a $PaCO_2$-$ETCO_2$ difference greater than 10 mm Hg. Since all intubated operative patients have real-time $ETCO_2$ monitors, all that is needed for this tool is a blood gas to determine the $PaCO_2$. It should be noted that there is no consensus as to the absolute physiologic cutoff points at which damage control surgery should be applied; however, once patients reach these critical values, the degree of metabolic derangement may be irreversible. Therefore, the decision to proceed with damage control should be made when the magnitude of the visceral damage is such that definitive repair is likely to exceed the patient's physiologic limits (Table 2-1). While this statement seems simple, it is difficult in practice, because the surgeon is conflicted with traditional teachings of the need for definitive repair coupled with the subtleties of recognizing a worsening physiologic state.

Table 2-1 Indications for Abbreviated Laparotomy	
Parameters	Findings
Physiologic	Shock plus hypothermia, acidosis, coagulopathy
Parameters	Suboptimal response to resuscitation Possibly increased $PaCO_2$-$ETCO_2$ difference
Injury Parameters	Severe hepatic hemorrhage/inaccessible IVC injury Hemorrhage control best accomplished by angioembolization Need for time-consuming repair (e.g., Whipple) Need for reevaluation (e.g., intestinal ischemia) Extra-abdominal life-threatening injuries

Technique of Damage Control Laparotomy

The goal of damage control laparotomy is to expeditiously control hemorrhage and intestinal contamination. Prior to surgery the operating room should be kept well above room temperature (approximately 80.6–84.2°F [27–29°C]) and be equipped with a rapid fluid warming infuser and cell saver. A large number of laparotomy sponges, vascular and thoracic instruments (e.g., sternal saw), and abdominal closure supplies should be readily available. The patient is placed supine with arms out and is prepped from the chin to the knees while a urinary catheter is placed. Upon entering the abdomen a rapid but systematic approach to evacuation of the hemoperitoneum, plus packing all four quadrants, are undertaken in less than 5 minutes. At this point, it should be clear which regions of the abdomen are most severely hemorrhaging. Active, ongoing exsanguinating hemorrhage in a patient with profound shock without a single, readily identifiable and easily controllable source may necessitate aortic inflow control at the hiatus until more definitive control at the injury site can be achieved. This control can be accomplished with manual compression or by using an aortic occlusion device to compress the aorta against the spine. If prolonged clamping is required to attain vascular control, the diaphragmatic crus should be split to permit placement of an aortic clamp to free the surgeon's hands and provide adequate space. After local control is obtained, the aortic clamp should be moved to a site just proximal to the injury to restore flow to the kidneys in the case of an infrarenal injury.

If packing alone controls the hemorrhage, then control of intestinal spillage is the next step. During this time, anesthesia can replete the intravascular volume, replace clotting factors, and prepare the patient for the subsequent insult of hemorrhage that will occur upon packing removal. Noncrushing bowel clamps, simple suture, or umbilical tapes can be used to contain spillage as perforations are identified. Restoration of gastrointestinal (GI) integrity, formation of ostomies, or placement of feeding tubes should not be performed at the initial operation, as this is time-consuming and unnecessary to the survival of the patient in the first hours of resuscitation. These procedures should be undertaken at subsequent operations after the metabolic derangements have been corrected. Once the bowel has been assessed from the ligament of Treitz to the rectum, the GI staplers can be used to resect devitalized areas or segments with multiple perforations in a short region. Packs are then removed, starting with the quadrant with the least amount of hemorrhage and the region assessed and controlled, before moving to the next region. Bleeding vessels that can be ligated without compromising viability of tissue should be ligated, whereas major vascular injuries should undergo definitive repair or temporary shunting if the patient's condition does not permit repair.

With respect to solid organ injuries, extensive efforts to repair these injuries should not be undertaken. The actively hemorrhaging spleen or kidney should be resected in the physiologically compromised patient. Hepatic hemorrhage should be managed with packing, balloon tamponade, and/or selective or common hepatic arterial ligation if necessary. In cases of deep parenchymal liver injuries or large pelvic hematomas, angioembolization after control of intra-abdominal hemorrhage and hollow viscous injuries has been useful.[33,38,39]

The choices for abdominal closure techniques and materials are extensive, therefore a routinely used strategy for temporary abdominal closure should be established to prevent delays in procuring necessary materials. There are three major concerns of abdominal closure in these patients: (1) the development of ACS, (2) preservation of abdominal fascia for subsequent closure, and (3) the length of time required to perform the closure. Since the majority of these patients will have significant resuscitation requirements combined with an ischemia-reperfusion syndrome that produces significant bowel wall edema, formal fascial closure is typically not performed, as this will likely lead to ACS, further compromising organ function in an already metabolically challenged patient. In cases of ongoing bleeding from coagulopathy, a period of abdominal tamponade may be desirable while clotting factors are replenished and the patient is warmed. This may be achieved by closing the skin with 30 to 40 piercing towel clips or a running #1 nylon suture. These patients are still at risk for ACS, so bladder pressures, the degree of hypoxia, inspiratory pressures, and urine output should be closely monitored.

If the skin cannot be closed without risking ACS, then temporary abdominal closure using the "vac pack" method, silicone elastomer sheeting (Silastic), mesh or plastic silos, or "Bogota Bag" techniques have been employed.[40–45] The method chosen must be expeditious and ideally prevent loss of control of the fascia to facilitate subsequent fascial closure when physiologically possible. Mesh, Silastic, silos, and the "Bogota Bag" (3-L genitourinary irrigation bag) can be sutured to the skin or fascia. Suturing to the skin is usually faster and prevents undue fascial damage for subsequent closure, while suturing to fascia prevents loss of abdominal domain and minimizes fascial retraction.

The relatively low number of cases per year at any one center has precluded a randomized trial comparing one technique over another to test the rates of complications and subsequent fascial closures. Furthermore, the variety of methods and variability in patient profiles between centers precludes comparison of one case series to another. Still, it is important to note the complications and closure rates

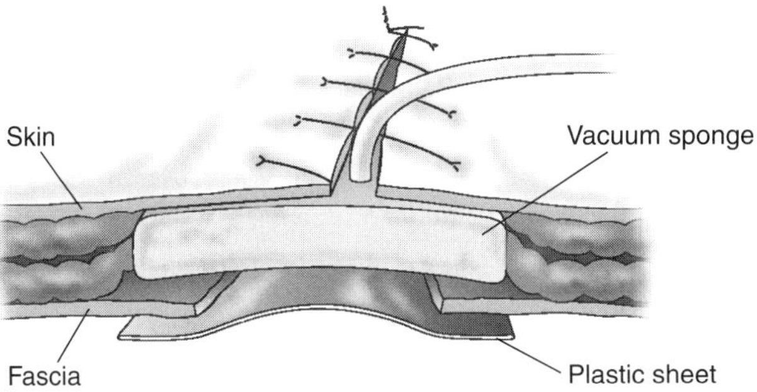

Figure 2-2 Vacuum-assisted temporary abdominal closure prevents adhesion of the fascia to the bowel while controlling fluid losses and maintaining wall tension. (Modified from Garner GB, Ware DN, Cocanour CS, et al. Vacuum-assisted wound closure provides early fascial reapproximation in trauma patients with open abdomens. Am J Surg 2001;182:630–638.)

in these series to determine any potential benefit of one technique over another. In a series of 181 patients with open abdomens employing a variety of temporary closure techniques the authors found a 52% rate of fascial closure among survivors. Despite temporary closure, 13% of patients still developed ACS, and there was a 14% incidence of gastrointestinal fistula.[40] In a series of 14 patients treated by vacuum-assisted wound closure techniques, 13 (92%) achieved fascial closure, with only 2 (14%) out of 14 developing wound infections; no fistulae or eviscerations occurred.[42] In this series, a vacuum sponge was placed over a plastic perforated drape, interposed between fascia and bowel, over which the skin is closed (Figure 2-2). The Harborview experience with Silastic sewn to the fascia or skin at the initial laparotomy consisted of 134 patients with 83 survivors. Drains were placed between moist Kerlix over the Silastic, and an Ioban drape covered the abdomen to create a seal for the closed suction drainage system. Among the survivors, 62 (75%) were successfully closed at the initial hospitalization, 4 (5%) of all patients developed fistulae, and 3 (4%) developed intra-abdominal abscesses. The approach consistently used in the vacuum-assisted and Harborview studies included returns to the operating room every 2 to 3 days for sequential tightening of the fascia to a physiologically accepted limit until closure. Using a hybrid technique of the vacuum-assisted and Silastic approaches, Sherck et al. reported a fascial closure rate of 88% during initial admission, and a fistula rate of 6%. In this technique, a perforated plastic sheet is placed over the bowel and under the fascia, on top of which drains and Ioban are placed and closed suction drainage applied. This approach does not require any suturing and therefore can be applied quickly in most cases.

Timing of Reoperation

Several factors must be considered prior to reoperation in the polytrauma patient. First, the metabolic consequences of the initial insult must be corrected with improvement of hypothermia, coagulopathy, and acidosis, indicating completion of the resuscitation phase. Typically this can be achieved within 24 to 36 hours unless a missed injury or surgical bleeding exists.[32] Other injuries must be considered before the return to the operating room. Open fractures may necessitate an earlier trip to the operating room once it is clear that the patient's physiologic status is normalizing and coagulopathy resolved, whereas worsening intracranial hypertension would generally be a contraindication for relaparotomy.

Once the decision has been made to reoperate, all packs should be removed and bleeding reassessed. By this point most bleeding should have ceased; however, repeat packing may occasionally be required for complex liver injuries. If the patient's resuscitation is complete and adequate oxygen delivery parameters exist without the use of pressors, then gastrointestinal continuity should be restored. Definitive vascular repairs should be undertaken as soon as the physiologic status of the patient permits, to avoid thromboembolic phenomena associated with temporary shunts. Any previous repairs performed at the initial operation should be reassessed for integrity and repaired accordingly. The abdominal fascia should be reapproximated from the superior and inferior edges of the wound as much as possible, so long as peak airway pressures and fascial tension are not excessive. Some advocate leaving the fascia open if the peak inspiratory pressure rises more than 10 cm H_2O with fascial apposition.[22] Most surgeons will return to the operating room every 1 to 2 days for sequential fascial tightening until closure is achieved. Diuresis on the third or fourth postinjury day, once the resuscitation phase is complete, may reduce bowel wall edema and facilitate fascial closure.

If fascial closure cannot be attained in the first 2 weeks, most will be left with a hernia defect.[22,44] In these instances Vicryl mesh can be used to close the defect and skin flaps can be raised to cover the wound. If the defect is too large to achieve skin coverage, then wet-to-dry dressings should be performed until a bed of granulation tissue has grown through the mesh. At that time, a skin graft can be placed over the defect and the patient can return for definitive hernia repair 6 to 12 months later, to allow skin graft maturation and separation from the underlying granulation bed.[22] Alternatively, a component separation technique or tensor fascia lata may be used to obtain visceral coverage, obviating the need for placement of prosthetic material.[46,47]

In some instances reoperation may be unplanned. For example, the damage-control patient with ongoing hemorrhage may require reexploration before full resuscitation if it is believed that there is surgical bleeding. Occasionally, angioembolization is useful in these patients, particularly if there is a known pelvic fracture or extensive hepatic injury.[45] The decision to reoperate for ongoing hemorrhage can be difficult. Generally, ongoing blood loss requiring 2 or more units/hour after coagulopathy has been corrected indicates the need for reoperation or angioembolization, depending on the injury.[32,36] The second indication for reoperation is ACS, which may develop in patients with open abdomens as well as those with primary wound closure.[40] As a result, most surgeons routinely measure bladder pressures during the resuscitation phase to minimize delayed recognition of ACS, since elevated pressures over 35 cm H_2O lead to decreased urine output, pulmonary hypertension, inability to ventilate, and decreased cardiac output.[36] If the

ACS is due to ongoing hemorrhage, the procedure must be performed in the operating theater to facilitate repair and/or repacking. ACS that develops secondary to ischemia-reperfusion edema and third-spacing can be decompressed in the ICU, as these patients are typically severely compromised and best not moved unnecessarily to the operating room.

Extension of Reoperative Strategies in Polytrauma

The use of the damage control approach during laparotomy has spread to include other surgical specialties with the development of innovative techniques to temporize the anatomic derangements of injuries. In general, these approaches are used when multiple life-threatening injuries exist that preclude definitive repair of any one specific injury or when surgical expertise for definitive repair is lacking.

VASCULAR TRAUMA

Isolated major vascular injuries, if quickly controlled, may be repaired primarily if the patient has not developed irreversible shock, acidosis, hypothermia, and coagulopathy. With other significant injuries or profound shock, it may be prudent to employ a planned reoperative strategy for a repair that is timely and of an exacting nature.

The literature includes several reports of temporizing shunts for arterial injuries in the extremities, aortoiliacs, and superior mesenteric artery.[12,15,48,49] Temporizing shunts in the extremities may be particularly useful if there is an associated fracture. In this case, vascular flow is restored with a shunt such as the Pruitt shunt while controlling arterial hemorrhage. The advantage of the Pruitt shunt is its side port, which permits infusion of contrast for angiography or of heparin locally to minimize thrombosis of the shunt and distal vessel. Alignment of the fracture can then be undertaken without risking disruption of a vascular repair. The fracture fixation method used may also be damage-control in nature in dire circumstances. When the physiologic status permits, definitive vascular repair can then be undertaken.

Intra-abdominal vascular injuries are often accompanied by other injuries, increasing the need for damage control techniques. Complex vascular repairs in the setting of acidosis and coagulopathy will not be well tolerated. In this circumstance, a temporizing shunt will restore flow and control hemorrhage. The shunt is placed intraluminally and secured with umbilical tape or vessel loops until resuscitation is complete.

ORTHOPEDIC SURGERY

Management of fractures in the trauma patient has evolved from the belief, in the 1950s and 1960s, that these patients were too sick to have their fractures fixed, to the current emphasis on early total care of fractures. This shift developed from the realization that early fixation of long-bone fractures led to improved pulmonary outcomes, improved pain control, and shorter lengths of stay.[50,51] Unfortunately, in the severely injured subset of patients undergoing early total care, requiring prolonged operative times that induce significant blood loss, outcomes were unexpectedly worsened. Studies investigating the effect of prolonged operations on the proinflammatory response demonstrated an exaggerated response with operations of greater duration. The use of reamed nails for femoral fracture fixation has similarly been associated with an impairment in immunoreactivity.[52,53] Therefore, the second hit model of multiple organ failure is believed to be at play in these patients.[54]

The damage control approach adopted by general surgeons for extensive abdominal injury was therefore applied to the polytrauma patient's orthopedic injuries.[11,55] Long-bone and pelvic fractures can await definitive open reduction and internal fixation, but can rapidly be stabilized with external fixators to minimize pain and local inflammatory response until physiologic derangements have been corrected. Similarly, open fractures can be washed out and externally stabilized with delayed definitive repair.

The timing of definitive orthopedic repair has been a subject of debate. Several studies report a higher incidence of organ failure if definitive repair is undertaken 2 to 4 days postinjury compared to delayed fixation.[56–58] It should be noted that these studies are retrospective in nature, so selection bias may influence the results. In general, any planned reoperative surgery should await restoration of physiologic derangements and then, in the absence of a randomized prospective trial, best clinical judgment must be used to determine the optimal timing of definitive fracture fixation, noting the potential for increased risk of multiple organ failure if fixation is undertaken too soon.

THORACIC SURGERY

Abbreviated thoracotomy in the polytrauma patient follows the same guidelines as with abbreviated laparotomy. Major vascular injuries can be temporarily shunted if the patient is facing metabolic exhaustion. Inaccessible vascular injuries can be occluded with a Fogarty catheter to be later removed once resuscitation is complete. Significant hemorrhage from bronchial arteries associated with rib fractures may be difficult to control surgically. In these instances, tamponade with packs or use of fibrin glue may temporize the hemorrhage until angiographic embolization can be performed. Packing in the chest is not always practical, since it may lead to cardiac tamponade, so it is often reserved for regions in the chest that can be isolated from the heart.[9] Reoperation and pack removal should be performed as soon as physiologic parameters permit, to reduce the risk of empyema.

Patients in extremis may benefit from cross-clamping the thoracic aorta. It may not be possible to immediately remove this clamp while resuscitation is ongoing. To reduce heat loss, the chest wall can be closed with the clamp in place. As resuscitation progresses, the clamp can be gradually weaned off the aorta. Temporary closure of the chest usually requires an en masse closure of the skin and chest wall muscles, since these will bleed significantly if only the skin is closed. Occasionally, attempts at closing lead to hypotension with significant rises in peak airway pressures and tamponade-like physiology. Silastic or mesh can be used in these instances to prevent thoracic compartment syndrome until edema has resolved or the chest can simply be packed open.[7] In a series of 11 patients requiring damage control thoracotomy, Vargo et al. noted a 36% mortality rate, which was significantly lower than that predicted based upon their Trauma and Injury Severity Scores (59%).[7] Another interesting maneuver reported in two patients with pulmonary hilar bleeding and extensive pulmonary lacerations is the pulmonary hilar twist. The inferior pulmonary ligament is released and the lung rotated 180°, thereby occluding the inflow to the lung and arresting hemorrhage. Packs are placed to keep the lung from untwisting, and the critical patient is returned to the operating room once other injuries and resuscitation have been addressed.[8] These findings indicate that damage control thoracotomy can be tolerated in severely injured patients and must be considered an important life-saving maneuver in the trauma surgeon's armamentarium.

Summary

Reoperation in the trauma patient revolves around the damage control approach to the critically injured. Early recognition of the metabolically exhausted patient permits the appropriate application of damage control techniques, followed by restoration of normal physiology. Only then should definitive repair be undertaken. This approach is now the standard of care to severely injured patients. Its application has extended beyond the scope of the abdomen, and surgeons responsible for care of the trauma patient must be aware of the indications and use of these techniques to optimize patient outcome.

REFERENCES

1. Pringle J. Notes on the arrest of hepatic hemorrhage due to trauma. Ann Surg 1908;48:541–549.
2. Sharp KW, Locicero RJ. Abdominal packing for surgically uncontrollable hemorrhage. Ann Surg 1992;215:467–475.
3. Stone HH, Strom PR, Mullins RJ. Management of the major coagulopathy with onset during laparotomy. Ann Surg 1983;197:532–535.
4. Rotondo MF, Zonies DH. The damage control sequence and underlying logic. Surg Clin North Am 1997;77:761–777.
5. Rotondo MF, Schwab CW, McGonigal MD, et al. "Damage control": an approach for improved survival in exsanguinating penetrating abdominal injury. J Trauma 1993;35:375–383.
6. Johnson JW, Gracias VH, Schwab CW, et al. Evolution in damage control for exsanguinating penetrating abdominal injury. J Trauma 2001;51:261–271.
7. Vargo DJ, Battistella FD. Abbreviated thoracotomy and temporary chest closure: an application of damage control after thoracic trauma. Arch Surg 2001;136:21–24.
8. Wilson A, Wall MJ Jr, Maxson R, Mattox K. The pulmonary hilum twist as a thoracic damage control procedure. Am J Surg 2003;186:49–52.

9. Wall MJ Jr, Soltero E. Damage control for thoracic injuries. Surg Clin North Am 1997;77:863–878.
10. Coburn M. Damage control for urologic injuries. Surg Clin North Am 1997;77:821–834.
11. Scalea TM, Boswell SA, Scott JD, et al. External fixation as a bridge to intramedullary nailing for patients with multiple injuries and with femur fractures: damage control orthopedics. J Trauma 2000;48:613–623.
12. Henry SM, Tornetta P 3rd, Scalea TM. Damage control for devastating pelvic and extremity injuries. Surg Clin North Am 1997;77:879–895.
13. Giannoudis PV. Surgical priorities in damage control in polytrauma. J Bone Joint Surg Br 2003;85:478–483.
14. Pape HC, Giannoudis P, Krettek C. The timing of fracture treatment in polytrauma patients: relevance of damage control orthopedic surgery. Am J Surg 2002;183:622–629.
15. Porter JM, Ivatury RR, Nassoura ZE. Extending the horizons of "damage control" in unstable trauma patients beyond the abdomen and gastrointestinal tract. J Trauma 1997;42:559–561.
16. Pourmoghadam KK, Fogler RJ, Shaftan GW. Ligation: an alternative for control of exsanguination in major vascular injuries. J Trauma 1997;43:126–130.
17. Aucar JA, Hirshberg A. Damage control for vascular injuries. Surg Clin North Am 1997;77:853–862.
18. Firoozmand E, Velmahos GC. Extending damage-control principles to the neck. J Trauma 2000;48:541–543.
19. Hoffer EK, Borsa JJ, Bloch RD, Fontaine AB. Endovascular techniques in the damage control setting. Radiographics 1999;19:1340–1348.
20. Slotman GJ, Jed EH, Burchard KW. Adverse effects of hypothermia in postoperative patients. Am J Surg 1985;149:495–501.
21. Gentilello LM, Jurkovich GJ, Stark MS, et al. Is hypothermia in the victim of major trauma protective or harmful? A randomized, prospective study. Ann Surg 1997;226:439–449.
22. Hoey BA, Schwab CW. Damage control surgery. Scand J Surg 2002;91:92–103.
23. Davis JW, Schackford SR, Mackersie RC, Hoyt DB. Base deficit as a guide to volume resuscitation. J Trauma 1988;28:1464–1467.
24. Husain FA, Martin MJ, Mullenix PS, et al. Serum lactate and base deficit as predictors of mortality and morbidity. Am J Surg 2003;185:485–491.
25. Chang MC, Meredith JW, Kincaid EH, Miller PR. Maintaining survivors' values of left ventricular power output during shock resuscitation: a prospective pilot study. J Trauma 2000;49:26–37.
26. Davis JW, Kaups KL, Parks SN. Base deficit is superior to pH in evaluating clearance of acidosis after traumatic shock. J Trauma 1998;44:114–118.
27. Abramson D, Scalea TM, Hitchcock R, et al. Lactate clearance and survival following injury. J Trauma 1993;35:584–589.

28. McNelis J, Marini CP, Jurkiewicz A, et al. Prolonged lactate clearance is associated with increased mortality in the surgical intensive care unit. Am J Surg 2001;182:481–485.

29. Aoki N, Wall MJ, Demsar J, et al. Predictive model for survival at the conclusion of a damage control laparotomy. Am J Surg 2000;180:540–545.

30. Rohrer MJ, Natale AM. Effect of hypothermia on the coagulation cascade. Crit Care Med 1992;20:1402–1405.

31. Reed RL 2nd, Bracey AW Jr, Hudson JD, et al. Hypothermia and blood coagulation: dissociation between enzyme activity and clotting factor levels. Circ Shock 1990;32:141–152.

32. Morris JA Jr, Eddy VA, Blinman TA, et al. The staged celiotomy for trauma. Issues in unpacking and reconstruction. Ann Surg 1993;217:576–586.

33. Hirshberg A, Walden R. Damage control for abdominal trauma. Surg Clin North Am 1997;77:813–820.

34. Krishna G, Sleigh JW, Rahman H. Physiological predictors of death in exsanguinating trauma patients undergoing conventional trauma surgery. Aust N Z J Surg 1998;68:826–829.

35. Cosgriff N, Moore EE, Sauaia A, et al. Predicting life-threatening coagulopathy in the massively transfused trauma patient: hypothermia and acidoses revisited. J Trauma 1997;42:857–862.

36. Moore EE, Burch JM, Franciose RJ, et al. Staged physiologic restoration and damage control surgery. World J Surg 1998;22:1184–1191.

37. Sanders AB, Kern KB, Otto CW, et al. End-tidal carbon dioxide monitoring during cardiopulmonary resuscitation. A prognostic indicator for survival. JAMA 1989;262:1347–1351.

38. Asensio JA, Roldan G, Petrone P, et al. Operative management and outcomes in 103 AAST-OIS grades IV and V complex hepatic injuries: trauma surgeons still need to operate, but angioembolization helps. J Trauma 2003;54:647–654.

39. Velmahos GC, Toutouzas KG, Vassiliu P, et al. A prospective study on the safety and efficacy of angiographic embolization for pelvic and visceral injuries. J Trauma 2002;53:303–308.

40. Tremblay LN, Feliciano DV, Schmidt J, et al. Skin only or silo closure in the critically ill patient with an open abdomen. Am J Surg 2001;182:670–675.

41. Myers JA, Latenser BA. Nonoperative progressive "Bogota bag" closure after abdominal decompression. Am Surg 2002;68:1029–1030.

42. Garner GB, Ware DN, Cocanour CS, et al. Vacuum-assisted wound closure provides early fascial reapproximation in trauma patients with open abdomens. Am J Surg 2001;182:630–638.

43. Sherck J, Seiver A, Shatney C, et al. Covering the "open abdomen": a better technique. Am Surg 1998;64:854–857.

44. Foy HM, Nathens AB, Maser B, et al. Reinforced silicone elastomer sheeting, an improved method of temporary abdominal closure in damage control laparotomy. Am J Surg 2003;185:498–501.

45. Brasel KJ, Weigelt JA. Damage control in trauma surgery. Curr Opin Crit Care 2000;6:276–280.

46. Steinwald PM, Mathes SJ. Management of the complex abdominal wall wound. Adv Surg 2001;35:77–108.

47. Sukkar SM, Dumanian GA, Szczerba SM, Tellez MG. Challenging abdominal wall defects. Am J Surg 2001;181:115–121.

48. Moldovan S, Granchi TS, Hirshberg A. Bilateral temporary aortoiliac shunts for vascular damage control. J Trauma 2003;55:592.

49. Reilly PM, Rotondo MF, Carpenter JP, et al. Temporary vascular continuity during damage control: intraluminal shunting for proximal superior mesenteric artery injury. J Trauma 1995;39:757–760.

50. Goris RJ, Gimbrere JS, van Niekerk JL, et al. Early osteosynthesis and prophylactic mechanical ventilation in the multitrauma patient. J Trauma 1982;22:895–903.

51. Talucci RC, Manning J, Lampard S, et al. Early intramedullary nailing of femoral shaft fractures: a cause of fat embolism syndrome. Am J Surg 1983;146:107–111.

52. Cruickshank AM, Fraser WD, Burns HJ, et al. Response of serum interleukin-6 in patients undergoing elective surgery of varying severity. Clin Sci (Lond) 1990;79:161–165.

53. Pape HC, Schmidt RE, Rice J, et al. Biochemical changes after trauma and skeletal surgery of the lower extremity: quantification of the operative burden. Crit Care Med 2000;28:3441–3448.

54. Moore FA, Moore EE. Evolving concepts in the pathogenesis of postinjury multiple organ failure. Surg Clin North Am 1995;75:257–277.

55. Nowotarski PJ, Turen CH, Brumback RJ, Scarboro JM. Conversion of external fixation to intramedullary nailing for fractures of the shaft of the femur in multiply injured patients. J Bone Joint Surg Am 2000;82:781–788.

56. Pape HC, van Griensven M, Rice J, et al. Major secondary surgery in blunt trauma patients and perioperative cytokine liberation: determination of the clinical relevance of biochemical markers. J Trauma 2001;50:989–1000.

57. Pape H, Stalp M, van Griensven M, et al. [Optimal timing for secondary surgery in polytrauma patients: an evaluation of 4,314 serious-injury cases]. Chirurg 1999;70:1287–1293.

58. Brundage SI, McGhan R, Jurkovich GJ, et al. Timing of femur fracture fixation: effect on outcome in patients with thoracic and head injuries. J Trauma 2002;52:299–307.

CHAPTER 3

Reoperative Gastric Surgery

Scott F. Gallagher, MD; Sharona B. Ross, MD;
Michel M. Murr, MD, FACS

Précis

Important principles of reoperative gastric surgery transcend the cyclical nature of surgical diseases of the stomach such as peptic ulcer. Lessons learned from peptic ulcer surgery and its associated complications are employed in reoperative gastric procedures. The current approach to revisional antireflux procedures is also discussed, as laparoscopic antireflux procedures continue to be undertaken with increasing frequency.

Introduction

Revisional operations are frequently a challenging technical endeavor. Much has been written about gastric reoperative procedures, especially for complications and sequelae of the treatment of peptic ulcer disease. However, most of that information has become nearly irrelevant and relegated to historical significance because of the paucity of peptic ulcer operations that are undertaken in this era. However, some important principles of reoperative gastric surgery transcend the cyclical nature of diseases and can be applied to the current approach to reoperative gastric surgery.

Recurrent Ulcer Disease and Its Complications

The management of peptic ulcer disease has paralleled the evolution and understanding of anatomy, physiology, and pathophysiology of acid secretion, and more recently, of *Helicobacter pylori* infection. Fortunately, the incidence of peptic ulcer disease has been steadily decreasing over the last 50 years.[1] This decrease is primarily related to improvements in medical therapy, the identification and treatment of *H. pylori*, and an awareness of the importance of ulcerogenic agents (e.g., nonsteroidal anti-inflammatory drugs [NSAIDs], etc.) in the etiology of peptic ulcer disease.

Currently, the necessity for primary, elective operations for peptic ulcer disease has become rare. Nonetheless, the incidence of operations for specific complications of peptic ulcer disease and of previous peptic ulcer operations has remained unchanged.[2] Definitive hemostasis of bleeding peptic ulcers can be almost universally (>90%) achieved through endoscopic treatment.[2] Angiographic embolization is another effective method of controlling hemorrhage from gastroduodenal ulcers, which is particularly useful in patients with prohibitive operative risk.[3]

In general, it is established that worse outcomes and worse quality of life are commonplace following reoperations for recurrent peptic ulcer disease, especially in women undergoing secondary procedures for recurrent peptic ulcer disease.[4] In fact, many in this subset of patients ultimately require additional operations because of various gastrointestinal complaints considered to be a failure of maximal medical therapy or a recurrence of disease.[4]

Although it is uncommon, as a rule the principal indication for operative treatment of recurrent peptic ulcer disease is the persistence or recurrence of ulcer complications—specifically, those that do not respond to maximal medical or endoscopic therapy, and complications of the previous acid-reducing operations.[5,6] Although this chapter provides a summary of the important highlights for reoperative gastric surgery following recurrent peptic ulcer disease, the best and most current evidence-based review for the evaluation and management of patients with recurrent peptic ulcer disease after acid-reducing operations was recently published by Turnage et al.[5]

EARLY COMPLICATIONS

Early complications following peptic ulcer operations include gastroparesis, rebleeding, gastric perforations, anastomotic leaks, and duodenal stump blowout. Duodenal stump blowout, gastric perforations, and anastomotic leaks usually require urgent reoperation, whereas rebleeding and gastroparesis can usually be managed nonoperatively.

Early gastroparesis (or delayed gastric emptying), particularly following operations for indications that included gastric outlet obstruction, should be managed nonoperatively and with the utmost patience, as it nearly always resolves with prolonged gastric decompression, with nasogastric tube, or, preferably, through a surgically placed gastrostomy tube.

Recurrent hemorrhage from the ulcer bed may be evaluated and controlled endoscopically or sometimes angiographically. Attention to technical considerations in placing hemostatic sutures may minimize bleeding from collateral vessels to the gastroduodenal artery (Figure 3-1).

Gastric perforation and anastomotic leaks are best treated with closure of the defect and decompression of the stomach either with a nasogastric tube or a surgically placed gastrostomy tube. The use of drains is controversial in uncomplicated leaks, but is required for intra-abdominal abscesses.

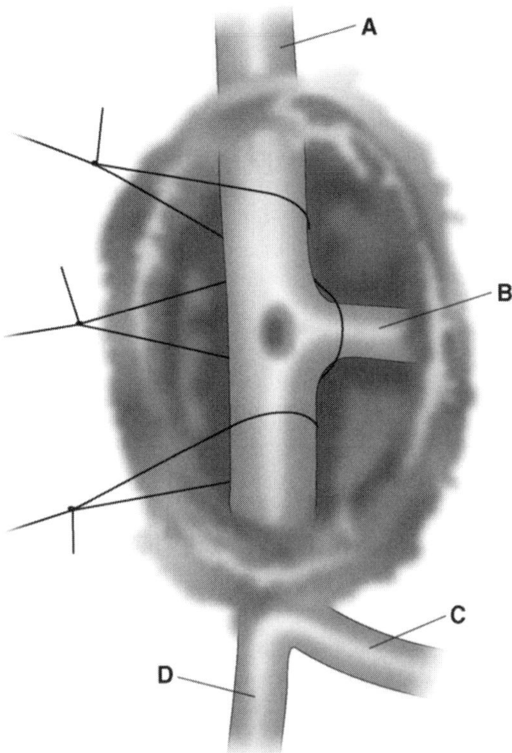

Figure 3-1 Technical considerations in controlling bleeding from an ulcer that eroded into the gastroduodenal artery. In addition to cephalad and caudad sutures to control the main trunk of the artery, a "U" stitch controls hemorrhage from often ignored collateral circulation (B).

Duodenal stump blowout is a dreaded complication of foregut operations and requires urgent celiotomy to prevent its usually severe sequelae. A duodenal stump blowout can result either from ischemia secondary to overly aggressive dissection of the duodenum during the initial operation, or as a result of complete obstruction of the aborad enteroenterostomy and ultimately a closed-loop obstruction that decompresses through the duodenal stump.

Primary closure of the dehisced duodenal stump may not be feasible because of friable or devitalized tissue. Alternatives include closing the stump around a duodenostomy tube with a purse string, or using tissue in approximation such as an omental patch or a jejunal serosal patch, otherwise known as a Thal patch. Routine use of drains is recommended to prevent or minimize the consequences of further (and common, problematic) leakage of duodenal contents. A gastrostomy and a feeding jejunostomy tube should be strongly considered. Inspection of the aborad enteroenterostomy should also be routine to ensure and document adequate patency.

Although a duodenal stump dehiscence may not be necessarily an indicator of poor surgical technique, it is appropriate to discuss various techniques to handle a difficult duodenum at the initial and revisional operations.

The best advice when considering the approach to a *difficult duodenum stump* is not to create one. Meticulous attention to technique and familiarity with this anatomically complex area cannot be overstated. Nevertheless, longstanding structuring ulcer disease and severe inflammatory changes can impose limitations to safe handling of the duodenum, especially in *posterior penetrating ulcers* that have eroded into the pancreas. In these instances, it is recommended that the duodenum be divided as close as possible to the pylorus, leaving sufficient anterior duodenal wall that can cover the ulcer bed, which may communicate with the duct of Santorini and can withstand sutures to the bed of the ulcer and pancreas, to close the duodenotomy. This procedure is otherwise known as a *Nissen's closure* (Figure 3-2).

In patients with severe inflammatory changes that preclude safe dissection of the duodenum, transecting the antrum in the context of an antrectomy proximal to the pylorus and undertaking a mucosectomy of the antrum *(Bancroft-Plenck procedure)* will avoid creating a difficult duodenal stump while removing all of the antral mucosa, thereby eliminating acid secretion and preserving adequate tissue to close the duodenum (Figure 3-3).

Alternatively, a *jejunal serosal patch* (Thal patch) can be undertaken by approximating the open edges of a duodenotomy to the serosal outer layer of the jejunum, using full thickness and water-tight sutures.

LATE COMPLICATIONS

Late complications following antiulcer operations include recurrent peptic ulceration, chronic postvagotomy postgastrectomy gastroparesis, alkaline reflux gastritis, dumping syndrome, postvagotomy diarrhea, afferent and efferent loop syndromes, and postgastrectomy cancer.

Recurrent Peptic Ulcer Disease—Initial evaluation of recurrent peptic ulcer disease begins with a thorough history and physical examination, specifically including a search for ulcerogenic substances and a family history of multiple endocrine neoplasia (MEN). Secondly, the details of the initial operations must be thoroughly reviewed, including indications, operative notes, pathology reports, prior contrast studies, and discussion with the operating surgeon, if possible. The incidence of recurrent peptic ulcers following vagotomy and drainage procedures is much higher than following vagotomy and antrectomy (2% to 27% and 0% to 5%, respectively).[5–7]

Likewise, recurrent peptic ulcerations can usually be attributed to either an incorrect or an incomplete primary operation. Ulcer recurrence was usually procedure-related (60% to 78%): large gastric remnant (56%), anastomotic stenosis (18%), and loop problems (4%); the remaining 22% of recurrent peptic ulcers could be attributed to ulcerogenic agents (10%), hyperacidity (6%), and Zollinger-Ellison syndrome (6%).[8–10] Clearly, the other most important etiologic association with ulcer disease and recurrence is chronic use of ulcerogenic agents, particularly NSAIDs (38%).[8–10]

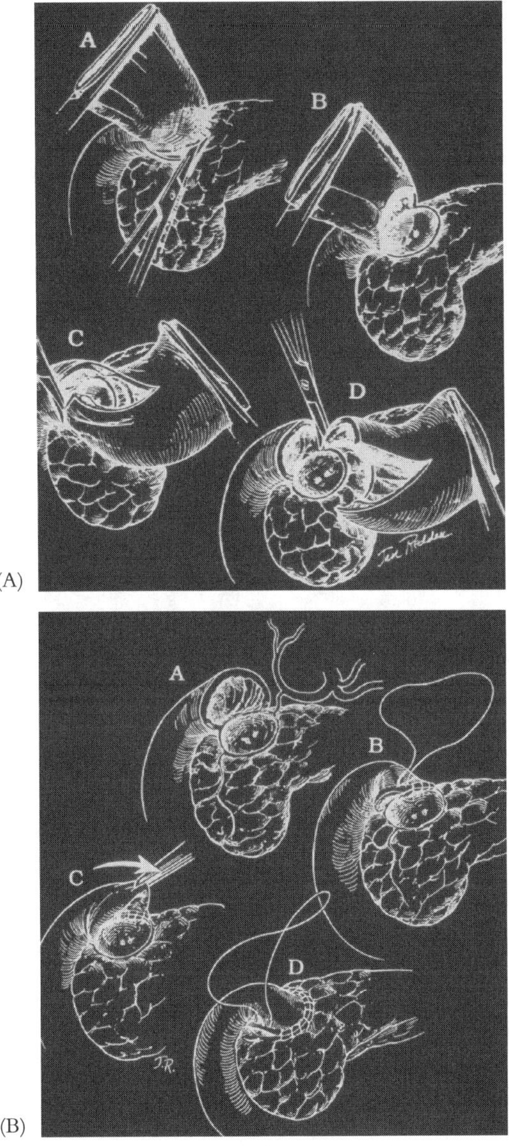

Figure 3-2 Initial dissection required for Nissen's closure. Large, posterior, penetrating ulcer may be safely managed by excising the duodenum but not the ulcer bed (A) and leaving adequate anterior duodenal wall to suture to the pancreas while closing the duodenotomy (B).

Following vagotomy and antrectomy, the evaluation algorithm and differential diagnosis are succinct. First and foremost, the most likely explanation is an intact vagus nerve *(incomplete vagotomy),* which can be attributed to aberrant nerve location or incomplete transection at the initial operation. Reoperation to completely divide the abdominal vagi may prove technically difficult and unrewarding; the

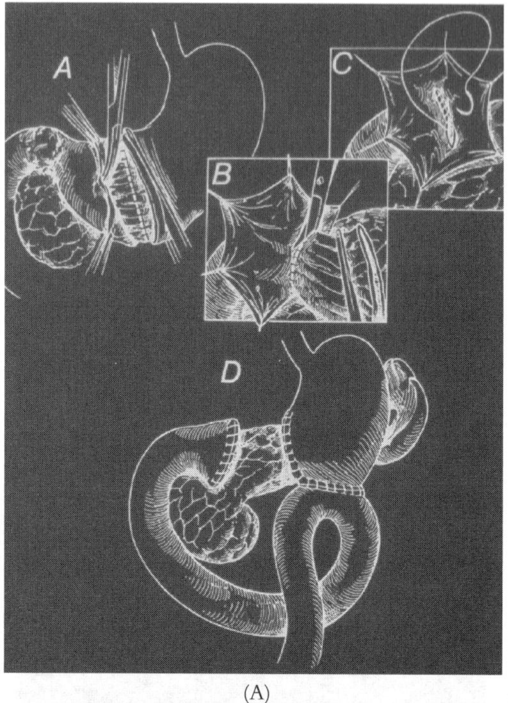

(A)

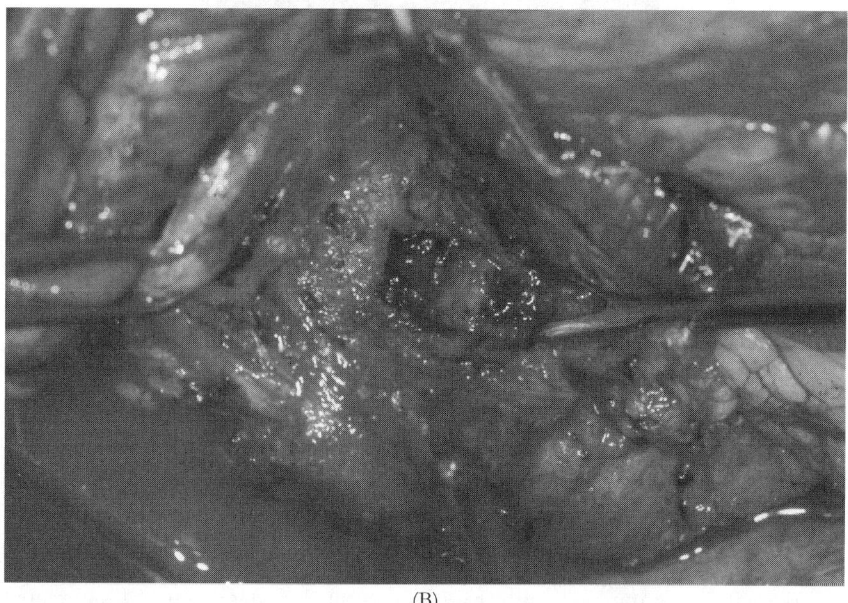

(B)

Figure 3-3 (A) Sketch demonstrating the technique of Bancroft's closure. (B) Intraoperative picture after an antral mucosectomy has been completed with electrocautery to the level of the pylorus. The Babcock clamps are at the cut edge of the antral muscle wall.

esophagus must be circumferentially skeletonized to ensure division of all vagal branches. Alternatively, a transthoracic vagotomy may be undertaken. A chemical vagotomy (proton pump inhibitor) may prove satisfactory and appealing to patients, and therefore many consider it as first-line therapy for uncomplicated recurrent peptic ulcers.

Retained gastric antrum is a rare but important consideration during the evaluation of recurrent peptic ulcer disease. When the excluded or retained antrum is continuously exposed to the alkaline duodenal and pancreatic fluids, gastrin inappropriately induces acid hypersecretion. The diagnosis can be confirmed with a sodium 99m-technetium pertechnetate scan that localizes retained antral mucosa within the closed end of the afferent loop.[5]

Zollinger-Ellison syndrome, although typically rare, becomes a more significant consideration in patients with recurrent peptic ulcer disease following an initial ulcer operation, especially when antrectomy was included. History of MEN, multiple or jejunal ulcerations often in atypical locations, and rugal hypertrophy are diagnostic clues.[5,11] Hence, a serum gastrin level should be included during the evaluation of recurrent peptic ulcer disease. Recommendations for serum gastrin as a screening tool have been summarized in a thought-provoking review by Ellison et al.[11] Early surgical resection of gastrinoma not only reduces metastases but also prolongs survival.[12–14]

Although rarely undertaken currently, revisional procedures for *intractable and recurrent ulcers* following technically satisfactory primary acid-reducing operations may involve either an antrectomy for patients with prior vagotomy and drainage procedure or a subtotal gastrectomy for patients with a prior vagotomy and antrectomy. Patients with proximal gastric vagotomy and recurrent ulcers may require an antrectomy with either a total abdominal or a transthoracic vagotomy.

Postvagotomy and Postgastrectomy Gastroparesis—The preponderance of postgastrectomy syndromes and the unpleasant side effects have driven a shift toward proximal gastric vagotomy as the preferred denervation procedure, with its lower incidence of these complications.[15,16]

Chronic postvagotomy postgastrectomy gastroparesis is one of the most incapacitating and difficult problems after gastric surgery. This syndrome occurs in patients, typically women (82%), as a consequence of denervating the proximal stomach and resecting the antral pump.[17] Initially, it was attributed to a dysmotility in the Roux limb (Roux stasis syndrome); however, evidence of clinical improvement after completion gastrectomy suggests that gastric stasis originates as a direct result of the paretic gastric remnant. Secondly, a large body of evidence from Roux-en-Y gastric bypass for obesity suggests that the Roux stasis syndrome is not clinically apparent or significant. Nevertheless, completion gastrectomy has been the most successful for relieving complaints of nausea, emesis, and postprandial pain; however, it had no significant effect on chronic pain.[17] Completion gastrectomy is recommended for patients who have clear and objective evidence of severe postvagotomy, postgastrectomy gastric stasis and have failed exhaustive attempts at nonoperative management.[17] The apparent hiatus from chronic pain up to 2 years subsequent to completion gastrectomy mandates an interdisciplinary approach, including pain specialists and psychiatrists, for long-term successful management of these patients.

Alkaline Reflux Gastritis—Otherwise known as bile acid reflux, is the most common postgastrectomy syndrome requiring reoperation.[16,18] It occurs commonly after loop gastrojejunostomy, but can occur following short limb Roux-en-Y reconstruction. A thorough evaluation, including endoscopy and radiography, is essential to correlate symptoms with the appropriate findings.

Conversion of a loop gastrojejunostomy (Billroth II) to Roux-en-Y anatomy will alleviate the symptoms of bile reflux. Because of concerns for dysmotility and delayed emptying, the technically cumbersome uncut Roux limb that interrupts luminal flow but maintains neuromuscular transmission, and hence eliminates the Roux stasis syndrome, can be constructed.[19] Alternatively, a Braun (distal) enteroenterostomy can be utilized to divert the bile from the gastric remnant in patients with a loop gastrojejunostomy.[18]

Dumping Syndrome—Dumping syndrome is thought to arise from a loss of the reservoir function of the stomach and contact of hyperosmolar foods with the jejunum. Early dumping symptoms occur within 15–30 minutes after a meal (both vasomotor and gastrointestinal symptoms), whereas late dumping symptoms occur within 2–4 hours after a meal, and are typically limited to vasomotor symptoms that are relieved by ingesting carbohydrates.[16] Maximal medical management as well as dietary education and manipulation (specifically avoiding carbohydrate-rich foods) are the mainstays of treatment and are usually satisfactory. With the development of octreotide, although expensive, few patients progress to operative management. Relief with operative treatment such as an antiperistaltic interposition is anecdotal.

Postvagotomy Diarrhea—Nonoperative and dietary manipulations have become the mainstay of treatment for postvagotomy diarrhea. In addition, fiber supplementation and cholestyramine are useful adjuncts. As with dumping syndrome, relief with operative treatment is anecdotal.

Afferent and Efferent Loop Syndromes—The afferent loop syndrome (projectile emesis of bile) and the efferent loop syndrome (emesis of gastric contents) are a consequence of anastomotic strictures of the gastrojejunostomy and respond to operative intervention. Similar complaints or symptoms that are not attributable to a correctable anatomic abnormality, such as a mechanical obstruction, usually do not respond to any of a multitude of interventions designed to relocate the anastomosis, since they typically have gastric stasis or paresis as the underlying etiology.[16,17]

Postgastrectomy Cancer—Postgastrectomy cancer is relatively uncommon, yet it is 3- to 5-fold more common than that observed in age- and sex-matched controls.[20] Malignancy associated with Billroth II reconstruction is significantly more predominant in the anastomotic areas within marginal ulcers, and, therefore, biopsy is required for any nonhealing anastomotic ulcer. Persistent, nonhealing ulcers should be excised.

DIAGNOSTIC STUDIES

The importance of endoscopy in the evaluation of recurrent peptic ulcer disease and its complications cannot be overemphasized. The location, number, and distribution of ulcers as well as retained food (gastric bezoar) or a stenotic anastomosis can be visualized. Endoscopic therapy for hemorrhage and stenotic anastomosis can be applied. Biopsy of all gastric ulcers is mandatory.

Upper gastrointestinal series radiography is also useful to evaluate gastric emptying and to clarify the details of the anatomic reconstruction. However, radiography is notoriously insensitive for detecting small or multiple ulcers, emphasizing the prior suggestion to routinely include endoscopy during the evaluation of recurrent ulcer disease.

TECHNICAL CONSIDERATIONS IN REOPERATIVE GASTRIC SURGERY FOR PEPTIC ULCER DISEASE

Knowledge of the index operative anatomy is of paramount importance to avoid surgical misadventures. Meticulous technique in adhesiolysis in the upper abdomen should be undertaken to delineate the anatomic reconstruction as usual landmarks are less apparent. The liver edge is usually one of the more consistent and early landmarks encountered. The liver edge (left lobe) can be followed to the gastroesophageal junction and anterior surface of the stomach. Caution should be exercised not to avulse the capsule of the liver or spleen, which can result in unnecessary and troublesome bleeding. However, it is better to dissect into the liver parenchyma to avoid multiple gastrotomies in the thin wall of the adherent fundus of the stomach.

Information about prior handling of the left gastric artery and short gastric vessels is important in planning resection of the gastric remnant. Liberal use of stapling devices will facilitate and expedite resection of the stomach and division of the duodenum.

The routine placement of drains during uncomplicated procedures is not warranted; however, placement of a jejunostomy feeding tube facilitates delivery of postoperative nutrition and is strongly recommended.

Revisional Antireflux Procedures

Laparoscopic fundoplication has emerged as an effective treatment for gastroesophageal reflux disease (GERD). Nevertheless, many studies have demonstrated a small group of patients in whom antireflux operations fail, thereby requiring revisional procedures for recurrent or persistent GERD symptoms.[21–23]

The majority of the patients can be managed nonoperatively with acid-reducing medications; nevertheless, approximately 4% to 6% will ultimately require revisional operations.[24–26] Notwithstanding the relatively short follow-up period, failure rates of laparoscopic fundoplication are similar to open procedures.[23]

The morbidity and mortality of patients who undergo revisional antireflux procedures is higher than those of primary fundoplication. Although the average mortality rate is 3%, with a range from 2.5% to 18%,[23,25,26] outcomes following revisional procedures are generally good, with success rates of 70% to 80% for the first reoperation.[25,27]

ANATOMIC CLASSIFICATION OF FAILED ANTIREFLUX OPERATIONS

Type 1 is present when the gastroesophageal junction is above the diaphragm, which can occur in two settings when the fundoplication as well as the gastroesophageal junction are above the diaphragm (Type 1a) or when the gastroesophageal junction migrates above the hiatus while the fundoplication remains below the hiatus (Type 1b)—akin to a "slipped Nissen" fundoplication. These patients generally experience symptoms consistent with delayed esophageal emptying: dysphagia and recurrence of GERD-like symptoms (Figure 3-4).

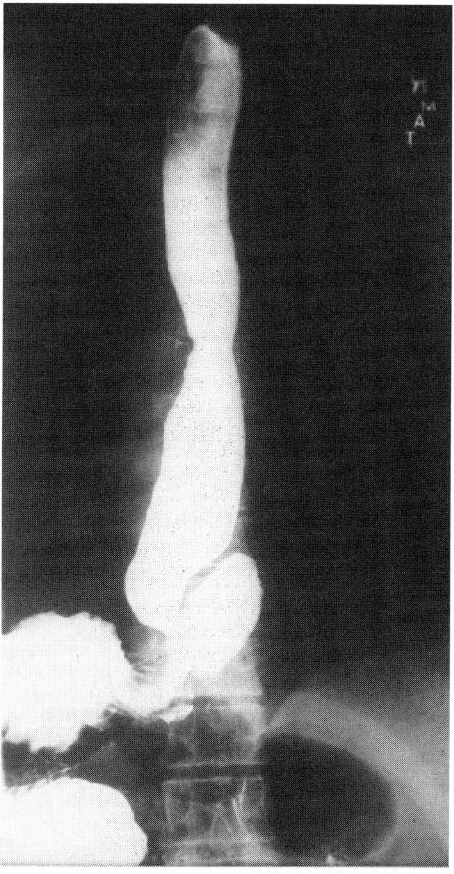

Figure 3-4 A contrast radiograph demonstrating the gastroesophageal junction below the diaphragm. A large portion of the fundus is present between the diaphragmatic hiatus and the opacified fundoplication wrap demonstrating a "slipped" Nissen.

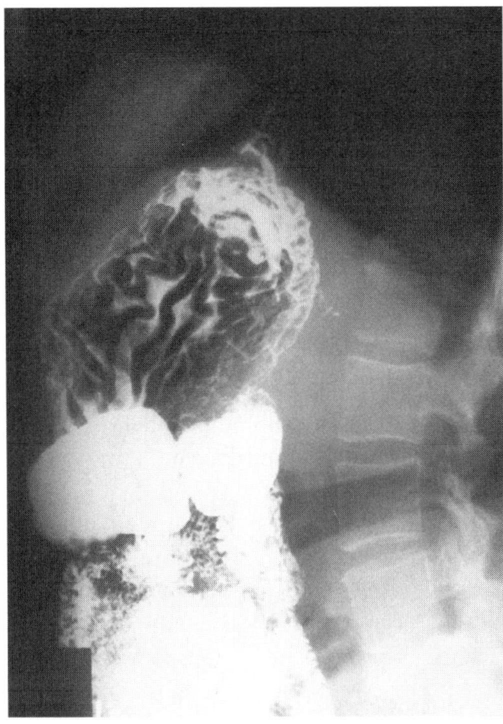

Figure 3-5 A contrast radiography showing a Type 2 failed Nissen fundoplication. The gastroesophageal junction and wrap are below the diaphragm; however, the posterior fundus migrated into the chest similar to a paraesophageal hernia.

Type 2 occurs when a portion of the stomach is above the diaphragmatic hiatus, commonly the posterior fundus. Given that the gastroesophageal junction in these patients is often in the normal position, these failures are sometimes misclassified as paraesophageal hernias (Figure 3-5). Because the herniated fundus leads to compression of the distal esophagus, dysphagia is a dominant compliant of these patients. Less commonly, patients complain of reflux-like symptoms.

Type 3 is used to describe a malformation of the fundic wrap. The malformation involves incorrect utilization of the midbody of the stomach in constructing the fundoplication instead of the true anterior fundus. This leads to redundant fundus and may promote delayed esophageal emptying.

In general, causes of failure of primary antireflux operations are different for open and laparoscopic procedures.[28] The major reasons for failure are summarized in Table 3-1. Failure of laparoscopic fundoplication is frequently associated with unwinding of the wrap, while open fundoplications frequently fail through disruption of the hiatal reconstruction.[28] Intraoperative findings during revisional

Table 3-1 Major Reasons for Fundoplication Failure

Reason for Failure	Patients (%)
Type 1a[31,33]	24–42
Type 1b[22,28,31,33]	13–25
Type 2[22,28,31,33]	16–29
Type 3[22,33]	7–16
Tight wrap[22,28,31]	4–6
Slipped Nissen with hiatus failure[28,31]	7–11
Missed diagnosis of achalasia[22,31]	4–5
Wrap breakdown and hiatus failure[28,31]	9–36

procedures after failed primary minimally invasive antireflux procedures reported from 1993–2000 include wrap herniation (36%), tight wrap (17%), slipped wrap (14%), disrupted wrap (13%), malpositioned wrap (11%), esophageal stricture (5%), loose wrap (2%), and other (6%).[29]

Because so many of these failures may be traced to suboptimal operative techniques (such as poor purchase of crural muscles, poor approximation of the diaphragmatic crura, or inadequate mobilization of the gastric fundus that result in tension along the wrap and ultimately promote unwinding of the fundoplication), we recommend dividing the short gastric vessels to fully mobilize the gastric fundus.[28] Additionally, putting tension on the wrap, from poor mobilization of the esophagus, can result in the fundoplication herniating into the chest. Consequently, we recommend mobilizing the esophagus to establish approximately 6–8 cm of intra-abdominal esophagus. In addition, patient selection is quite important and worth noting here. Obesity should be considered a relative contraindication for primary and reoperative antireflux procedures, given its frequent association with failure.

DIAGNOSTIC STUDIES

Evaluation of persistent or recurrent symptoms following fundoplication should include endoscopy and upper gastrointestinal radiography.[28] In addition to determining the presence and position of the wrap, a barium meal is also important to determine the adequacy of gastric emptying.

Endoscopy is more accurate than radiography in determining the anatomic location of the wrap and distinguishing whether a slipped Nissen or a tight fundoplication is present.[28] Endoscopic examination can also provide additional information, such as whether Barrett's changes exist in the esophagus or whether any other pathology is present in the esophagus, stomach, or duodenum.[28]

An ambulatory 24-hour pH study should be undertaken if radiography and endoscopy are not diagnostic. These studies are particularly important in patients who do not have an apparent anatomic cause for their symptoms. Results of the most recent pH studies should be compared to the prefundoplication studies, because some patients will have persistent symptoms of reflux despite an anatomically intact fundoplication, and this will be reflected through a remarkable improvement in their pH studies.

Similarly, esophageal manometry can be used to locate the lower esophageal sphincter (LES) and confirm the presence of an excessively tight wrap, changes consistent with achalasia, or generalized, poor esophageal motility. Manometrically, an LES constructed via fundoplication should not relax, as would be expected with a normally functioning sphincter mechanism.

CANDIDATES FOR REVISIONAL OPERATIONS

Patients with a surgically correctable anatomic or functional disorder corresponding to their symptoms are candidates for revisional procedures. Patients with recurrent or new symptoms following an antireflux operation are initially treated nonoperatively; however, symptoms of dysphagia will ultimately require revision. Patients who present with symptoms other than reflux or dysphagia rarely require or benefit from reoperation. This was confirmed in a recent review of the complications and results of 10,735 primary minimally invasive antireflux procedures, as the indications for reoperation after failed primary minimally invasive antireflux procedures from 1993–2000 included reflux (43%), dysphagia (24%), wrap herniation (18%), and others (14%).[29]

As mentioned previously, overweight patients should be encouraged to lose weight prior to surgery, because obesity increases intra-abdominal pressure which may predispose to breakdown of the crural reconstruction. Detailed information from the previous abdominal operations and the previous fundoplication is essential to the conduct of the revisional operation and should be sought as part of the initial evaluation.

TECHNICAL CONSIDERATIONS IN REOPERATIVE ANTIREFLUX OPERATIONS

Although technically challenging, laparoscopic revisions are feasible even after primary, open operations.[30] The laparoscopic approach begins with the placement of a Hassan cannula at the umbilicus under direct visualization.[28] After adequate pneumoperitoneum is established with maximum pressure of 12 to 14 mm Hg, four additional trocars are inserted along the right anterior axillary line, along the right and left midclavicular lines as they cross the subcostal margins and the subxyphoid area.[28]

The stomach is dissected off the liver bed and surrounding structures followed by identification of both the left and right crura. The left crus is more easily and safely approached along the greater curvature of the stomach, taking down the short gastric vessels if not already divided during the primary operation. Once the hiatus and the esophagus are identified, the distal esophagus is mobilized up into the mediastinum in order to reestablish 6–8 cm of intra-abdominal esophagus while reducing any hiatal hernia.[28] The gastroesophageal junction is located by repositioning the stomach into the abdomen.[31] Finally, the wrap should be completely mobilized and dissected from the surrounding adhesions. Once the anatomy of the stomach, hiatus, esophagus, and the wrap is defined, the cause for the failure of the primary fundoplication can be confirmed.[31,32] We utilize a bougie dilator (54 Fr for women and 60 Fr for men) to standardize the tightness of the wrap and to minimize postoperative dysphagia.

Revision is tailored to correct the anatomic cause of the failed fundoplication. If the wrap was completely disrupted or incorrectly constructed, a new fundoplication is created over a bougie dilator. If the wrap was partially undone, then the original wrap is repaired over a bougie dilator.[28]

The decision regarding whether construct a total (360°) or partial (270° or less) fundoplication is made in view of the anatomy and the preoperative manometric studies; patients with disordered esophageal motility usually require a partial wrap. For posterior wraps, the posterior fundus of the fundoplication is sewn to the diaphragmatic crura to secure the wrap in the abdomen and to minimize tension.[24]

In the presence of a sliding or paraesophageal hernia, which occurs because of a redundant fundoplication or a defective crural closure, the wrap is positioned into the abdominal cavity and the crura reapproximated behind the esophagus with interrupted sutures.[28] While mesh can be used to repair large defects in which the diaphragmatic tissues are significantly attenuated, the use of prosthetic material should be minimized, particularly if the gastrointestinal tract was entered during the course of the operation.

If a slipped Nissen is present, the wrap must be taken down, the gastroesophageal junction identified, and the fundoplication reconstructed around the esophagus. Occasionally, the original wrap is too tight and, therefore, needs to be converted to a 270° Toupet fundoplication. A pyloroplasty may be added when preoperative gastric emptying studies indicate delayed emptying.

Not uncommonly, incidental gastrotomies are made during dissection of the wrap, from either vigorous dissection or retraction. All gastrotomies are closed primarily. Air can be insufflated in the stomach under water seal to locate any unidentified defects. Drains and nasogastric tubes are utilized at the discretion of the operating surgeon.

COMPLICATIONS

As expected, complications after revisional antireflux operations are more frequent than they are after primary operations. The complications of revisional surgery are summarized in Table 3-2.

Incidental gastrotomies and esophagotomies are not uncommon and require immediate attention and closure. Similarly, pneumothorax is common, especially with extensive dissection into the chest where the pleura is adherent to the herniated stomach; it can be evacuated intraoperatively at the conclusion of the operation with a small-caliber catheter. The most dreaded long-term sequelae of revisional surgery is recurrence of symptoms or the onset of new symptoms such as dysphagia as a consequence of a tight wrap. Severe dysphagia may not be amenable to endoscopic dilatation and may require operative intervention.

Table 3-2 Complications of Fundoplication

Complications	Laparoscopic (%)	Open (%)
Gastrostomy[28]	25	44
Dysphagia[22,31,34]	2–27	NR
Esophagotomy[28,31]	0–2	NR
Pneumothorax[28,31,34]	2–19	25
Intra-abdominal bleeding[28,31]	6–8	0
Esophageal or gastric leak[28,34]	4–8	13
Myocardial infarction[28]	0	6.3
Recurrent reflux[32,35]	7	7
Delayed gastric emptying[34]	4	3
Stroke[28]	0	6
Pneumonia[22]	0	6
Wound infection[22]	0	3
Persistent nausea[22]	5	0

ND, not defined.

Summary and Future Directions

Reoperative gastric surgery is being revived by the explosion in antireflux surgery and bariatric surgery. Understanding the principles of gastric physiology and its anatomical considerations is paramount to successful outcomes. Lessons learned from peptic ulcer surgery should guide surgeons in revisional gastric procedures. Selection of patients based on objective and reproducible diagnostic studies may improve long-term outcomes. Clear understanding of the endpoints of treatment by both surgeons and patients may be achievable with nonoperative treatment and should be considered in the context of an interdisciplinary approach. The application of minimally invasive surgery may reduce the morbidity of reoperative gastric surgery and should be undertaken by technically adept surgeons.

REFERENCES

1. Gustavsson G, Kelly KA, Melton LJ, et al. Trends in peptic ulcer surgery: a population-based study in Rochester, Minnesota, 1956–1985. Gastroenterology 1988;94:688–694.
2. Zittel TT, Jehle EC, Becker HD. Surgical management of peptic ulcer disease today—indication, technique and outcome. Langenbecks Arch Surg 2000;385: 84–96.
3. Ljungdahl M, Eriksson LG, Nyman R, Gustavsson S. Arterial embolisation in management of massive bleeding from gastric and duodenal ulcers. Eur J Surg 2000;168:384–390.
4. Gonzalez-Stawinski GV, Rovak JM, Seigler HF, et al. Poor outcome and quality of life in female patients undergoing secondary surgery for recurrent peptic ulcer disease. J Gastrointest Surg 2002;6:396–402.

5. Turnage RH, Sarosi G, Cryer B, et al. Evaluation and management of patients with recurrent peptic ulcer disease after acid-reducing operations: a systematic review. J Gastrointest Surg 2003;7:606–626.
6. Browder W, Thompson J, Younberg G, Walters D. Delayed ulcer recurrence after gastric resection: a new postgastrectomy syndrome? Am Surg 1997;63:1091–1096.
7. Trout HH. Ulcer occurrence morbidity and mortality after operations for duodenal ulcer. Am J Surg 1982;144:570–572.
8. Stabile BE, Passaro E. Duodenal ulcer: a disease in evolution. Curr Prob Surg 1984;21:6.
9. Holscher AH, Klingele C, Bollschweiler E, et al. Postoperative recurrent ulcer after gastric resection—results of surgical treatment. Chirurg 1996;67:814–820.
10. Hirschowitz BI, Lanas A. Intractable upper gastrointestinal ulceration due to aspirin in patients who have undergone surgery for peptic ulcer. Gastroenterology 1998;114:883–892.
11. Ellison EC, Sparks J. Zollinger-Ellison syndrome in the era of effective acid suppression: are we unknowingly growing tumors? Am J Surg 2003;186:245–248.
12. Ellison EC, Carey LC, Sparks J, et al. Early surgical treatment of gastrinoma. Am J Med 1987;83(suppl 5B):17–24.
13. Ellison EC. Forty year appraisal of gastrinoma: back to the future. Ann Surg 1995;222:511–524.
14. Norton JA, Fraker KL, Alexander HR, et al. Surgery to cure Zollinger-Ellison syndrome. N Engl J Med 1999;341:635–644.
15. Johnston D, Blackett RL. A new look at selective vagotomies. Am J Surg 1988;156:416–427.
16. Delcore R, Cheung LY. Surgical options in postgastrectomy syndromes. Surg Clin North Am 1991;71:57–75.
17. Forstner-Barthell AW, Murr MM, Sarr MG, et al. Near-total completion gastrectomy for severe postvagotomy gastric stasis: analysis of early and long-term results in 62 patients. J Gastrointest Surg 1999;3:15–23.
18. Vogel SB, Braun WE, Woodward ER. Clinical and radionuclide evaluation of bile diversion by Braun enterostomy: prevention and treatment of alkaline reflux gastritis. Ann Surg 1994;219:458–466.
19. Tu BL, Kelly KA. Surgical treatment of Roux stasis syndrome. J Gastrointest Surg 1999;3:613–617.
20. Toftgaard C. Gastric cancer after peptic ulcer surgery. A historic prospective cohort investigation. Ann Surg 1989;210:159–164.
21. Watson DI, DeBeaux AC. Complications of laparoscopic antireflux surgery. Surg Endosc 2001;15:344–352.
22. Hunter JG, Smith CD, Branum GD, et al. Laparoscopic fundoplication failures: patterns of failure and response to fundoplication revision. Ann Surg 1999;230:595–604.

23. Hinder RA, Klingler PJ, Perdikis G, Smith SL. Management of the failed antireflux operation: surgery of the esophagus. Surg Clin North Am 1997;77: 1083–1098.

24. O'Hanrahan T, Marples M, Bancewicz J. Recurrent reflux and wrap disruption after Nissen fundoplication: detection, incidence and timing. Br J Surg 1990;77: 544–547.

25. Reiger NA, Jamieson GG, Britten-Jones R, Tew S. Reoperation after failed antireflux surgery. Br J Surg 1994;81:1159–1161.

26. Siewert JR, Isolauri J, Feussner H. Reoperation following failed fundoplication. World J Surg 1989;13:791–797.

27. Skinner DB. Surgical management after failed antireflux operations. World J Surg 1992;16:359–363.

28. Serafini FM, Bloomston M, Zervos E, et al. Laparoscopic revision of failed antireflux operations. J Surg Res 2001;95:13–18.

29. Carlson MA, Frantzides CT. Complications and results of primary minimally invasive antireflux procedures: a review of 10,735 reported cases. J Am Coll Surg 2001;193:428–439.

30. Rosemurgy AS. What's new in surgery: gastrointestinal conditions. J Am Coll Surg 2003;197:792–801.

31. Floch NR, Hinder RA, Klingler PJ, et al. Is laparoscopic reoperation for failed antireflux surgery feasible? Arch Surg 1999;134:733–737.

32. Granderath FA, Kamolz T, Schweiger UM, Pointner R. Laparoscopic refundoplication with prosthetic hiatal closure for recurrent hiatal hernia after primary failed antireflux surgery. Arch Surg 2003;138:902–907.

33. Pellegrini C, Horgan S, Pohl D, et al. Failed antireflux surgery: What have we learned from reoperations? Arch Surg 1999;134:809–817.

34. Curet MJ, Josleff RK, Schoeb O, Zucker KA. Laparoscopic reoperation for failed antireflux procedures. Arch Surg 1999;134:559–563.

35. Bais JE, Horbach TL, Masclee AA, et al. Surgical treatment for recurrent gastro-oesophageal reflux disease after failed antireflux surgery. Br J Surg 2000; 87:243–249.

CHAPTER 4

Reopérative Surgery for Inflammatory Bowel Disease

Tonia M. Young-Fadok, MD, MS, FACS, FASCRS

Précis

Although there are, of course, exceptions, in general reoperative surgery for Crohn's disease involves the complexities associated with recurrence of the disease, whereas reoperative intervention for ulcerative colitis entails management of complications from a preceding operation.

Introduction

Inflammatory bowel disease (IBD) comprises Crohn's disease (CD) and ulcerative colitis (UC). Both are often challenging disease entities in the operating room—Crohn's because of the associated features of fistula, stricture, abscess, phlegmon, and the propensity for multiple areas of disease, and UC as a result of the extent of the disease coupled with the complexity of procedures that restore intestinal continuity after excision of the entire colon and rectum. Reoperative surgery is even more challenging. In general, reoperative surgery for CD involves the complexities associated with recurrence of the disease, whereas reoperative intervention for UC entails management of complications from a preceding operation. Many series detail the frequency of reoperative procedures, and somewhat sparser data are available regarding outcomes. There is, however, a dearth of practical "how-to" information on the thought processes used as patients are evaluated for operation, the practicalities of re-do surgery, and the intraoperative decision-making that often is required as the procedure unfolds. This review is thus not an encyclopedic review of every topic, but hopefully a collection of practical advice gleaned from wise colleagues and patients with complex operative problems. In addition are included pointers regarding technical aspects at the initial procedure that may help to avoid a reoperation or facilitate a subsequent procedure.

Crohn's Disease

PRIOR OPERATION

General Principles—Most patients with CD ultimately require operative intervention. With current measures, the disease is incurable by medical or surgical means, and thus the goals of therapy are control of symptoms with minimal morbidity, while maintaining quality of life and continuity of the gastrointestinal tract when possible. Up to 90% of patients with CD ultimately fail medical therapy and undergo operation, and the majority of this group experience recurrence of disease. The need for reoperation is greatest within the first 5 years postoperatively, with 40% to 70% requiring one or more operations in the next 15 years.[1–3] The indications for reoperation are the same as for an initial procedure. Emergent indications include high-grade obstruction, uncontrolled sepsis, toxic megacolon, hemorrhage, or perforation. Medical therapy has failed and surgical intervention is warranted if the response to medical treatment is incomplete, maintenance medications cannot be discontinued as planned, or significant medication-related side effects develop.

In the absence of obstructive symptoms, a standard bowel preparation of one's choosing (usually either polyethylene glycol or Fleet phospho-soda) is used. If a laparoscopic approach is being considered, this author adds two tablets (10 mg) of bisacodyl, to minimize the amount of retained fluid that makes loops of small bowel difficult to handle. With chronic obstructive symptoms, a modified preparation consists of clear liquids and nutritional supplements for 2 to 3 days preoperatively. Magnesium citrate or phospho-soda may be used in small amounts.

Other preoperative preparation includes consideration of the position of a colostomy or ileostomy. Potential sites should be marked, preferably by an enterostomal therapist. If time allows, immunosuppressives such as 6-mercaptopurine, azathioprine, and cyclosporine should be stopped 2 weeks prior to operation. Stress dosing of corticosteroids is necessary if the patient has used corticosteroids within the preceding 6 months, and should follow published guidelines.[4]

Multiple Prior Operations—Care on entering the abdomen is essential in any patient with a previous laparotomy. Starting the midline incision either cephalad or caudad to the prior incision may help to identify a portion of the midline that is free of adhesions. CD is often additionally complicated by the presence of fistulas or phlegmon, and careful dissection is necessary to identify and protect adjacent structures. As CD often affects the small bowel diffusely, it is important to lyse all adhesions completely to evaluate the small bowel in its entirety, unless the risk of doing so (in terms of creating enterotomies) is considered to outweigh the potential risk of leaving an unidentified stricture. Review of the prior operative reports can be very helpful in identifying unexpected anatomy, as may exist, for example, after a previous bypass, and review of pathology reports indicate how much small bowel has already been resected.

Defunct Procedures—Internal bypass, once relatively commonly used, is now rarely recommended due to relatively high recurrence rates and the risk of malignancy.

The 15-year recurrence rates of CD treated by exclusion bypass, bypass in continuity, or resection were 82%, 94%, and 65% in one series, respectively.[5] A review of the literature showed that 30% of small bowel carcinomas occurring in the presence of CD were in bypassed segments. Bypass is acceptable if a phlegmon is densely adherent to other structures such as the retroperitoneum, when dissection is considered hazardous to retroperitoneal structures. Definitive resection and anastomosis should be planned for about 6 months later.[6]

RECURRENT SMALL BOWEL DISEASE

The management of recurrent small bowel or ileocolic disease is similar to that of primary disease in terms of intraoperative decision-making regarding whether to perform small bowel resection or strictureplasty. There is, however, a greater imperative to preserve small bowel length at reoperation, and limited areas of disease that might have been treated with resection at a primary procedure are more likely to be treated with strictureplasty. The total length of small bowel remaining at the end of the procedure should be measured and documented in the operative note. Marking the sites of resection and strictureplasty with metal clips may later be helpful in terms of identifying likely areas of recurrent disease on imaging studies.

Laparoscopic resection has an increasing role in the management of these patients. Isolated ileocolic CD is readily approached laparoscopically and has been shown in multiple series to have benefits of more rapid resolution of ileus, shorter hospital stays, reduced costs, and improved cosmetic results.[7–10] The small bowel can be inspected in its entirety, facilitated by a periumbilical extraction incision, so that proximal disease is not missed. An additional benefit is that the laparoscopic approach appears to result in fewer adhesions than laparotomy, thus facilitating a subsequent laparoscopic procedure. In addition, a laparoscopic approach is frequently possible even after a prior laparotomy.[10–12] In such cases, placement of the first port is safest by cutdown in an area distant from the prior midline incision, to avoid the likely presence of adhesions to the incision.

Small Bowel Resection—The length of unaffected bowel that should be resected proximal and distal to an area of CD is no longer the subject of controversy. Using frozen section evaluation of resection margins versus margins chosen after macroscopic inspection, case control studies have demonstrated no significant difference in clinical recurrence rates (60% versus 66%) and reoperative rates (36% versus 32%) at 10 years.[13] A randomized trial[14] of macroscopically disease-free margins of 2 cm versus 12 cm also showed no significant difference in clinical recurrence and reoperative rates. Thus, an anastomosis should be created with bowel that is soft, supple, and free of the macroscopic hallmarks of CD: wall thickening, fat creeping, serositis marked by corkscrew appearance of serosal vessels, and thickening of the mesenteric margin of the intestine. The mucosal surface should be inspected and should be free of frank ulceration; the presence of aphthous ulcers alone in supple bowel does not preclude an anastomosis.[6]

Strictureplasty—Strictureplasty is indicated as a means of bowel conservation. It is used for diffuse small bowel involvement with multiple strictures, strictures after prior major resection or in the presence of short bowel syndrome, and nonphlegmonous fibrotic stricture. At initial operation, resection is often preferred even for short segment disease if it allows complete resection of all disease. At repeat operation, resection is usually reserved for extensive segments of disease, multiple strictures within a short segment, or a stricture close to a site already requiring resection. Whether the procedure is performed open or laparoscopically, it is important to evaluate the entire small bowel to rule out other sites of disease. This is particularly important in patients who have been on immunosuppression and may have few if any serosal manifestations of the disease at the site of a short stricture. Passing a Baker tube (a long tube with an inflatable balloon) helps both in identification of other strictures and also in decompressing distended bowel proximal to a stricture.

RECURRENT COLONIC DISEASE

CD affecting a single segment of colon has been successfully approached with a limited resection and colocolonic or colorectal anastomosis.[15,16] The majority of patients will develop a symptomatic recurrence, but in a series of 49 patients undergoing segmental colonic resection, 86% maintained intestinal continuity and avoided a stoma with a mean follow-up of 14 years after the first resection. Recurrence is often limited to the anastomosis itself, and further resection or even strictureplasty may continue to avoid the need for a stoma.

COMPLICATIONS OF PRIOR OPERATION—NONHEALING PERINEAL WOUND

Pancolitis with perianal disease can result in proctocolectomy with ileostomy, and isolated severe perianal disease may result in proctectomy with colostomy. Both involve resection of the rectum and anal sphincter complex and can lead to an unhealed perineal wound. Attention to certain details at the time of the primary procedure can reduce the risk of this complication. An intersphincteric dissection leaves the muscle of the external sphincter in place, allowing approximation of muscle-to-muscle with attendant improved blood supply and healing, compared with the fat-to-fat apposition necessary if the entire sphincter is excised. Primary closure of the perineal wound, if possible, demonstrates improved healing compared with leaving the wound open to heal by secondary intention.[6] The muscles of the pelvic floor are approximated, and all abscesses and fistulae are unroofed and curetted free of debris and chronic granulation tissue. Then the relatively superficial wound can be packed, or, in the absence of perianal sepsis, the external sphincter and skin are also approximated. From the abdominal aspect, an omental flap can be raised and used to fill the dead space in the pelvis. Placement of pelvic drains with postoperative irrigation may result in fewer perineal wound infections (and thus chronic open wounds),[17,18] especially if the drains are brought out transabdominally rather than transperineally.[19] It is the author's preference, especially in young patients, to remove the entire rectum down to the pelvic floor, but leave the sphincter complex in place, with or without mucosectomy depending on the degree of anal canal involvement. In this manner, the possibility of subsequent reconstruction remains, in the event that improved medications at some point in the future allow for ileal pouch-anal reconstruction in the patient with CD.

In the early postoperative period, an unhealed perineal wound may respond to careful wound care at home combined with repeated curettage of the fibrotic walls in the operating room. If a perineal sinus persists after 6 months, more aggressive investigation and management are indicated. A sinogram, small bowel series, or computed tomography (CT) will exclude an enteroperineal fistula. Examination under anesthesia may be necessary to evaluate the wound adequately, as the patent skin opening is frequently smaller than the underlying chronic cavity. Previously, the mainstay of therapy for large chronic wounds would be a muscle or musculocutaneous flap, using gracilis, gluteus maximus, or rectus abdominis.[20,21] Current wound vacuum dressings would now be the preferred option,[22] with flaps reserved for failure of this technique.

Ulcerative Colitis

The gold standard procedure for surgical management of ulcerative colitis is proctocolectomy and ileal J-pouch-anal anastomosis (IPAA). In the majority of cases this is performed electively as a two-stage operation, with a diverting loop ileostomy to protect the pouch at the first stage, and stoma closure at the second. Occasionally, in the elective setting, a single-stage operation is performed without the addition of the loop ileostomy. When the initial indication is for emergent surgical intervention, the standard three-stage approach commences with an emergent subtotal colectomy, leaving an end (Brooke) ileostomy, and the proximal rectal stump either is stapled over or a mucus fistula is created at the rectosigmoid, thus avoiding pelvic dissection in the sick or unstable patient.

PRIOR ELECTIVE OPERATION (PROCTOCOLECTOMY AND IPAA)

Ileostomy Closure—Ileostomy closure after IPAA is usually performed 8 to 12 weeks after the first stage. As this is a planned second stage procedure, measures may be taken during the first procedure to facilitate this operation. The use of a hyaluronic acid adhesion-prevention membrane (Seprafilm) is becoming widespread, and the two-stage model of proctocolectomy followed by ileostomy closure was the model chosen to demonstrate a reduction in incidence of midline adhesions from 94% in the control group to 49% in the treatment group.[23] In addition to placement of the film over areas of dissection and between the bowel and abdominal wall, wrapping a half-sheet of the barrier around the chosen loop of ileum prior to bringing it up through the ileostomy site may result in easier mobilization of the stoma at the time of closure. In the event of extensive peristomal adhesions, adequate mobilization may not be possible via the ileostomy site. Although often discussed in preoperative counseling, this is a relatively unusual occurrence, and may be addressed either by utilizing the patient's prior midline incision or by extending the incision in the right lower quadrant. If the first procedure were performed laparoscopically, extensive adhesions are highly unlikely, as preliminary experience with this approach appears to result in reduced adhesion formation.[24,25]

The ileostomy may be closed in one of several fashions: unfolding the spout and closing the anterior defect; resecting the spout and creating a sutured end-to-end anastomosis; or performing a side-to-side stapled anastomosis. The author's preference is for the latter, as this appears to reduce the incidence of delayed return of bowel function secondary to suture line edema. A stapled anastomosis is facilitated if, at the first procedure, a loop of ileum of adequate mobility is chosen when creating the ileostomy; this may require slightly more proximal placement than usual, but should not compromise function.

PRIOR EMERGENT OPERATION (SUBTOTAL COLECTOMY AND RECTAL STUMP)

Completion Proctectomy and IPAA—Subtotal colectomy with retention of the rectum is the procedure of choice in the emergent setting in which ulcerative colitis presents with perforation, toxic megacolon, or bleeding, and in the semiemergent setting in the nutritionally compromised patient whose disease is refractory to medical therapy. Bowel is excised from the terminal ileum close to the ileocecal valve and preserving the ileocolic vascular pedicle, to the rectosigmoid junction, which is divided by stapling or brought up as a mucous fistula. Dissection in the pelvis in the presacral plane is avoided, to facilitate subsequent completion proctectomy. The stapled edge of rectum can be tagged with a permanent monofilament suture to aid later identification. The extensive adhesions often encountered at completion proctectomy can probably be reduced, as noted above, by using Seprafilm. It is the author's experience that adhesions are reduced even further, and are frequently minimal or even absent, if the first procedure is performed laparoscopically.

EARLY COMPLICATIONS OF IPAA

These complications of ileal pouch-anal construction occur within hours to 2 weeks postoperatively.

Pouch Bleeding—Minor oozing is common from the staple lines of the linear staplers used to construct the J-pouch, as the staples are not hemostatic; in most cases, this is self-limited. Some surgeons prefer to evert the pouch if bleeding continues, a practice the author does not advocate, as this can lead to separation of the staple lines. Alternatively, with illumination provided by a cable light source, the pouch can be irrigated and aspirated, and the bleeding point controlled by careful cautery or suture. If bleeding manifests itself postoperatively, it is best to take the patient back to the operating room for careful endoscopic (preferably flexible) evaluation of the pouch, with irrigation and cautery.

Pouch Ischemia—This complication is rare (it occurred in five of 101 patients undergoing pouch revision at the Cleveland Clinic[26]), but it is potentially devastating. The arrangement of the vascular arcades to the terminal ileum protects against ischemia in most cases, even if one branch of the arcade has been divided to produce extra length of the mesentery for creation of the pouch-anal anastomosis.

This diagnosis should be considered in the patient with features of septic shock, such as tachycardia, hypotension, and abdominal pain, within the first 24 to 48 hours, when peritonitis is still unlikely. The diagnosis is confirmed by gentle flexible endoscopy. At laparotomy, the pouch should be disconnected and examined, in case relieving tension on the mesentery improves blood flow. If the pouch requires excision, it is prudent not to attempt further pouch creation at this time, and instead leave the blind limb distal to the existing loop ileostomy after excision of the ischemic bowel, and return at a later date to attempt pouch creation again. Where the pouch has been disconnected, the anus may be closed with a mucosal purse-string suture, so that the sphincter mechanism is preserved. Seprafilm may be placed in the pelvis.

Pouch Sepsis—Rates of pelvic sepsis after IPAA range from 3% to 25%.[27–34] Several factors explain the variability of this rate, the most influential probably being differences in definition.[35] Some authors record any septic complication, whereas others confine the definition to the need for surgical intervention. Experience is another factor, as the incidence decreases as surgical experience increases. This applies both to experience gained over time, as the procedure has been modified, but also individual and institutional experience.

Early pelvic sepsis is signaled by fever, anal pain, tenesmus, and discharge of pus or secondary hemorrhage via the anus. Peritonitis generally indicates significant disruption of the pouch anal anastomosis. A combination of tests will establish the diagnosis: digital examination (under anesthesia if indicated), pouchogram with water soluble contrast, CT and magnetic resonance imaging (MRI). A localized abscess can generally be approached with CT-guided drainage. If this is not possible, or is unsuccessful, operative endoanal drainage may be considered via the anastomosis, thus creating a communication between the abscess and the pouch—the aim is to establish drainage and salvage the pouch. Later, once sepsis is controlled, if a defect remains at the anastomosis, and the patient is symptomatic (he or she may not be), then a transanal repair or advancement of the ileum and resuturing of the ileoanal anastomosis should be performed. In one series of patients with partial anastomotic disruption, success was obtained in three of seven patients treated with resuturing of the anastomotic defect and counter-drainage, and successful outcomes were seen in five of seven who underwent pouch advancement flap.[36]

Rarely, for example when peritonitis is present, laparotomy is indicated. Pouch excision is common when indications of extensive anastomotic breakdown exist. It is, however, worth salvaging the pouch if it can be disconnected from the anus without significant damage to the pouch, and bringing the distal end of the pouch up as an ileostomy. This then allows a subsequent attempt at reconnecting the pouch, without compromising function by having excised the 30 cm of distal ileum employed to construct the pouch.

LATE COMPLICATIONS OF IPAA

Small Bowel Obstruction—Small bowel obstruction (SBO) has traditionally been one of the more common of the late complications after IPAA, with an incidence of up to 30% at 10 years.[29,37] Up to 7.5% of patients require operative intervention for relief of obstruction.[37] The Seprafilm randomized trial demonstrated that, after laparotomy, 94% of control patients had adhesions to the midline incision at the time of ileostomy closure, compared with 49% of those treated with Seprafilm.[23] Whether this reduction in adhesions ultimately translates into a reduced incidence of SBO is the subject of a second multicenter randomized trial, currently in the process of accruing longer term follow-up. Given that the risk of bowel obstruction is so high, many surgeons performing this procedure routinely use this adhesion barrier, paying attention to placement of the membrane in the pelvis in addition to other surfaces of dissection. Interestingly, preliminary evidence suggests that a laparoscopic approach to the initial proctocolectomy and IPAA reduces adhesions to a greater extent than use of an adhesion barrier. Long-term impact on SBO is unknown for this procedure, although series of other, less extensive colectomies suggest a reduction in SBO.[24,25]

At laparotomy for SBO unresponsive to conservative management, it is often easiest to enter the abdomen above the upper limit of the prior incision, as the incision probably extended to the pubis at the initial procedure, making it inadvisable to enter the abdomen below this point. There are often extensive adhesions throughout the abdomen, requiring meticulous division. The point of obstruction is frequently a loop of small bowel adherent within the pelvis, either to the pouch or to the presacral area, which was exposed at the preceding pelvic dissection. Careful dissection is mandatory to avoid damage to the pouch. An obturator or sponge stick placed inside the pouch may aid in identification.

Delayed Pouch Sepsis—Delayed pelvic sepsis presents as abscess formation, with or without a fistulous connection to the pouch. These chronic, thick-walled abscesses often have few of the normal signs of sepsis, such as fever and elevated white cell count, as they have a means of partial egress via a pouch fistula. Instead, they often present with continued pain and poor pouch function, with frequent, loose, small-volume stools. If drainage can be established, and there is no continuing connection with the pouch, resolution may be achieved. In persistent sepsis there are three surgical options: the perineal approaches described above for acute sepsis, excision of the pouch, or an attempt at salvage, usually via an abdominal approach.

Multiple factors must be considered during discussion of whether pouch salvage or pouch excision is appropriate. Discussion should cover likelihood of success, magnitude of the operation in light of any comorbidities, and the patient's own wishes and lifestyle. Although many patients will opt to salvage the pouch if possible, excision of the pouch and ileostomy may not be considered a failure by the patient who is able to return to a normal life. Complications of attempted pouch salvage include damage to the pouch and loss of small bowel, pelvic nerve injury, enterotomy, and potential loss of the pouch if it cannot be salvaged. Potential complications from pouch excision include high-output ileostomy and nonhealing perineal wound.

Pouch sepsis is one of the most common serious complications after IPAA, and is also one of the most common indications for attempted pouch salvage.

Heuschen et al have described criteria for classifying patients into those with septic and nonseptic indications.[38] This classification was employed in a series of 101 patients undergoing repeat IPAA at Cleveland Clinic.[26] Anastomotic leak and any abscess or fistula were considered to be septic indications. Chronic anastomotic leak was defined as a chronic sinus, generally a presacral sinus commencing at the anastomotic line. One or more septic complications were found in 65 patients. Thirty patients had an IPAA leak and five a pouch body or tip leak; 21 had pouch- or anovaginal fistula; 21 a pouch or perianal fistula, a pouch-urethral fistula, or a pouch-cutaneous fistula; in addition, 46 patients had a chronic sinus or abscess. Repeat IPAA was performed in all patients in this series, and was defined as laparotomy, disconnection of the ileoanal anastomosis by either an abdominal or combined abdominoperineal approach, repair or refashioning of the pouch, and repeat pouch-anal anastomosis. Additional procedures were performed as indicated, including curettage of chronic sinuses and abscesses, and repair of fistulas.

As noted above for SBO, extensive adhesions are often encountered at laparotomy for salvage. These may be dense in the pelvis, particularly when salvage is being attempted for sepsis. Ureteral stents are helpful in identifying the course of the ureters, which may be drawn more medially than expected secondary to chronic inflammatory changes. Placing an obturator (e.g., a rigid proctoscope) in the pouch may assist with its identification. A sponge stick in the vagina helps to identify the correct plane anterior to the pouch. If possible, the integrity of the pouch is maintained, but in the presence of a known fistula or sinus, entry into the pouch at some point during the dissection must be expected. Given the dense peripouch inflammation that is usually present in chronic sepsis, identification of fistulas or pouch enterotomies can be facilitated by prior intrapouch instillation of diluted methylene blue. Distally, the pouch may be disconnected in one of two manners. Occasionally it is possible to staple below a prior staple line, but in general, it is easier to use a combined abdominoperineal approach and add a mucosectomy in the patient with a prior stapled anastomosis.[26] In the patient who previously has a mucosectomy, the perineal dissection is commenced at the anastomotic line. The pouch is salvaged if possible, or excised and another pouch created. Large pelvic drains are brought out through the lower anterior abdominal wall. Use of an omental flap can also be considered to fill dead space in the pelvis.

Results of abdominal salvage for chronic sepsis are highly variable. Outcome may be determined by severity of sepsis, level of sepsis in relation to the pouch (upper pouch, lower pouch, or pouch-anal anastomosis),[38] salvage procedure used, and length of follow-up.[35]

POUCH-VAGINAL FISTULA Pouch-vaginal fistula occurs in 0.6% to 16% of patients. The fistula may present before ileostomy closure (in which case, closure is delayed until the fistula is successfully treated), but about three-quarters present afterward.[39,40] Symptoms include vaginal discharge or passage of air or stool. Clinical examination frequently reveals the fistula, but it is occasionally found unexpectedly on pouchogram performed prior to ileostomy closure. In the patient in whom a fistula is suspected on the basis of symptoms, but cannot be demonstrated, instillation of dilute methylene blue in the pouch while the patient wears a vaginal tampon is a very useful test and may prevent the need for examination under anesthesia.

The fistula is usually at the level of the ileoanal anastomosis. Some series have, however, reported it as being at the dentate line. This may be reasonable in one series where two of 17 patients had the fistula at the dentate line,[39] but seems inordinately high in another series, where 14 of 59 were at the dentate line. Obviously, in the patient with a mucosectomy commencing at the dentate line, the distinction is spurious. Factors may include injury to the vagina during dissection in the rectovaginal septum, anastomotic dehiscence and sepsis, or incorporation of the posterior wall of the vagina during stapled pouch-anal anastomosis. It is thus extremely important at the time of the initial procedure to perform digital examination to ensure that the posterior wall of the vagina is free of the stapler.

Management is influenced by degree of symptoms and location of the fistula. If symptoms are not troublesome, intervention may not be necessary. In the symptomatic patient, imaging should assess whether there is evidence of undrained sepsis; usually there is not. Although some authors recommend defunctioning ileostomy at this point,[35] many surgeons would attempt at least one local (perineal) repair without subjecting the patient to another stoma. Defunctioning alone does not result in closure of the fistula.[41]

The distance of the fistula (at the ileoanal anastomosis) from the anal verge determines the surgical approach, either perineal alone or combined abdominoperineal. A perineal approach is feasible for a fistula arising from an ileoanal anastomosis within the anal canal or just above the sphincter. Ileal or vaginal advancement flaps may be options. An ileal advancement flap has a 51% success rate,[39,42–44] and a transvaginal flap achieves closure in 60% of patients.[39,45–47] If a muscle transposition (gracilis, rectus abdominis) is considered (usually after a prior failed repair), then a diverting ileostomy should be considered to protect this more complex approach. A pouch-vaginal fistula above the anorectal junction is approached via laparotomy, pouch revision, and repair of the vaginal aspect of the fistula. Combining series, salvage is obtained in 80% of patients.[48,49]

Poor Pouch Function—On average, patients with IPAA will have four to six bowel movements during the day, and up to two at night. The subjective impression of pouch dysfunction will change from patient to patient, and is often dependent on expectations. Many patients cheerfully accept up to 10 bowel movements daily, if the urgency, cramping, and bleeding previously associated with their disease is now resolved. Most would consider pouch dysfunction to exist if there are more than 10 stools per day, particularly if associated with urgency, cramping, or the need to strain to evacuate. Fecal incontinence is another cause of dissatisfaction with the pouch. Dysfunction is the cause of 20% to 40% of pouch failures.[31,45,50–52] Causes include mechanical outlet obstruction, sphincter dysfunction, and a small volume reservoir.

POUCH-ANAL ANASTOMOTIC STRICTURE Mechanical outlet obstruction is the result of either pouch-anal anastomotic stricture or a long efferent loop from an S-pouch. Stricture requiring dilation under anesthesia occurs in 4% to 40% of patients.[45,53–56] It is important to distinguish this from the web-like stricture that the vast majority of patients have at the time of ileostomy closure, and which responds to dilation under the same anesthetic. Stenosis may be more common after a stapled anastomosis than a sutured one (40% versus 14% in one series[56]), but studies do not control for the size of the stapler. Other contributing factors include sepsis, anastomotic separation, and ischemia.[55,57]

Most studies describe repeated dilations under anesthesia, and in this group of patients reasonable function is achieved in about 50%.[45,56,57] The problem in this setting is that patients frequently return when the stricture has recurred and there are no interval attempts to maintain patency and prevent restricturing. My preference, when a patient has required a second dilation under anesthesia, is to instruct them in self-dilation and send then home with several dilators of increasing sizes, to be used on a daily basis. In this manner, further operative dilations have been avoided in most patients. In short strictures, stricturotomy has been described, but experience with this is minimal, as it is for pouch advancement, which is difficult in the setting of stricture.[58] In the setting of a long stricture, pouch salvage, with mobilization via laparotomy, excision of stricture, and reanastomosis may be possible.[59]

OUTLET OBSTRUCTION SECONDARY TO LONG EFFERENT LIMB The S-pouch,[60] although infrequently used (fewer than 5% of pouches in the first 1000 patients at the Mayo Clinic, and almost nonexistent in the subsequent procedures in the new series of more than 2400 patients), is associated with evacuation difficulties secondary to a long efferent limb. In early series, 50% of patients with an efferent limb of 8 cm required pouch catheterization to evacuate the pouch; this decreased to 10% with a shorter (2-cm) limb. Some patients will tolerate self-catheterization, but many do not. Endoanal approaches are rarely possible, thus revision requires abdominoanal salvage, with pouch mobilization, division of the anastomosis, excision of the efferent limb, and creation of a new anastomosis. Improvement in function was obtained in 18 of 26 patients from five series using this approach.[61–65]

Small Volume Reservoir—Function appears to be related to pouch size and compliance. Frequency of defecation is inversely related to maximal tolerated volume of the pouch.[66–68] Contrast radiology can directly measure the dimensions of the pouch, and balloon volumetry measures maximal tolerated volume and urge. Although a small pouch may occasionally be the problem, with the solution being revision and augmentation of the pouch, this is usually not the issue with the currently accepted standard pouch size of 15 cm. Instead, the most common cause of a small reservoir is prior peripouch sepsis that has resulted in a contracted, noncompliant pouch. The solution here is the same as for chronic sepsis, namely mobilization and excision of the pouch, with revision versus reconstruction as indicated.

Pouchitis—Acute or chronic inflammation of the pouch occurs in 9% to 50% of patients[69,70] and increases with duration of follow-up. As a cause of frank pouch failure, however, this is an infrequent cause, accounting for only 7% to 15% of failures.[52] Treatment is medical. Defunctioning may provide temporary relief of symptoms, but further attacks resume when the stoma is closed.[71] For pouchitis refractory to medical therapy, pouch excision is one option, whereas a loop ileostomy offers the potential to reestablish continuity, should improved treatments for pouchitis be developed.

Retained Rectum/Cuffitis—The aim of proctocolectomy and IPAA is to eliminate symptoms by removing all mucosal disease. The earliest descriptions included mucosectomy of the upper anal canal with a sutured anastomosis at the dentate line. With stapling techniques, the anastomosis is created at the top of the anal canal and potentially leaves 1 to 2 cm of diseased mucosa. Some evidence supports retention of the transition zone at the dentate line, in terms of improved function, especially night-time continence; plus, a stapled anastomosis is easier to create. Symptomatic disease in the retained cuff of mucosa in the proximal anal canal is referred to as cuffitis. Many believe that if the anastomosis is truly at the level of the top of the anal canal, the amount of mucosa retained is so minimal that cuffitis is unlikely to be a true entity. Symptomatic disease is the result of an anastomosis performed too high, in the distal rectum, rather than at the top of the anal canal, leading to retention of too much rectum and its associated mucosal disease. Symptoms are those of proctitis. The level of the anastomosis is identified by digital examination; endoscopy with biopsies confirms the diagnosis. Topical treatments are attempted first, but if these fail, surgical intervention is indicated. An endoanal approach with mucosectomy and advancement of the pouch is rarely possible, as the nature of the diagnosis generally means the anastomosis is too high to reach from this approach. A combined abdominoanal approach is best, with mobilization of the pouch past the level of the anastomosis, ensuring that full mobilization is performed to the level of the pelvic floor. A mucosectomy and hand-sewn anastomosis is then performed. In a series of 22 patients, successful outcomes with reduced frequency and improved quality of life occurred in 15 of 22 patients.[72] The most successful approach to this problem is to ensure that it does not occur in the first place, by creating a stapled anastomosis truly at the top of the anal canal, or by performing a mucosectomy. Some features predispose to difficulties in performing the anastomosis—a narrow male pelvis, but most especially obesity. In the obese patient who is sufficiently symptomatic to be considering a surgical revision, chances of success are improved by insisting on preoperative weight loss.

CANCER

Patients with chronic UC will occasionally present with colon or rectal cancer. Concomitant colorectal cancer was present in 77 of 1616 patients undergoing IPAA at Mayo Clinic.[73] In the presence of resectable colon cancer, IPAA proceeds as usual; closure of the ileostomy is delayed until chemotherapy is completed. In the setting of rectal cancer, management choices made at the initial operation can facilitate subsequent surgery in the case of delayed pouch construction, and can reduce the risk of reoperative surgery for recurrent cancer. A rectal cancer that is stage II or III at presentation requires chemoradiation. This is preferably performed preoperatively to avoid subsequent radiation of the pouch. Despite preoperative imaging studies such as CT, endoanal ultrasound, and MRI, preoperative staging may be inaccurate. If intraoperative frozen section reveals more advanced disease than previously suspected in a patient who had had no radiation therapy preoperatively, it may be best to staple at the appropriate level below the tumor, place Seprafilm in the pelvis, and leave a Brooke ileostomy with the intent of returning after chemoradiation to create the ileal J-pouch. Either an omental flap placed in the pelvis or an omental sling may help to keep small bowel out of the pelvis and the field of radiation. Principles of resection for rectal cancer should be fulfilled with an appropriate total mesorectal excision and no compromise of the distal margin—the sphincter should be sacrificed if indicated by standard oncologic principles.

CESAREAN SECTION AFTER IPAA

As UC is a disease of young people, many female patients are capable of becoming pregnant after IPAA. Certain fallacies among patient and obstetrician alike must be dispelled. The pouch takes up no more room in the pelvis than the rectum did previously, and thus cannot obstruct the development of the uterus, nor can it obstruct labor. Likewise, the remainder of the small bowel remains in its normal anatomic position and does not fall in front of the uterus. The few series available have shown that pregnancy is safe in women with IPAA with minimal effect on postpartum pouch function, although this may be altered during the pregnancy.[74,75] Vaginal delivery is safe and obstetric reasons should determine whether a caesarian section is performed.[76] Approximately half of pouch patients have a vaginal delivery and half have a cesarean section.[74–76] Possibly the one pouch-related indication for cesarean section is the presence of a scarred perineum that will not dilate sufficiently to allow delivery. Additionally, in those patients in whom an episiotomy is indicated, the preference would be for a posterolateral incision rather than a midline episiotomy, to reduce the potential for tearing into the sphincter.

LIVER TRANSPLANTATION AND IPAA

A small subset of patients with UC and primary sclerosing cholangitis (PSC) will develop liver failure requiring transplantation. In a series from Mayo Clinic, 81 (75%) of 108 patients undergoing liver transplantation for PSC had concomitant IBD (all except one had UC).[77] Proctocolectomy had been performed prior to transplantation in 24 (22%). Among the 57 patients who retained their colons, three (5.3%) developed colorectal cancer, an incidence of approximately 1% per person per year, and the cumulative incidence of dysplasia was 15% at 5 years and 21% at 8 years. The authors concluded that the risk of colorectal neoplasia (dysplasia and cancer) after liver transplantation in patients with PSC and UC was not sufficient to mandate prophylactic proctocolectomy, but annual surveillance colonoscopy was recommended.

In one series of 16 patients with PSC undergoing surgical intervention for UC, the authors concluded that patients with significant PSC and requiring colectomy can undergo simultaneous orthotopic liver transplantation/total abdominal colectomy and then be candidates for subsequent ileal pouch-anal anastomosis reconstruction once liver function has improved.[78] Patients with well-controlled primary sclerosing cholangitis can undergo ileal pouch-anal anastomosis surgery safely. In another series of 30 patients undergoing liver transplantation for PSC, preexisting

UC was found to have an aggressive course in 15 (50%) of the patients, while de novo UC may develop after transplant for PSC when treated without long-term steroids.[79] Whether IPAA or liver transplantation is the first procedure performed in the patient with PSC and UC, the risk of requiring a second procedure merits placement of an antiadhesion barrier at the first procedure to facilitate the second should the need arise. The incidence of adhesions may be reduced even further if the initial IPAA is performed laparoscopically.

REFERENCES

1. De Dombal FT, Burton I, Goligher JC. Recurrence of Crohn's disease after primary excisional surgery. Gut 1971;12:519–527.
2. Farmer RG, Hawk WA, Turnbull RB. Clinical patterns in Crohn's disease: a statistical study of 615 cases. Gastroenterol 1975;668:627–635.
3. Himal HS, Belliveau P. Prognosis after surgical treatment for granulomatous enteritis and colitis. Am J Surg 1981;142:347–349.
4. Coursin DB, Wood KE. Corticosteroid supplementation for adrenal insufficiency. JAMA 2002;287:236–240.
5. Homan WP, Dineen P. Comparison of the results of resection, bypass and bypass with exclusion for ileocecal Crohn's disease Ann Surg 1978;187:530–538.
6. Strong SA. Crohn's Disease. In: Nicholls RJ, Dozois RR, eds. Surgery of the Colon and Rectum. New York, NY: Churchill Livingstone;1997:617–644.
7. Duepree HJ, Senagore AJ, Delaney CP, et al. Advantages of laparoscopic resection for ileocecal Crohn's disease. Dis Colon Rectum 2002;45:605–610.
8. Milsom JW, Hammerhofer KA, Bohm B, et al. Prospective, randomized trial comparing laparoscopic vs. conventional surgery for refractory ileocolic Crohn's disease. Dis Colon Rectum 2001;44:1–9.
9. Young-Fadok TM, Hall Long K, McConnell EJ, et al. Advantages of laparoscopic resection for ileocolic Crohn's disease. Improved outcomes and reduced costs. Surg Endosc 2001;15:450–454.
10. Wu JS, Birnbaum EH, Kodner IJ, et al. Laparoscopic-assisted ileocolic resections in patients with Crohn's disease: are abscesses, phlegmons, or recurrent disease contraindications? Surg 1997;122:682–688.
11. Young-Fadok T, Potenti F, Nelson H, et al. Laparoscopic resection of inflammatory bowel disease. Gastroenterol 1998;114:G459.
12. Hasegawa H, Watanabe M, Nishibori H, et al. Laparoscopic surgery for recurrent Crohn's disease. Brit J Surg 2003;90:970–973.
13. Hamilton SR, Reese J, Pennington L, et al. The role of resection margin frozen section in the surgical management of Crohn's disease. Surg Gynecol Obstet 1985;160:57–62.
14. Fazio VW, Marchetti F, Church JM, et al. Effect of resection margins on the recurrence of Crohn's disease in the small bowel. A randomized controlled trial. Ann Surg 1996;224:563–573.

15. Allan A, Andrews MB, Hilton CJ, et al. Segmental colonic resection is an appropriate option for short skip lesions due to Crohn's disease in the colon. World J Surg 1989;13:611–616.

16. Prabhakar LP, Laramee C, Nelson H, et al. Avoiding a stoma: role for segmental or abdominal colectomy in Crohn's colitis. Dis Colon Rectum 1997;40:71–78.

17. Fingerhut A, Hay JM, Delalande JP, et al. Passive vs. closed suction drainage after perineal wound closure following abdominoperineal rectal excision for carcinoma. A multicenter, controlled trial. The French Association for Surgical Research. Dis Colon Rectum 1995;38:926–932.

18. Robles Campos R, Garcia Ayllon J, Parrila Paricio P, et al. Management of the perineal wound following abdominoperineal resection: prospective study of three methods. Brit J Surg 1992;79:29–31.

19. Pahlman L, Enblad P, Stahle E. Abdominal vs. perineal drainage in rectal surgery. Dis Colon Rectum 1987;30:372–375.

20. Hurst RD, Gottlieb LJ, Crucitti P, et al. Primary closure of complicated perineal wounds with myocutaneous and fasciocutaneous flaps after proctectomy for Crohn's disease. Surgery 2001;130:767–773.

21. Loessin SJ, Meland NB, Devine RM, et al. Management of sacral and perineal defects following abdominoperineal resection and radiation with transpelvic muscle flaps. Dis Colon Rectum 1995;38:940–945.

22. Argenta LC, Morykwas MJ. Vacuum-assisted closure: A new method for wound control and treatment. Clinical experience. Ann Plast Surg 1997;38:563–576.

23. Becker JM, Dayton MT, Fazio VW, et al. Prevention of postoperative abdominal adhesions by a sodium hyaluronate-based bioresorbable membrane: a prospective, randomized, double-blind multicenter study. J Am Coll Surg 1996;183:297–306.

24. Reissman P, Tiong A, Skinner K, et al. Adhesion formation after laparoscopic anterior resection in a porcine model: a pilot study. Surg Laparosc Endosc Percutaneous Tech 1996;6:136–139.

25. Martz J, Marcello P, Braveman J, et al. Does laparoscopic colectomy prevent small-bowel obstruction? A long-term analysis. Dis Colon Rectum 2002;44: A48–A49.

26. Baixauli J, Delaney CP, Wu JS, et al. Functional outcome and quality of life after repeat ileal pouch-anal anastomosis for complications of ileoanal surgery. Dis Colon Rectum 2004;47:2–11.

27. Pemberton JH, Kelly KA, Beart RW Jr, et al. Ileal pouch–anal anastomosis for chronic ulcerative colitis. Long-term results. Ann Surg 1987;206:504–513.

28. McMullen K, Hicks TC, Ray JE, et al. Complications associated with ileal pouch-anal anastomosis. World J Surg 1991;15:763–767.

29. Meagher AP, Farouk R, Dozois RR, et al. J ileal pouch–anal anastomosis for chronic ulcerative colitis: complications and long-term outcome in 1310 patients. Br J Surg 1998;85:800–803.

30. Fazio VW, Ziv Y, Church JM, et al. Ileal pouch–anal anastomoses: complications and function in 1005 patients. Ann Surg 1995;222:120–127.

31. Gemlo BT, Wong WD, Rothenberger DA, et al. Ileal pouch–anal anastomosis. Patterns of failure. Arch Surg 1992;127:784–787.

32. Breen EM, Schoetz DJ Jr, Marcello PW, et al. Functional results after perineal complications of ileal pouch–anal anastomosis. Dis Colon Rectum 1998;41: 691–695.

33. Farouk R, Dozois RR, Pemberton JH, et al. Incidence and subsequent impact of pelvic abscess after ileal pouch–anal anastomosis for chronic ulcerative colitis. Dis Colon Rectum 1998;41:1239–1243.

34. Poggioli G, Marchetti F, Selleri S, et al. Redo pouches: salvaging of failed ileal pouch–anal anastomoses. Dis Colon Rectum 1993;36:492–496.

35. Tulchinsky H, Cohen CRG, Nicholls RJ. Salvage surgery after restorative proctocolectomy. Br J Surg 2003;90:909–921.

36. Fleshman J, McLeod RS, Cohen Z, et al. Improved results following use of an advancement technique in the treatment of ileoanal anastomotic complications. Int J Colorectal Dis 1988;3:161–165.

37. MacLean AR, Cohen Z, MacRae HM, et al. Risk of small bowel obstruction after the ileal pouch-anal anastomosis. Ann Surg 2002;235:200–206.

38. Heuschen UA, Allemeyer EH, Hinz U, et al. Outcome after septic complications in J pouch procedures. Br J Surg 2002;89:194–200.

39. Groom JS, Nicholls RJ, Hawley PR, et al. Pouch–vaginal fistula. Br J Surg 1993;80:936–940.

40. Carraro PS, Nicholls RJ, Groom J. Pouch–vaginal fistula occurring 13 years after restorative proctocolectomy. Br J Surg 1992;79:716–717.

41. Paye F, Penna C, Chiche L, et al. Pouch-related fistula following restorative proctocolectomy. Br J Surg 1996;83:1574–1577.

42. Ozuner G, Hull T, Lee P, et al. What happens to a pelvic pouch when a fistula develops? Dis Colon Rectum 1997;40:543–547.

43. Wexner SD, Rothenberger DA, Jensen L, et al. Ileal pouch vaginal fistulas: incidence, etiology, and management. Dis Colon Rectum 1989;32:460–465.

44. Lee PY, Fazio VW, Church JM, et al. Vaginal fistula following restorative proctocolectomy. Dis Colon Rectum 1997;40:752–759.

45. Galandiuk S, Scott NA, Dozois RR, et al. Ileal pouch–anal anastomosis. Reoperation for pouch-related complications. Ann Surg 1990;212:446–454.

46. Keighley MR, Grobler SP. Fistula complicating restorative proctocolectomy. Br J Surg 1993;80:1065–1067.

47. Burke D, van Laarhoven CJ, Herbst F, et al. Transvaginal repair of pouch–vaginal fistula. Br J Surg 2001;88:241–245.

48. MacLean AR, O'Connor B, Parkes R, et al. Reconstructive surgery for failed ileal pouch-anal anastomosis: a viable surgical option with acceptable results. Dis Colon Rectum 2002;45:880–886.

49. Shah NS, Remzi FH, Baixauli J, et al. Management and treatment outcome of pouch–vaginal fistula following restorative proctocolectomy. Colorectal Dis 2002;4(suppl 1):17.

50. Foley EF, Schoetz DJ Jr, Roberts PL, et al. Rediversion after ileal pouch–anal anastomosis. Causes of failures and predictors of subsequent pouch salvage. Dis Colon Rectum 1995;38:793–798.

51. MacRae HM, McLeod RS, Cohen Z, et al. Risk factors for pelvic pouch failure. Dis Colon Rectum 1997;40:257–262.

52. Tulchinsky H, Nicholls RJ. Long term failure after restorative proctocolectomy for ulcerative colitis. Dis Colon Rectum 2001;(suppl 3):19.

53. Marcello PW, Roberts PL, Schoetz DJ Jr, et al. Long-term results of the ileoanal pouch procedure. Arch Surg 1993;128:500–504.

54. Fleshman JW, Cohen Z, McLeod RS, et al. The ileal reservoir and ileoanal anastomosis procedure. Factors affecting technical and functional outcome. Dis Colon Rectum 1988;31:10–16.

55. Breen EM, Schoetz DJ Jr, Marcello PW, et al. Functional results after perineal complications of ileal pouch–anal anastomosis. Dis Colon Rectum 1998;41: 691–695.

56. Senapati A, Tibbs CJ, Ritchie JK, et al. Stenosis of the pouch anal anastomosis following restorative proctocolectomy. Int J Colorectal Dis 1996;11:57–59.

57. Lewis WG, Kuzu A, Sagar PM, et al. Stricture at the pouch-anal anastomosis after restorative proctocolectomy. Dis Colon Rectum 1994;37:120–125.

58. Fazio VW, Tjandra JJ. Pouch advancement and neoileoanal anastomosis for anastomotic stricture and anovaginal fistula complicating restorative proctocolectomy. Br J Surg 1992;79:694–696.

59. Fazio VW, Wu JS, Lavery IC. Repeat ileal pouch–anal anastomosis to salvage septic complications of pelvic pouches: clinical outcome and quality of life assessment. Ann Surg 1998;228:588–597.

60. Parks AG, Nicholls RJ. Proctocolectomy without ileostomy for ulcerative colitis. BMJ 1978;ii:85–88.

61. Ogunbiyi OA, Korsgen S, Keighley MR. Pouch salvage. Long-term outcome. Dis Colon Rectum 1997;40:548–552.

62. Nicholls RJ, Gilbert JM. Surgical correction of the efferent ileal limb for disordered defecation following restorative proctocolectomy with the J ileal reservoir. Br J Surg 1990;77:152–154.

63. Liljeqvist L, Lindquist K. A reconstructive operation in malfunctioning S-shaped pelvic reservoirs. Dis Colon Rectum 1985;28:506–511.

64. Sagar PM, Dozois RR, Wolff BG, et al. Disconnection, pouch revision and reconnection of the ileal pouch–anal anastomosis. Br J Surg 1996;83:1401–1405.

65. Herbst F, Sielezneff I, Nicholls RJ. Salvage surgery for ileal pouch outlet obstruction. Br J Surg 1996;83:368–371.

66. Oresland T, Fasth S, Nordgren S, et al. Pouch size: the important functional determinant after restorative proctocolectomy. Br J Surg 1990;77:265–269.

67. Heppell J, Kelly KA, Phillips SF, et al. Physiologic aspects of continence after colectomy, mucosal proctectomy and endorectal ileo-anal anastomosis. Ann Surg 1982;195:435–443.

68. Nicholls RJ, Pezim ME. Restorative proctocolectomy with ileal reservoir for ulcerative colitis and familial adenomatous polyposis: a comparison of three reservoir designs. Br J Surg 1985;72:470–474.

69. Moskowitz RL, Shepherd NA, Nicholls RJ. An assessment of inflammation in the reservoir after restorative proctocolectomy with ileoanal ileal reservoir. Int J Colorectal Dis 1986;1:167–174.

70. Heuschen UA, Autschbach F, Allemeyer EH, et al. Long-term follow-up after ileoanal pouch procedure: algorithm for diagnosis, classification, and management of pouchitis. Dis Colon Rectum 2001;44:487–499.

71. Shepherd NA, Hulten L, Tytgat GN, et al. Pouchitis. Int J Colorectal Dis 1989;4:205–229.

72. Tulchinsky H, McCourtney JS, Rao KV, et al. Salvage abdominal surgery in patients with a retained rectal stump after restorative proctocolectomy and stapled anastomosis. Br J Surg 2001;88:1602–1606.

73. Radice E, Nelson H, Devine RM, et al. Ileal pouch-anal anastomosis in patients with colorectal cancer: long-term functional and oncologic outcomes. Dis Colon Rectum 1998;4:11–17.

74. Nelson H, Dozois RR, Kelly KA, et al. The effect of pregnancy and delivery on the ileal pouch-anal anastomosis functions. Dis Colon Rectum 1989;32:384–388.

75. Juhasz ES, Fozard B, Dozois RR, et al. Ileal pouch-anal anastomosis function following childbirth. Dis Colon Rectum 1995;38:159–165.

76. Scott HJ, McLeod RS, Blair J, et al. Ileal pouch-anal anastomosis: pregnancy, delivery and pouch function. Int J Colorect Dis 1996;11:84–87.

77. Loftus EV Jr, Aguilar HI, Sandborn WJ, et al. Risk of colorectal neoplasia in patients with primary sclerosing cholangitis and ulcerative colitis following orthotopic liver transplantation. Hepatol 1998;27:685–690.

78. Poritz LS, Koltun WA. Surgical management of ulcerative colitis in the presence of primary sclerosing cholangitis. Dis Colon Rectum 2003;46:173–178.

79. Papatheodoridis GV, Hamilton M, Mistry PK, et al. Ulcerative colitis has an aggressive course after orthotopic liver transplantation for primary sclerosing cholangitis. Gut 1998;43:639–644.

CHAPTER 5

Reoperative Bariatric Surgery

Vivian M. Sanchez, MD; Eric J. DeMaria, MD, FACS;
David A. Provost, MD, FACS; George Blackburn, MD, PhD, FACS;
Daniel B. Jones, MD, FACS

Précis

With obesity now a national epidemic in the United States, bariatric surgery is becoming commonplace. Reoperative bariatric surgery requires familiarity with various weight loss operations, surgical principles, and lessons learned. This chapter covers information about the procedure, and emphasizes the importance of experienced bariatric surgeons performing the procedure in settings able to provide a comprehensive lifelong program—preferably by the surgeon who performed the original operation.

Introduction

Obesity is a major medical epidemic in the United States. More than 64% of Americans are overweight or obese and nearly 31% of all adults in the United States meet criteria for obesity. This totals nearly 61 million people in the United States alone.[1] Obesity leads to major health problems such as type 2 diabetes, heart disease, stroke, certain cancers, osteoarthritis, liver disease, obstructive sleep apnea and depression.[2] Obesity also shortens life expectancy by 2 to 5 years for those that are moderately obese, or by 5 to 20 years for those that are severely obese.[3] For these reasons, bariatric surgery has emerged as a growing field. It is the only effective treatment for the long-term reversal of obesity and its associated comorbidities. With nearly 100,000 bariatric procedures performed annually in the United States, experience with reoperative bariatric surgery is growing.

Overall, between 10% to 25% of patients who have undergone a bariatric surgical procedure will require a revision.[4] The exact indications for revisional surgery and the management of weight loss failure following obesity surgery remain controversial. Current indications for reoperative bariatric surgery include: treatment of bariatric surgical complications or technical failures, failed weight loss, excessive weight loss leading to malnutrition, or psychological reasons. The most common

Table 5-1 Re-operative Bariatric Surgery Series

Author	Patients	Deaths	Complications	Leaks
Yale 1989[5]	120	1%	—	—
Cates 1990[6]	32	13%	—	—
Linner 1992[7]	100	1%	—	—
Behrns 1993[8]	61	2%	11%	—
Kfoury 1993[9]	45	0%	33%	0%
Benotti 1996[10]	53	0%	49%	6%
Sugarman 1996[11]	58	0%	48%	3%
Capella 1998[12]	60	0%	5%	0%
van Gemert 1998[13]	48	0%	33%	13%
O'Brien 2000[14]	50	0%	17%	0%
Jones 2001[15]	141	0%	13%	3%
Vassallo 2001[16]	60	0%	5%	2%
Cariani 2001[17]	47	0%	54%	13%
Kyzer 2001[18]	37	—	32%	0%
de Csepel 2001[19]	7	0%	43%	0%
Gagner 2002[4]	27	0%	22%	0%
Westling 2002[20]	44	0%	—	0%
Total	990	1%	22%	3%

reason for revisional bariatric surgery is insufficient weight loss, although the reasons for reoperation vary greatly depending on the original procedure performed. Contraindications to elective revision for insufficient weight loss may include severe malnutrition impeding healing, ongoing sepsis, uncontrolled heart failure, recent myocardial infarction, recent pneumonia or other pulmonary exacerbation, binge eating disorder, or uncontrolled anxiety/psychological issues.

Patients undergoing bariatric surgical revisions can be expected to experience more complications, require longer operative times and longer hospitalizations[4] (Table 5-1). For example, approximately, 5% to 54% of patients will have complications ranging from wound infections, intra-abdominal abscesses, and leaks.[4,13,17] The leak rate on revisional surgeries varies between 0% to 13%, higher than on primary procedures where the quoted leak rates are between 0.5% to 5%.[21] The published mortality rates range from 0% to 13%, with an average mortality rate of at least 1.0%.

Not all patients are candidates for revisional bariatric surgery. Patient selection should be based on debilitating complications following a previous bariatric procedure, or failure of weight loss in a patient with persistent, significant comorbidities. Patients with failure of weight loss and non-life-threatening comorbidities such as back pain, dyslipidemias, depression, gastroesophageal reflux disease (GERD), or urinary incontinence should not be subjected to the increased perioperative risk given the small return on improvement in comorbidities after revisional bariatric procedures.

Prior to undertaking a reoperative surgical procedure it is imperative to understand the anatomy of the patient through endoscopy, radiographs, original/prior operative notes, and medical and hospital records. Upper endoscopy is essential to understanding the gastric pouch, its size, and problems within it such as ulcers, esophageal dilatation, esophagitis, staple line disruption, and anastamotic problems both proximally and distally. An upper gastrointestinal series (UGI) can clarify the overall anatomic picture and detect problems such as small fistulas or distal obstruction. Abdominal computed tomography (CT) scans can also be a useful tool in detecting a possible transition point, fluid collection, or fistula. A surgeon should obtain a copy of the old operative note, if one is available, to further understand alterations in the gastrointestinal anatomy. Knowledge of the anatomy influences the choice of surgical technique. Having no operative revisional plan prior to starting a reoperative case can only prolong operative time and potentially lead to oversight. For these reasons, we feel that the original surgeon is often the best to undertake a revision, when warranted.

Patients approaching a reoperative surgical procedure should undergo rigorous nutritional and psychological evaluation looking for nutritional deficiencies or behaviors such as binge eating that may compromise postsurgical outcomes.[22] Food logs, exercise logs, and detailed assessment evaluating for associated vomiting, heartburn, and pain are important. Patients must be forewarned that reoperative procedures carry greater risks and that the postsurgical course may be complicated. Most patients, if reversed, may regain all of their weight and more. Furthermore, diabetes mellitus, sleep apnea, and other associated comorbidities may return or worsen.

The surgical consent discussion must clearly outline all of the risks, especially death, leak, pulmonary embolus, prolonged intubation, gastrostomy tube placement, bleeding, fistulas, sepsis, failure of weight loss, weight gain, and need for further revisions. The detailed nature of the discussion should be clearly documented in the chart. Moreover, the surgeon should document understanding of these risks by spouse and family members.

For these reasons, reoperative bariatric surgery is best performed by a highly experienced bariatric surgeon, at a center with intensive care units, radiology, and nutritional and psychological support staff that can accommodate bariatric patients.

Reoperation for Complications

Patients with complications following bariatric surgery typically present with a constellation of symptoms. Nausea, vomiting, abdominal pain, failure to tolerate oral intake, fatigue, dizziness, weakness, and/or reflux are some of the more common physical ailments. Other times, more subclinical complications such as esophagitis, GERD, staple line disruption, or malnutrition present in a more obscure manner. Each surgery will be discussed based on indications, common presentations of failures followed by reoperative techniques, and finally technical points.

Box 5-1 General Principles for Reoperative Bariatric Surgery

1. Obtain preoperative medical and psychological clearance and ensure patient has realistic expectations.
2. Obtain a detailed consent form with firm understanding of increased risks.
3. If considering operating for failed weight loss, evaluate comorbidities. Consider behavioral, nutritional, and exercise regimens for those who do not have significant comorbidities.
4. Obtain careful dietary and exercise logs for those with failed weight loss.
5. Know current anatomy of a patient. Use radiographs, endoscopy, and old operative notes.
6. Perform revisions open unless you are a highly experienced laparoscopic surgeon.
7. Take down adhesions between the stomach and the liver carefully, using sharp dissection to avoid blood loss. Find plane between Glissen's capsule and the serosa of the stomach. May have to take down short gastrics to expose lesser curvature.
8. Avoid crossing staple lines. Oversew those that do cross.
9. If leaving an old band in, open the band or remove excess stomach above it to prevent a gastric sequestrum.
10. Make liberal use of gastrotomy tubes.
11. Make liberal use of drains.
12. Do not staple across foreign objects such as mesh.
13. The original surgeon may be the best to undertake the reoperation.

REVISIONS FOR COMPLICATIONS OF VERTICAL BANDED GASTROPLASTY

Vertical banded gastroplasty (VBG) is uncommon today because of the lack of sustained/desired weight loss and the high incidence of complications requiring revision. The incidence of VBGs requiring revision is between 20% and 56%.[10,13] The majority of these revisions are required for staple line disruption, stomal stenosis, band erosion, band disruption, pouch dilatation, and GERD.[4]

Staple line disruption has an incidence of 27% to 31% and can be as high as 48% if assessed on routine postoperative endoscopy.[23] Staple line disruption typically leads to weight gain. Conversely, stomal stenosis occurs in approximately 31% to 33% and leads to food intolerance, reflux, and often weight regain due to dietary shifts to calorically dense liquids and softer foods. Band erosion is another frequent late complication of VBG occurring with an incidence of 1% to 11%. The band can erode along either the lesser curvature or the circular staple line.[24] External band erosion along the lesser curvature leads to more adhesions. Gastroesophageal reflux after VBG presents with classic symptoms such as burning pain, heartburn, aspiration, and cough. It typically occurs as a late complication as a result of stomal stenosis and pouch dilatation. GERD not responsive to comprehensive antireflux medical therapy will often require reversal of the VBG. Esophagitis is more indolent in presentation, and in a recent review of 25 patients undergoing a revision of a VBG for symptomatic reflux, esophagitis was present in 58% of patients and Barrett's esophagus in 28%.[25]

Recurrent vomiting will present in approximately 8% to 21% of all patients following VBG.[26] It can be a result of maladaptive dietary patterns such as eating too quickly or not chewing properly, but can also be secondary to functional problems such as stomal stenosis, pouch dilatation, staple line disruption, or GERD. Oftentimes, these patients will become sweet eaters in an attempt to ingest calories in a form that does not cause vomiting. Not all of these patients with recurrent vomiting will require an operative revision. Initial treatment should consist of dietary modification and radiologic/endoscopic assessment evaluating for structural problems. If the vomiting persists and leads to malnutrition, operative revision should be considered.

Stomal stenosis following VBG can be initially managed nonoperatively with the aid of endoscopic dilatation, with surgery reserved for failures. Some argue that dilatation, especially early postoperatively, is unsuccessful due to the rigid nature of the band. One series reports a success rate of 68% for endoscopic dilatation of stomal stenosis.[27] Symptomatic relief following endoscopic dilatation is often of short duration, and operative revision should be considered when symptoms such as persistent vomiting recur. A negative consequence of dilatation is the formation of scar tissue, making eventual revision more difficult. Overall, there is no unified consensus on the management of stomal stenosis. Initial management should consist of a trial of stage 2–3 diets. A gastrostomy tube for nutritional supplementation can also be helpful.

Band erosion can also be managed nonoperatively via endoscopic extraction. Some authors suggest that endoscopic band extraction has lower morbidity and mortality rates than surgery. Band extraction, however, leads to weight regain.

Vertical banded gastroplasty can be revised in a variety of ways. A simple alternative is to revise the staple lines and/or the band.[13,15,16,24] Another approach is to take down the gastroplasty and perform a formal Roux-en-Y gastric bypass (RYGB) or other malabsorptive procedure.[10,11,15,28,29] Several groups have described even converting a VBG into an adjustable gastric band.[14,30] Although there is no formal consensus on revision of a gastroplasty, most studies suggest that revision of a VBG alone leads to more complications and less weight loss than when gastroplasties are converted to a formal gastric bypass.[11] In the literature, conversion of a VBG to a RYGB decreases the reoperation rate from 68% to 0% and leads to sustained weight loss and improvements in symptoms in the majority of patients.[13] Morbidity rates are lower when gastroplasties are converted to open RYGB than when revised (11% versus 36%); leak rates are also lower (3% versus 7%).[15]

Conversion of a VBG to a RYGB can usually be performed safely via an open approach. Laparoscopic revisions should be reserved for experienced laparoscopic bariatric surgeons.[31] The band may or may not be removed, the stomach transected beyond the gastroplasty, and then a gastrojejunostomy constructed (Figure 5-1). Many surgeons have performed this with little mortality, sustained weight loss, and resolution of symptoms; but complication rates are high (20% to 33%).[9,13,20,25,29] These complications are usually related to leaks, wound infections, incisional hernias, and pulmonary issues. The leak rate in one series is as high as 20%,[13] the etiology of which has been attributed to tissue ischemia. This leak rate appears to

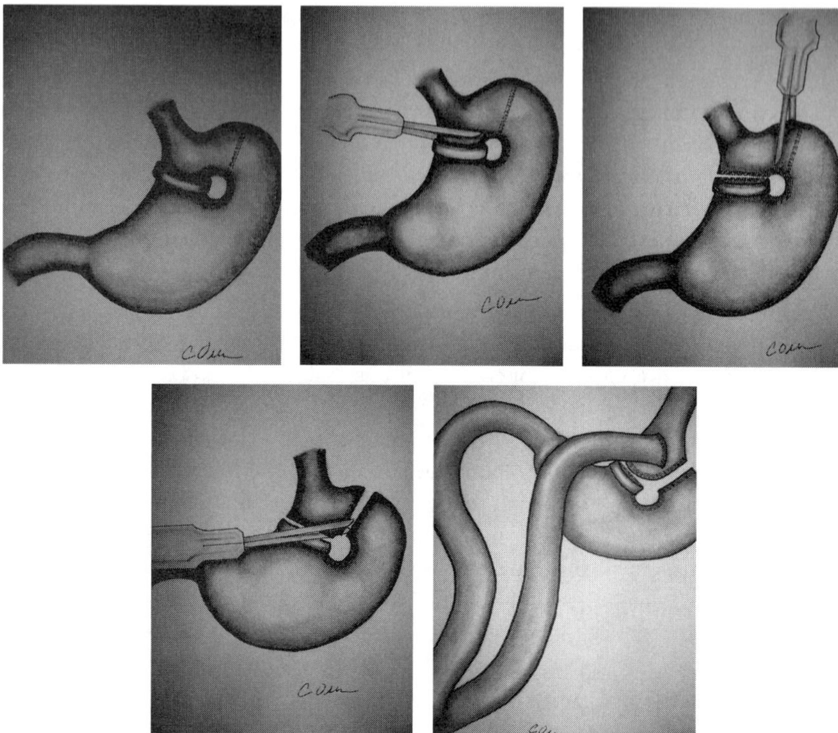

Figure 5-1 Conversion of a vertical banded gastroplasty to a Roux-en-Y gastric bypass.
Previous staple lines must be resected
New gastric pouch is formed, avoiding crossing staple lines or blind gastric sequestrums
Band can be either left in situ or removed completely
If band is left in place, it must be opened
Creation of a gastrojejunostomy and jejunojejunostomy

Acknowledgement: The authors kindly thank Christeen Osborn, a surgical resident at the BIDMC, for her talented illustrative work.

decrease dramatically if a lesser curvature pouch is made, preserving the rich vasculature along the lesser curvature.[12]

Technical points for conversion of a VBG to a RYGB include the complete mobilization of the pouch from the liver capsule up to the gastroesophageal (GE) junction, mobilization of the greater curvature to allow access to the lesser sac, removal of the band completely if technically feasible or opening it if unable to remove it secondary to dense fibrosis, division of the stomach above the band toward the angle of His, complete separation of the pouch from the gastric remnant, oversewing of any crossed staple lines, removal of any remaining stomach above the band (if left in situ), and formation of a gastrojejunostomy.[32,33] Many surgeons report extensive fibrosis and adhesions along the lesser curvature up to the liver.

These must be taken down gently to avoid excessive blood loss. Silastic rings can usually be removed, because they lie within a pseudocapsule, whereas Marlex or Prolene bands require more dissection due to dense fibrosis. It is important to remove any pouch remnants that are nonviable or excluded from the remaining stomach. Many report that the high incidence of leaks after revision of VBG is due to poor blood supply or an inadequately drained "blind" gastric pouch that develops between two staple lines.[34] It is also important to open the ring if leaving a remnant of the gastroplasty pouch above it to facilitate drainage. If removing the ring, it is important to evaluate the stomach for any evidence of serosal tears.

In general, we favor the use of a gastrostomy tube during reoperative bariatric procedures to help prevent postoperative gastric dilatation and gastric remnant rupture. Relative indications for a gastrostomy tube include patients who are beyond the weight limit for radiographic assessment or those who require nutritional support in the setting of a postoperative leak (again, as these patients are at a higher risk of developing a leak). Intraoperative testing of the anastomosis to exclude leaks can be useful in detecting leaks with methylene blue, saline, or air insufflation. Liberal use of drains is also recommended, even if intraoperative testing of the integrity of the anastomosis fails to reveal a leak, as small leaks can be missed. The timing of removal of a drain is more controversial; some surgeons advocate leaving a drain in as long as 10 days.[35] Other surgeons believe that drains can be a source of infection or a cause of erosion and remove them as soon as a patient has started oral intake.

REVISIONS FOR COMPLICATIONS OF ROUX-EN-Y GASTRIC BYPASS

Complications of RYGB are diverse and vary based on the technique utilized. The overall published reoperation rate varies from 6% to 23%.[10,36] If patients are followed to 12 years, Kaplan-Meier analysis predicts the incidence to be 12%.[13] Common complications requiring reoperation are internal hernias, bleeding, leak, marginal ulcers, strictures, and incisional hernias.

Internal hernias occur with a frequency between 0% and 5% in bariatric series.[21] Most hernias occur through the transverse mesocolon in cases where the anastomosis is constructed in a retrocolic manner. Hernias through the transverse mesocolon are not amenable to nonoperative treatment and must be repaired laparoscopically or via open surgery. The transverse colon must first be lifted cranially to expose the transverse mesocolon, the herniated bowel reduced, and the mesenteric defect reapproximated in a circumferential manner. Nonabsorbable sutures such as silk should be utilized to close this defect, decreasing the internal hernia rate by 50%.[37] Before securing the jejunum through the transverse mesocolon, one must ensure that the jejunum above the colon is not overly redundant, potentially leading to further intussusception. In addition, Peterson's space is closed to prevent herniation through this potential space.

Bleeding after gastric bypass occurs after 0.6% to 4.0% of all bariatric procedures.[21] Early bleeding typically occurs from one of the various staple lines, and can develop intra-abdominally or intraluminally. These bleeds typically resolve with conservative management, but may require a blood transfusion. Discontinuation of perioperative anticoagulation therapy used for prophylaxis of thromboembolic events may aid in cessation of bleeding. Surgery is reserved for hemodynamic instability or uncontrolled bleeding not responsive to conservative measures. These cases can be approached laparoscopically, especially if the patient is stable. All staple lines should be assessed and any areas with active oozing oversewn. Upper endoscopy can be utilized if the bleeding is intraluminal in nature. If the bleeding is localized to the pouch, sclerosing agents have been utilized successfully. Bleeding from the gastrojejunostomy occasionally occurs after RYGB and may occur more frequently in cases where the anastomosis is constructed with a stapler rather than by hand-sewn technique. Intraoperative intervention for a bleed may include oversewing the anastomosis in its entirety over an endoscope placed under direct visualization as a stent. Reexamination of the bleeding site via endoscopy can then be utilized to confirm cessation of bleeding. If the bleeding is suspected to originate from the enteroenterostomy, the entire anastomosis may be opened and inspected. Early postoperative bleeding from the gastric remnant is likely from the staple line. Opening the remnant may be helpful if oversewing the staple line fails to control the bleeding. Intraoperative endoscopy through the gastric remnant via a gastrotomy may help identify the location of bleeding.

Late bleeding after gastric bypass may be investigated with bleeding scans or angiography, after excluding pouch or marginal ulcer bleeding by endoscopy. Bleeding from the gastric remnant may be approached in several ways. If a patient is stable, a percutaneous gastrostomy can be placed and the patient scoped through a dilated gastrostomy. If a patient is unstable, bleeding recurs, or gastrostomy is not possible, operative gastrostomy extending through the pylorus permits evaluation of the gastric remnant and duodenum. If indicated, duodenal ulcers are oversewn, and completion gastrectomy performed to control acute hemorrhage.

Gastrojejunal stenosis occurs commonly with an incidence of 4% to 8% and is usually treated successfully by endoscopic balloon dilatation. Failures of medical management require revision in very few cases. Treatment of persistent stenosis despite repeated dilatations requires reconstruction of the entire gastrojejunostomy. The main objective in these revisions is to provide an anastomosis where there is little tension and good blood supply. These revisions may even require returning to the base of the jejunal mesentery to release it further. Repositioning an antecolic or antegastric Roux limb to a retrogastric, retrocolic position is often sufficient to eliminate tension on the anastomosis.

Revisions for marginal ulcers are relatively uncommon. Ulcers may be a complication of poor tissue vascularity, staple line disruption, gastrogastric fistulas resulting in chronic exposure of the gastrojejunal anastomosis to acid, anastomotic tension, or nonsteroidal anti-inflammatory use.[21] Medical management with acid suppression should be attempted as first-line therapy. Carafate may be a useful addition. Revision of marginal ulcers may require complete division of the remnant from the pouch, as well as resection of the ulcer and revision of the gastrojejunal anastomosis, in the manner described above.[10] Some groups advocate truncal vagotomy at the time of revision for marginal ulcers.

Incisional hernias occur with an incidence of 0% to 1.8% in laparoscopic series and at least as high as 20% in open series.[21] Repair of incisional hernias may fail if the patient is still significantly obese. Many surgeons postpone a formal repair until significant weight loss occurs (more than 1 year) and nutritional status is stabilized. Indications for early repair are pain, signs of obstruction, or rapid enlargement of the hernia. Mesh may be utilized to close the defect, or, if the procedure is combined with an abdominoplasty, primary closure or plication may suffice.

Reoperation for leak requires clinical vigilance of signs such as respiratory compromise or unexplained tachycardia greater than 120 bpm.[38] Treatment consists of percutaneous drainage of the fluid collection if the patient is stable, or operative drainage for instability. Operative drainage can be performed open or laparoscopically, but must include copious irrigation, wide drainage, possible repair of the defect (if tissue is viable), and broad-spectrum intravenous antibiotics. All gastric staple lines as well as the jejunojejunostomy must be assessed for integrity. Intraoperative testing for leaks with methylene blue, saline, or endoscopy is helpful to locate the area of leak. Some surgeons perform this laparoscopically, but often conversion to an open procedure may be necessary to find and repair the leak, if it is not clinically obvious.

Revisions for strictures at the jejunojejunostomy are also indicated in patients with gastric remnant distension or afferent loop syndrome to avoid gastric rupture, a highly lethal complication. Early postoperative strictures at the enteroenterostomy may result from technical error in creation of the anastomosis from narrowing of the efferent limb. Repair may include formation of an enteroenterostomy proximal to the stricture, but often the entire anastomosis will have to be redone. These strictures may also occur late postoperatively as a result of tissue ischemia from dividing the mesentery during the initial operation, narrowing of the common channel during JJ closure, or kinking of the common channel despite placement of a Brolin stitch. There are even some reports of adhesions formed at the JJ leading to a bowel obstruction with resultant gastric remnant rupture.

Overall, revisions of RYGB are associated with much higher leak rates of 19% to 37%.[35] Revisional surgery increases the predicted complication rate following gastric bypass by 67% to an incidence of 33%.[39] The use of gastrostomy tubes is advocated in the bypassed stomach to prevent postoperative gastric dilatation. Liberal utilization of drains may better identify and manage leaks postoperatively, if they occur.

REVISIONS FOR COMPLICATIONS OF LAPAROSCOPIC ADJUSTABLE GASTRIC BAND

Complications following laparoscopic adjustable gastric band (LAGB) are infrequently based on European, Australian, and United States FDA B trials. On average, approximately 6% to 8% of patients will require reoperation, although some have quoted rates as high as 50%.[40] New standards for training and certification should improve these outcomes. The majority of these reoperations are for acute stomal obstruction, band slippage, erosion, port problems, tube problems, pouch/esophageal dilatation, and infection.

Reoperations for acute stomal obstruction are early events, within the first few postoperative days. Acute stomal obstruction manifests as persistent nausea, vomiting, inability to tolerate oral secretions or oral intake. It may be caused by a band that is too tight, either from inclusion of excess tissue or secondary to tissue edema. The diagnosis is confirmed with a UGI. Acute stomal obstruction can be treated conservatively with nasogastric tube decompression until the edema subsides or it can be taken to the operating room, where the band is disengaged and the fat near the gastric cardia is defatted. Experts on the band describe defatting several areas along the lesser curvature, the angle of His, the GE junction, and posterior to the stomach to prevent acute stomal obstruction.[41] Conservative management, however, is not without risks. A surgeon should be aware of the potential for aspiration and tissue ischemia with management of acute stomal obstruction with nasogastric tube decompression.[42]

Later complications of the LAGB are erosions, prolapse, esophagitis, reflux, or tube/port problems. Similarly to the VBG, LAGB erosions can sometimes be removed endoscopically, but the laparoscopic approach may allow better assessment and tissue repair. Tube problems such as disconnects can be managed laparoscopically by reuniting the tubes and connectors. In the case of a port flip, the port must be reanchored to the anterior abdominal fascia. If a tube or port leak is suspected, the location should first be confirmed via radiologic contrast injection through the port. Later, the port and tubing should be exchanged.

Port infections pose a more difficult problem. Band erosion must first be ruled out via upper endoscopy. If there is no erosion, the port should be removed, the tube disconnected and tied, and then placed within the peritoneal cavity. Local wound care is accomplished with dressing changes and antibiotics until the infection is cleared. A new port can then be reimplanted several weeks later. If this conservative approach fails, it will usually require complete removal of the band. If an erosion is suspected because of persistent port infections despite a negative workup, band removal should also be considered.

Band prolapses occurred more frequently after the perigastric technique and before the utilization of the pars flaccida technique. These problems may be related to the position of the band at time of placement, large food consumption by the patient, or excessive vomiting. Symptoms of gastric prolapse include food intolerance, epigastric pain, and reflux.[42] Treatment of posterior prolapse consists of taking down the gastrogastric imbrication sutures, releasing the band, and rethreading the band through the angle of His, via a new retrogastric tunnel. Another alternative is to replace the band with a new one. Some surgeons will simply remove the band altogether,[42] especially if significant inflammation is found.

The presence of gastric/esophageal dilatation may develop in 10% or more of patients with the LAGB in long-term follow-up in some series. Overinflation of the band due to repeated adjustments precipitated by poor weight loss or excessive amounts of food intake may be the cause. The first maneuver is to completely deflate the LAGB. Deflation alone is usually successful.[42] If a trial of less restriction is unsuccessful, some would replace the band in a new location through a new tunnel. Another alternative is to convert the LAGB to an RYGB in cases of severe esophageal/pouch dilatation.[43] Some groups routinely convert failed bands in duodenal switch (DS) procedure,[34] especially in cases where there is extensive scar tissue around the band.

Problems such as esophagitis/GERD can usually be treated by deflating the band and placing the patient on acid suppression therapy. If this is unsuccessful, the patient may require band removal or conversion to a RYGB (if weight is still an issue).

REVISIONS FOR COMPLICATIONS OF MALABSORPTIVE PROCEDURES

Nutritional deficiencies and their complications are the most frequent indications for revision or reversal of malabsorptive weight loss operations. Although no longer performed as a primary weight loss operation, as many as 25,000 jejunoileal bypasses (JIBs) were performed in the United States through the early 1980s. The incidence of hepatic and renal failure following JIB increases linearly with time, and liver function tests are unreliable in detecting the development of hepatic disease.[44] As a result, many surgeons recommend reversal of JIB in appropriate operative candidates. Simultaneous revision to RYGB has been reported with success to prevent weight regain, and was better tolerated than VBG.[8]

Nutritional complications are less frequent following biliopancreatic diversion (BPD), with or without DS, although revision for protein malnutrition, excessive diarrhea, or excessive weight loss is required in 2% to 12%.[45,46] Revision of the enteroenterostomy to provide a common channel of at least 150 cm is usually sufficient, although weight regain may occur.

Reoperation for Failure of Weight Loss

Many studies indicate that the most common reason for revision of bariatric surgical procedures is failed weight loss. In series of patients undergoing revisional bariatric procedures, insufficient weight loss was the primary cause of revision in 35% to 91% of patients.[4,10,25] Interpreting the data on revisions for failed weight loss is difficult because of the lack of consistent criteria for defining insufficient weight loss. The definition for failure of weight loss varies from less than 50% EWL, to less than 30% EWL in some series. Other studies use weight regain as a criterion for revision. Perhaps the single most important criterion for consideration of a revision is the continued presence of serious comorbidities.

REVISIONS FOR INSUFFICIENT WEIGHT LOSS FOLLOWING VERTICAL BANDED GASTROPLASTY

The most common reason for weight gain after VBG is staple line disruption. Many of these staple line dehiscences occur at the angle of His by UGI,[16] but can occur at multiple points as well. Revisions of VBG can be performed in a variety of ways; however, if the indication is for failed weight loss, a conversion to a RYGB is often recommended. The reason for this includes the superior weight loss following conversion to a gastric bypass. Patients undergoing conversion of a VBG to a RYGB lost on average between 54% and 77% of EWL as compared to patients who had redo-VBGs who lost only between 24% and 33% of EWL.[8,47,48] In addition, 46% of patients undergoing a redo-VBG will require a third operation, usually for failed weight loss,[5] further stressing the importance of converting a failed VBG into a gastric bypass if the indication is for failed weight loss. It is important to note that some surgeons report successful conversion of a failed VBG into LAGB with excellent weight loss.[18]

REVISIONS FOR INSUFFICIENT WEIGHT LOSS FOLLOWING ROUX-EN-Y GASTRIC BYPASS

Modification of RYGB for insufficient weight loss is based on two principles. One approach is to modify the restrictive component by modifying pouch size. Another approach relies on increasing the malabsorptive component. It is believed that the pouch stretches from overeating, and thus patients can eat more without a sense of satiety. By making a smaller pouch, a surgeon may increase the restrictive component and possibly affect satiety. While initial weight loss occurs following reduction of pouch size or revision of a dilated gastrojejunal stoma, weight regain is common as the disordered eating behaviors that led to the initial failure persist making weight loss marginal. More effectively, RYGB can be converted to a distal RYGB by shortening the common channel to 150 cm from the ileocecal valve.[49] This technique increases EWL from 30% at 1 year to 69% at 5 years, but can be limited by malnutrition, requiring nutritional support.

REVISIONS FOR INSUFFICIENT WEIGHT LOSS FOLLOWING LAPAROSCOPIC ADJUSTABLE GASTRIC BYPASS

Failure to lose weight after LAGB must be carefully studied before undertaking revisional surgery. Often a careful dietary and exercise log with nutrition and psychological evaluation to investigate eating and exercise activity will lead a surgeon to elucidate the etiologies leading to weight gain. Counseling may help restore compliance and weight loss outcomes. Some surgeons specializing in LAGB advocate more frequent follow-up visits and band fills with a strict algorithm for these patients who fail to lose weight. The belief is that the failure of weight loss is more related to insufficient band fills.

Surgical revision is reserved for patients who have failed all of these maneuvers and who still have persistent serious comorbidities. Conversion to RYGB is our procedure of choice to date for failure of weight loss after LAGB. Alternative revisional approaches, such as DS with the band left in situ, may reduce the perioperative risk by avoiding the previously operated stomach with its thickened tissue and scarring. Patients revised to another band did not lose weight, indicating perhaps a maladaptive eating or psychological component.[50,51]

Conclusion

Revisional bariatric surgeries are performed most commonly for insufficient weight loss with lack of resolution of comorbidities or for complications of the original bariatric procedure. Before revising a patient, it is important to carefully evaluate the anatomy and screen patients for dietary, psychological, and medical issues. Patients need to commit preoperatively to lifestyle and dietary modifications, including daily exercise, monthly support groups, and lifetime follow-up. Reoperative bariatric surgery carries higher morbidity and mortality rates than the original bariatric procedure and should be undertaken primarily in patients with significant medical comorbidities due to obesity and by surgeons specialized in bariatric surgery who are aware of the technical nuances involved in such difficult procedures.

REFERENCES

1. Flegal KM, Carroll MD, Ogden CL, et al. Prevalence and trends in obesity among US adults, 1999–2000. JAMA 2002;288:1723–1727.
2. Statistics related to overweight and obesity. NIH publication No. 03-4158. July 2003.
3. Fontaine KR, Redden DT, Wang C, et al. Years of life lost due to obesity. JAMA 2003;289:187–193.
4. Gagner M, Gentileschi P, de Csepel J, et al. Laparoscopic reoperative bariatric surgery: experience from 27 consecutive patients. Obes Surg 2002;12:254–260.
5. Yale CE. Conversion surgery for morbid obesity: complications and long-term weight control. Surgery 1989;106:474–480.
6. Cates JA, Drenick EJ, Abedin MZ, Doty JF, Roslyn JJ. Reoperative surgery for the morbidly obese: a university experience. Arch Surg 1990;125:1400–1404.
7. Linner HL, Drew RL. Reoperative surgery: indications, efficacy and long-term follow-up. Am J Clin Nutr 1992;55(suppl):606S–670S.
8. Behrns KE, Smith CD, Kelly KA, Sarr MG. Reoperative bariatric surgery: lessons learned to improve patient selection and results. Ann Surg 1993;218: 646–653.
9. Kfoury E, Vanguri A. Distal Roux-en-Y gastric bypass conversion for failed vertical banded gastroplasty. Obes Surg 1993;3:41–43.
10. Benotti PN, Forse RA. Safety and long term efficacy of revisional surgery in severe obesity. Am J Surg 1996;172:232–235.
11. Sugarman HJ, Kellum JM, Demaria EJ, et al. Conversion of failed or complicated vertical banded gastroplasty to gastric bypass in morbid obesity. Am J Surg 1996;171:263–267.
12. Capella RF, Capella JF. Converting vertical banded gastroplasty to a lesser curvature gastric bypass: technical considerations. Obes Surg 1998;8:218–224.
13. van Gemert WG, Van Wersch MM, Greve JWM, et al. Revisional surgery after failed vertical banded gastroplasty or conversion to gastric bypass. Obesity Surg 1998;8:21–28.
14. O'Brien P, Brown W, Dixon J. Revisional surgery for morbid obesity-conversion to the LapBand system. Obes Surg 2000;10:557–563.

15. Jones KB. Revisional bariatric surgery—safe and effective. Obes Surg 2001;11:183–189.

16. Vassallo C, Andreoli M, LaManna A, et al. 60 reoperations on 890 patients after gastric restrictive surgery. Obes Surg 2001;11:752–756.

17. Cariani S, Nottola D, Grani S, et al. Complications after gastroplasty and gastric bypass as a primary operation and as a reoperation. Obes Surg 2001;11: 487–490.

18. Kyzer S, Raziel A, Landau O, et al. Use of adjustable silicone gastric banding for revision of failed gastric bariatric operations. Obes Surg 2001;11:66–69.

19. de Csepel J, Nahouraii R, Gagner M. Laparoscopic gastric bypass as a reoperative bariatric surgery for failed open restrictive procedures. Surg Endosc 2001;15: 393–397.

20. Westling A, Ohrvall M, Gustavsson S. Roux-en-Y gastric bypass after previous unsuccessful gastric restrictive surgery. J Gastrointest Surg 2002;6:206–211.

21. Schneider BE, Villegas L, Blackburn GL, et al. Laparoscopic gastric bypass surgery: outcomes. J Laparoendo & Adv Surg Tech 2003;13:247–255.

22. Hsu LK, Benotti PN, Dwyer J, et al. Nonsurgical factors that influence the outcome of bariatric surgery: a review. Psychosomatic Med 1998;60: 338–346.

23. Maclean LD, Rhode BM, Force RA. Late results of vertical banded gastroplasty for morbid obesity and super obesity. Surgery 1990;107:20–27.

24. Moreno P, Alastue A, Rull M, et al. Band erosion in patients who have undergone vertical banded gastroplasty: incidence and technical solutions. Arch Surg 1998;133:189–193.

25. Balsiger BM, Murr MM, Mai J, et al. Gastroesophageal reflux after intact vertical banded gastroplasty: correction by conversion to Roux-en-Y gastric bypass. J Gastrointest Surg 2000;4:276–281.

26. Balsinger BM, Poggio JL, Mai J, et al. Ten and more years after vertical banded gastroplasty as primary operation for morbid obesity. J Gastroint Surg 2000;4: 598–605.

27. Sataloff DM, Lieber CP, Seinige UL. Strictures following gastric stapling for morbid obesity. Results of endoscopic dilatation. Am Surg 1990;56: 167–174.

28. Salmon PA. Salvage of failed horizontal gastroplasty by the addition of a distal gastric bypass. Obes Surg 1993;3:45–51.

29. Denoel C, Denoel A, Coimbra C, et al. Lesser curvature Roux-en-Y gastric bypass as an alternative procedure to failed vertical banded gastroplasty: surgical technique and short term results. Acta Chir Belg 2001;101:179–184.

30. Szold A, Abu-Abeid. Laparoscopic adjustable silicone gastric banding for morbid obesity: results and complications in 715 patients. Surg Endosc 2002;16:230–233.

31. Bloomberg RD, Urback DR. Laparoscopic Roux-en-Y gastric bypass for severe gastroesophageal reflux disease after vertical banded gastroplasty. Obesity Surg 2002;12:4.

32. Torres JC, Oca CF, Honer HM. Gastroplasty conversion to Roux-en-Y gastric bypass at the lesser curvature due to weight loss failure. Am Surg 1985;51:559–562.

33. Sapala JA, Bolar RJ, Bell JP, et al. Technical strategies for converting the failed vertical banded gastroplasty to the Roux-en-Y gastric bypass. Obes Surg 1993;3:400–440.

34. de Csepel J, Quinn T, Pomp A, et al. Conversion to a laparoscopic biliopancreatic diversion with a duodenal switch for failed laparoscopic adjustable gastric banding. J Laparoendosc Adv Surg Tech 2002;12:237–240.

35. Marshall JS, Srivastava A, Gupta SK, et al. Roux-en-Y gastric bypass leak complications. Arch Surg 2003;138:520–524.

36. Schwartz RW, Strodel WE, Simpson WS, et al. Gastric bypass revision: lessons learned from 920 cases. Surgery 1988;104:806–812.

37. Higa KD, Boone KB, Ho T. Complications of the laparoscopic Roux-en-Y gastric bypass: 1,040 patients—what have we learned? Obes Surg 2000;10: 509–513.

38. Hamilton EC, Sims TL, Jones DB, et al. Clinical predictors of leak after laparoscopic Roux-en-Y gastric bypass for morbid obesity. Surg Endosc 2003;17:679–684.

39. Livingston EH, Ko CY. Assessing the relative contribution of individual risk factors on surgical outcome for gastric bypass surgery: a baseline probability analysis. J Surg Res 2002;105:48–52.

40. Kothari SN, Demaria EJ, Sugerman HJ, et al. LapBand failures: conversion to gastric bypass and their preliminary outcomes. Surgery 2002;131:625–629.

41. Shen R, Ren CJ. Removal of perigastric fat prevents acute obstruction after LapBand surgery. Obes Surg 2004;14:224–229.

42. Spivak H, Favretti F. Avoiding postoperative complications with the LapBand system. Am J Surg 2002;184:31S–37S.

43. Angrisani L, Borrelli V, Lorenzo M, et al. Conversion of LapBand to gastric bypass for dilated gastric pouch. Obes Surg 2001;11:232–234.

44. Requarth JA, Burchard KW, Colacchio TA, et al. Long-term morbidity following jejunoileal bypass. The continuing potential need for surgical reversal. Arch Surg 1995;130:318–325.

45. Hess DS, Hess DW. Biliopancreatic diversion with a duodenal switch. Obes Surg 1998;8:267–282.

46. Scopinaro N, Gianetta E, Adami GF. Biliopancreatic diversion for obesity at eighteen years. Surgery 1996;119:261–268.

47. Buckwalter JA, Herbst CA, Khouri RK. Morbid obesity: second gastric operations for poor weight loss. Am Surg 1985;51:208–211.

48. Sugarman HJ, Wolper JL. Failed gastroplasty for morbid obesity: revised gastroplasty versus Roux-en-Y gastric bypass. Am J Surg 1984;148:331–336.

49. Sugarman HJ, Kellum JM, Demaria EJ. Conversion of proximal to distal gastric bypass for failed gastric bypass for superobesity. J Gastrointest Surg 1997;1: 517–525.

50. Fobi MAL, Lee H, Igwe D, et al. Revision of failed gastric bypass to distal Roux-en-Y gastric bypass: a review of 65 cases. Obes Surg 2001;11:190–195.

51. Weber M, Muller MK, Michel JM, et al. Laparoscopic Roux-en-Y gastric bypass, not rebanding, should be proposed as rescue procedure for patients with failed laparoscopic gastric banding. Ann Surg 2003;238:827–833.

CHAPTER 6

Reoperative Inguinal Hernia Surgery

Kathrin L. Mayer, MD

Précis

Recurrent inguinal hernias constitute a significant problem. In the United States alone, over 70,000 recurrent inguinal herniorrhaphies are done each year. There is a general consensus in favor of the use of mesh in the treatment of recurrent inguinal hernias to minimize rerecurrence rates. For most patients, preperitoneal placement of a mesh (open or laparoscopic) circumvents the use of scarred and devascularized tissue for the repair, and prevents herniation of the visceral sac through all hernia defects in the inguinal region.

Hernia Repair Today

Within the last 10 years, the management of primary and recurrent groin hernias has stimulated new interest and undergone extensive reevaluation. This is in large part due to the advent of the laparoscopic approach and to increased scrutiny by health insurance companies. The introduction of new techniques has mandated that the surgeon possesses a good understanding of the anatomy and pathophysiology of primary and recurrent inguinal hernias, regardless of the approach used for repair.

Epidemiology of Inguinal Hernias

Inguinal herniorrhaphies constitute 15% of all general surgical procedures. According to data from the National Center for Health Statistics, it is the most common surgical operation performed by general surgeons in the United States.[1] Approximately 700,000 inguinal herniorrhaphies are performed as outpatient procedures per year.[2] This number would be even greater if it were to include the estimated 800,000 people with inguinal hernias who decline surgical intervention.[1]

It is estimated that 75% of all hernias occur in the inguinal region. Approximately 50% of all hernias are indirect inguinal hernias and 24% are direct inguinal hernias. Femoral hernias account for 3% of hernias and the remainder are incisional and rarer hernias (e.g., lumbar, epigastric). Twenty-five percent of all males and 2% of all females will develop inguinal hernias during their lifetimes.

Epidemiology of Recurrent Inguinal Hernias

Recurrent inguinal hernias constitute a significant problem for the surgical community. The exact incidence of recurrent hernias is not known, because many patients are not prospectively followed up over a long period of time.

Approximately 10% to 15% of all inguinal hernia repairs in the United States are performed to treat recurrent hernias.[1] Despite the fact that the inguinal anatomy and the various techniques of inguinal hernia repair have been described extensively in the literature, the inguinal canal is the most common location of recurrent herniation. The most common type of recurrence occurs in Hesselbach's triangle (direct hernia), and the recurrence rate is higher in patients who initially presented with bilateral hernias. Recurrence after repair of an inguinal hernia occurs mainly in men over 50 and is relatively rare in women and children.

An audit from Sweden has shown an incidence of recurrence of 16% to 18% after primary repair using varying techniques.[3] Another report predicts that the actual 5-year recurrence rate for modern inguinal hernia repair is 1% to 3% for primary hernias and 3% to 5% for recurrent hernias.[4]

Rerecurrence rates range from 2% to 36.8%, and some patients eventually undergo multiple, technically challenging repairs.[5] Given the overall relatively high recurrence rate, from a patient's point of view, prevention of recurrence is more important than the speed of recovery.[6]

Etiology and Risk Factors

The etiologies of groin hernias are traditionally divided into two categories: congenital and acquired defects. Congenital factors are responsible for the majority of primary groin hernias. A patent processus vaginalis is the main factor leading to formation of an indirect inguinal hernia. Direct hernias are attributed to the physical stresses on the inguinal canal that increase intra-abdominal pressure and, possibly, collagen matrix defects.

Some hernias recur despite good surgical judgment and a technically sound primary hernia repair. Recurrences within the first year are more likely the result of technical errors, whereas those that occur later are more likely due to progressive weakening of the tissues, an imbalance of collagen metabolism, or other poorly characterized factors.

Recurrence because of a technically inadequate primary repair is the most common cause for recurrence of inguinal hernias. The success of hernia surgery depends primarily on the skill and experience of the surgeon. This is more important than the type of repair used. Technical reasons for recurrence are numerous, including a missed sac or defect at the time of the primary repair; inadequate exposure of an indirect hernia sac to the internal ring; incorrect closure of the internal ring during a conventional repair; insufficient reinforcement of the inguinal canal floor; undue tissue tension causing new defects; and improper suturing and/or fixation of mesh.

At 6 months, the wound will have gained approximately 80% of its final strength, and suture material that will not hold the tissue for at least 6 months should, therefore, not be used for repair. Monofilament polyamide or polypropylene sutures are strong, nonabsorbable, and inert and are therefore recommended.

With regard to the suturing technique, the Shouldice Hospital has always stressed the importance of using a continuous suture and taking large bites of the tissue with each suture.[7] Continuous suturing techniques have a greater wound-bursting pressure than simple, interrupted suturing techniques.

The type of repair may also affect recurrence rates. Numerous studies have evaluated the recurrence rates of myoaponeurotic repairs and mesh repairs. Some authors report low rerecurrence rates with the Shouldice repair (3% to 7%), yet others report rerecurrence of 36.8% with the same technique.[5] Dudda and Schunk report rerecurrence rates of 11% with the McVay procedure.[8] Lichtenstein reports a low rerecurrence rate of less than 1%.[17] For open preperitoneal repairs with mesh, the rerecurrence rate ranges from 1.1% to 12%.

The European Union Hernia Trialists Collaboration in 2002 evaluated the effects of the use of synthetic mesh on recurrence and persisting pain after groin hernia repair.[10] A meta-analysis included 11,174 participants in randomized and quasirandomized trials. Recurrence and persistent pain incidence after mesh repair were approximately half that of the nonmesh techniques. As a result of the high recurrence rates with the nonmesh techniques, there is currently a general acceptance for the use of mesh in the treatment of recurrent inguinal hernias.

Infected tissue repairs made without mesh are four times more likely to fail than those in uninfected repairs. Fortunately, infection is now a rare cause of recurrence, underscoring the importance of strict antiseptic technique, hemostasis, and preoperative antibiotics. Hematomas and infection are more likely following the repair of larger hernias and repeated attempts at repair.

Patient factors may precipitate recurrence, and all efforts should be made to minimize the recurrence risk factors prior to repair. Risk factors include excessive intra-abdominal pressure due to chronic cough/chronic obstructive pulmonary disease, prostatic obstruction, ascites, constipation, and pregnancy. A poor general state of health of the patient may increase the risk of recurrence of hernia by adversely influencing wound healing. Contributing factors include poor nutrition, hypoproteinemia, infections, and chronic diseases.

Unfortunately, many patients presenting with recurrence today are debilitated and have poor intrinsic tissue strength. Mesenchymal metabolic defects and hereditary connective tissue disorders may cause a higher incidence of primary and recurrent hernias. Zheng et al found a decreased ratio of collagen types I to III in patients with recurrent hernias.[11] He suggested that the increase of collagen type III may change the cross-linking with collagen type I and result in decreased tensile strength of the abdominal wall.

A reduction in the collagen amino acid hydroxyproline was noted in the aponeurosis of patients with inguinal hernias. Additionally, rectus sheath collagen was found to contain irregular microfibrils in patients with direct hernias.[12] Read evaluated rectus sheath collagen and showed a reduced hydroxyproline ratio, suggesting impaired hydroxylation and lysyl oxidase activity.[13] Synthesis of hydroxyproline, and therefore collagen, were noted to be inhibited under those circumstances.

An association between cigarette smoking and groin hernias has been reported. A higher percentage of smokers than nonsmokers develop groin hernias and recurrences.[14] Some patients suffer from collagenolysis brought on by smoking. Smokers have higher serum elastolytic levels than controls, as well as more uninhibited proteolysis.[15]

It is interesting to note that the recurrence rate is higher following repair of primary or recurrent inguinal hernias in younger than in older patients.[16] Additionally, for those with a sedentary occupation, recurrence incidence is twice as high as for those performing heavy manual labor.[17]

Variables that do not affect recurrence rates include gender and type of anesthesia used at the time of primary repair. Surprisingly, markedly overweight patients are not at increased risk for recurrent inguinal hernias.[16] In fact, a slightly greater proportion of patients with recurrent hernias are near or below ideal body weight.

Types of Recurrence

RECURRENT HERNIA IS A DIRECT INGUINAL HERNIA

After Repair of a Direct Inguinal Hernia—This is the most common type of recurrence after primary inguinal herniorrhaphy. Patients tend to be elderly or have had previous bilateral or rerecurrent inguinal hernias. Many patients with direct recurrences are prone to hernia formation in other locations as well. Some recurrences are associated with risk factors that increase intra-abdominal pressure.

A technical reason for recurrence that is frequently encountered in these patients is failure to include the inferomedial portion over the pubic tubercle when reinforcing the posterior wall in a myoaponeurotic repair. Similarly, patients may experience a recurrence due to failure to secure the mesh inferomedially during a Lichtenstein repair. Clinically, the patients often present with a small tender nonreducible mass of trapped preperitoneal fat deep to the external ring.

After Repair of an Indirect Inguinal Hernia—Most of these recurrences occur years after the initial repair and present as a new bulge medially in the groin. An indirect sac was usually removed at the initial operation and frequently there is a history of a cord lipoma. A direct hernia may have been missed at the initial repair or a new direct hernia may have developed since the initial surgery. Neither of these cases are recurrent hernias per se.

RECURRENT HERNIA IS AN INDIRECT INGUINAL HERNIA

After Repair of an Indirect Inguinal Hernia—An indirect recurrence after repair of an indirect hernia often occurs within months of the repair. The recurrence is typically found at the lateral aspect of the deep inguinal ring, in contrast to a primary indirect hernia that is usually located anteromedial to the cord structures. Most of these recurrences are due to improper ligation of the sac, incomplete invagination of an intact sac, or incomplete dissection of the cord. To prevent this type of recurrence, the cord must be skeletonized down to the vessels, lipomas of the cord excised or reduced, the cremaster fibers excised or retracted, and the internal ring appropriately narrowed around the cord structures. Also, the inferior epigastric vessels in the preperitoneal fat deep to and medial to the internal ring must be visualized.

After Repair of a Direct Inguinal Hernia—The previous operative report usually states that the cord structures were examined and no processus vaginalis was found. Nevertheless, at the time of the recurrent repair, a sac can be easily dissected off of the cord and likely represents a previously missed indirect hernia. In some instances, lipomas of the cord were documented. Alternatively, a true, new indirect hernia may have developed.

RECURRENT HERNIA IS A FEMORAL HERNIA

After Repair of Femoral Hernia—Primary femoral hernias are uncommon and rarely recur after repair.

After Repair of an Inguinal Hernia—More commonly, a femoral hernia presents after an inguinal defect (primary or recurrent) has been operated on. Use of the inguinal ligament in classic inguinal repairs leads to cephalad displacement of the inguinal ligament and opens the femoral canal to protrusions of preperitoneal structures. Use of the Cooper's ligament repair of McVay for primary repair, or fixating the mesh to Cooper's ligament in a prosthetic repair, can prevent femoral hernias following inguinal hernia repairs.

Anatomy—The distortion of normal anatomical relationships and weakening of tissues often results in extreme technical challenges to the surgeon. It is important to know the underlying, "normal" anatomy in order to understand the abnormal anatomy and to safely perform an appropriate recurrent hernia repair (Figures 6-1 and 6-2).

The complex anatomy of the inguinal canal must be understood as a three-dimensional structure with convergence of tissue planes. The transversalis fascia and the aponeurosis of the transversus abdominis muscle constitute the posterior wall of the inguinal canal. Hesselbach's triangle, one of the canal's weak areas, is directly subject to changes in intra-abdominal pressure. It is thickened at its inferolateral margin where it becomes the iliopubic tract. It is a wedge-shaped planar layer surrounded superiorly by the transversus abdominis and internal oblique muscles,

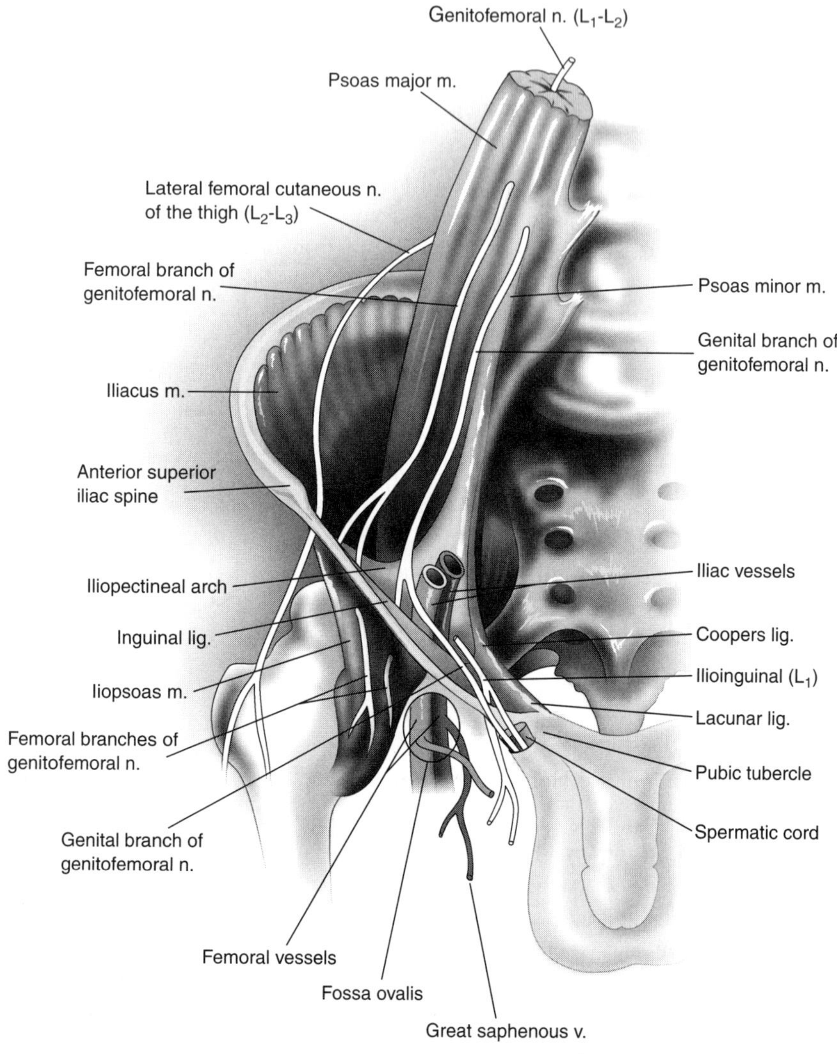

Figure 6-1 The neuroanatomy of the inguinal canal (the iliohypogastric nerve is not shown). (From Gray SW, Skandalakis JE, McClusky DA. Anatomy for General Surgeons. Baltimore: Williams & Wilkins, 1985.)

medially by the rectus muscle, and inferolaterally by the iliopubic tract and inguinal ligament. The iliopubic tract is located posterior to the inguinal ligament. Staples should not be placed inferior (dorsal) to the lateral iliopubic tract (lateral to the internal inguinal ring). The lateral femoral cutaneous and genitofemoral nerves are located in this region and may be injured during a laparoscopic inguinal hernia repair.

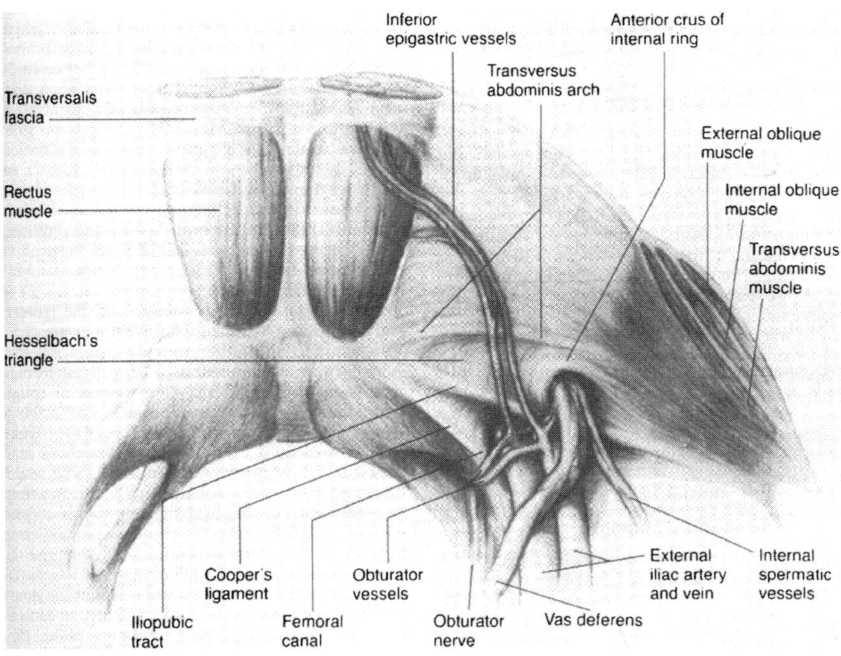

Figure 6-2 The preperitoneal inguinal anatomy (peritoneum and preperitoneal fat removed). (From Madden JL: Abdominal Wall Hernias: An Atlas of Anatomy and Repair. Philadelphia: WB Saunders, 1989.)

The surgeon must also be aware of the location of the ilioinguinal nerve, iliohypogastric nerve, genital branch of the genitofemoral nerve (particularly important in anterior repairs), the femoral nerve, lateral femoral cutaneous nerve, and femoral branch of the genitofemoral nerve (particularly important during posterior repairs), to avoid injury and chronic pain.[9]

Surgical Management of Recurrent Inguinal Hernias

Recurrent inguinal hernias do not resolve spontaneously and are likely to progressively enlarge, resulting in further weakening of the tissues. Due to the potential for incarceration, intestinal obstruction, and strangulation, all recurrent inguinal hernias should be considered, in principle, for repair. Special considerations may apply, however, to the elderly and patients with comorbid conditions. In those cases, the surgeon may elect to defer repair.

TIMING OF SURGERY

Unless painful incarceration or strangulation is present, repair can be done electively. All risk factors should be minimized and corrected, if possible. Long delays carry additional risks that include a higher rate of testicular problems and hernia enlargement. Any evidence of enlargement, discomfort, or inability to easily reduce the hernia should mandate immediate repair.

REPAIR TECHNIQUES FOR RECURRENT GROIN HERNIA

In 1884, Bassini first described a technique for repairing inguinal hernias by reinforcing the inguinal floor and performing high ligation of the sac.[18] This repair was fraught with a high recurrence rate. Since then, many techniques have been described to try to decrease recurrence. Lichtenstein set forth five cardinal principles to prevent recurrence:[19]

1. Do not depend on fascial structures to close or reinforce the defect.
2. Reinforce the entire inguinal floor irrespective of the type of hernia.
3. Avoid tension on suture lines.
4. Avoid the use of scarred or devascularized tissue in the repair of recurrent hernias.
5. Use a large piece of prosthetic material to reinforce the entire inguinal floor permanently.

Recurrent hernias are most successfully repaired using prosthetic material, either by an open anterior, preperitoneal open, or preperitoneal laparoscopic approach. The approach for recurrent hernia (anterior versus preperitoneal) depends on the type of hernia repair performed initially and the experience of the surgeon.

The ideal mesh is one that is strong and nonabsorbable, allows for tissue ingrowth, resists infection, conforms to the curves of the pelvis, and is pliable. The knitted polypropylene and polyester meshes are as close to ideal as are available today. Polyester mesh has traditionally been the mesh of choice for the giant prosthetic reinforcement of the visceral sac (GPRVS) of Stoppa, since the polypropylene was thought to be too stiff to conform to the contour of the pelvis when used in large pieces. However, a recent study showed that polyester mesh has a higher incidence of infection than knitted polypropylene meshes.[20] Expanded polytetrafluoroethylene is only partially incorporated into the tissues and is primarily used today as a composite mesh with polypropylene when the peritoneal lining has been disrupted in the preperitoneal repair. Under selected circumstances (e.g., in the presence of infection) absorbable mesh can be used for recurrent hernia repairs. The hernia will recur a few months after repair. Thereafter, a permanent mesh can be placed when bacterial load is minimized (usually 1 year after gross infection). Recently, an allogeneic matrix (Alloderm) made from cadaver skin has become available. This mesh could conceivably be used in cases of large, complex, infected hernias. No long-term data is available, but the product is promising.

To avoid recurrence, certain general principles must be followed when using mesh to repair primary or recurrent hernias. The sheet of mesh must be large enough to overlap the hernia defect with a few centimeters margin, which allows for tissue ingrowth. The wider the areas of overlap the stronger the force holding the mesh against the force of the intra-abdominal pressure. In certain circumstances (e.g., preperitoneal repair) the mesh does not need to be fixed at all, since it is kept in the proper position by the force of the intra-abdominal pressure. During laparoscopic preperitoneal repairs, I like to use one or two tacking staples to Cooper's ligament or the pubic tubercle to prevent dislodgment at the time of implantation.

Anterior Repair with Mesh—Originally used for the repair of incisional hernias, synthetic mesh was thereafter applied to the repair of recurrent inguinal hernias. A popular and frequently performed open herniorrhaphy technique is the Lichtenstein tension-free repair, popularized by Irving L. Lichtenstein. He emphasized that a tension-free hernia repair performed with mesh reinforcement of the inguinal floor significantly decreases the recurrence rate. The Lichtenstein repair can also be used to repair a recurrent hernia that was previously repaired without mesh. An advantage to using the anterior-tension free approach for treatment of recurrence after the open myoaponeurotic repair is its relative safety and familiarity. The disadvantage consists of the necessity of dissecting through scarred tissue and risk of cord injury.

The Lichtenstein repair is usually performed in an outpatient setting with local, regional, or general anesthesia. If no mesh was previously used, the old incision can be used. The techniques of repair, once the hernia has been identified, are very similar as for primary repair.

The initial step involves reduction of the hernia, or ligation of the sac if it extends into the scrotum. Experience with the laparoscopic approach has shown us that the sac does not need to be excised and needs merely to be reduced. Next, the margins of the hernia defect are cleared of adherent tissue. A mesh patch is sutured to the aponeurotic tissue overlying the pubic bone, with continuation of this suture in a running fashion along the shelving edge of the inguinal ligament beyond the internal ring. A slit is made into the lateral edge of the mesh to allow passage of the cord structures. The cephalad mesh edge is sewn to the conjoined tendon. The lateral tails are then sewn together laterally to the internal ring and cord structures.

This method was further improved with Gilbert's "tensionless and sutureless" repair of inguinal hernia.[21] Rutkow combined these two principles in his "open-mesh plug hernioplasty" for primary and recurrent hernias.[22] The plug-and-patch technique uses an additional bloom-like plug that is inserted into the preperitoneal space from the anterior approach. The plug is secured with nonabsorbable interrupted sutures, either through the internal ring (indirect defect) or into Hesselbach's triangle (direct defect). These new methods are simple and reinforce the transversalis fascia, allowing for a lower recurrence rate, at least for primary repairs.[23]

The Danish and Swedish Hernia Databases were used to evaluate operative findings in recurrent hernia after a previous Lichtenstein procedure.[24] In all, 87 records from operations for recurrence were reviewed. Direct recurrences were found in 62%; the remaining recurrences were indirect (17%), femoral (13%), or other (8%). For direct recurrences, the most common causes were insufficient medial mesh fixation and inadequate overlap over the pubic tubercle. These findings are likely also relevant when using the Lichtenstein technique for repair of recurrent hernias.

Gianetta evaluated a 7-year experience of anterior tension-free repair of recurrent hernia under local anesthesia.[25] One hundred forty-five elective and one emergency herniorrhaphy, all for recurrent inguinal hernias, were performed in 141 patients. The mean length of hospital stay was 1.5 days, and complications consisted of one case of intestinal bleeding and two cases of urinary retention. Local complications consisted of eight (5.5%) minor complications and one case of orchitis (0.7%) followed by testicular atrophy. No postoperative neuralgia or chronic pain was reported. Only two rerecurrences occurred. The authors concluded that anterior mesh repair is a low-cost alternative that can be used safely and effectively for the treatment of recurrent groin hernias.

The Swedish Hernia Register prospectively documented all reoperations for recurrent or primary inguinal hernias from 1996 to 1998. They studied variables associated with increased or decreased relative risk for reoperation after recurrent hernia.[26] During the time period, they operated on 17,985 patients with groin hernias; 2698 (15%) of these were performed for recurrences. At 24 months, the incidence for re-operation was 4.6% after recurrent hernia repair, and 1.7% after primary hernia repair. The relative risk for reoperation was significantly lower following laparoscopic or anterior tension-free repairs. No group of "pure" preperitoneal open repairs was analyzed. Postoperative complications (e.g., hematomas, infection) and direct hernias were significant risk factors for reoperation. Ambulatory surgery and local anesthesia were less frequently used for recurrent hernia.

The authors stressed that, when choosing between the laparoscopic and anterior tension free repair, the higher cost and longer learning curve of the laparoscopic repair should be taken into consideration.

Preperitoneal Repairs with Mesh—During the repair of a recurrent hernia that was previously repaired through an anterior approach, dissection through fresh tissue in the preperitoneal space is, in principle, preferable to another anterior repair. The scarred and damaged contents of the inguinal canal are avoided. The risk of hematoma formation, injury to canal structures, and missed defects is minimized. It is particularly advantageous to use the preperitoneal approach if the previous anterior repair was infected (regardless of whether mesh was used).

OPEN PREPERITONEAL REPAIRS FOR RECURRENT INGUINAL HERNIAS Regardless of whether a bilateral or unilateral open preperitoneal repair is done, the principles for both are the same. The key aspect of these repairs is the entry into the preperitoneal space for insertion of a mesh to prevent herniation of the visceral sac and any of its contents. The inguinal canal is never entered. The technique for the open preperitoneal management of bilateral recurrent inguinal hernias with mesh was described by Stoppa in 1984 and is known as the GPRVS[27] (Figure 6-3). It is a particularly useful approach for very large, complex hernias, for bilateral recurrences that are to be repaired simultaneously, and for unilateral recurrences with a contralateral primary hernia. Approaches for the bilateral repair include a midline

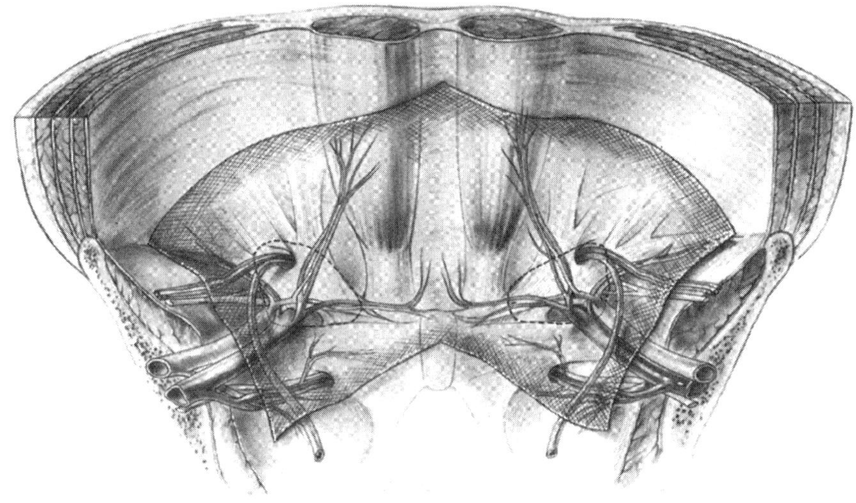

Figure 6-3 Bilateral giant prosthetic reinforcement of the visceral sac (GPRVS), the Stoppa procedure.

(From Wantz GE. Atlas of Hernia Surgery. New York: Raven Press, 1991.)

infra-umbilical incision (as described by Stoppa), or a Pfannenstiel incision. Attempting to locally anesthetize the peritoneum next to the pelvic wall may be difficult, and thus epidural, spinal, or general anesthesia should be used.

Dissection is carried down to the preperitoneal space, which is widely opened in all directions, exposing the superior pubic ramus, the iliac vessels, and the iliopsoas muscle. The vas deferens and testicular vessels are naturally adherent to the peritoneum. They must be dissected away from the peritoneum (i.e., parietalized). The inferior epigastric vessels should be left in place on the posterior aspect of the rectus muscle. Infrequently, the epigastric vessels may need to be divided to allow better access to the preperitoneal space when large hernias are present.

The hernia sacs of indirect, direct, sliding, and femoral hernias are easily visualized and are dissected from the adjacent tissues. If the indirect sac is large and extends to the scrotum, the cephalad pedicle of the hernia is divided and the proximal peritoneum oversewn. The distal sac is left in place to minimize bleeding. Large incarcerated recurrent hernias may require an anterior incision for reduction. For bilateral hernias, two separate meshes or one, large chevron-shaped mesh can be used. It is tailored to the patient and should measure transversely 2 cm less than the distance between the anterior iliac spines, and vertically should correspond to the distance between the umbilicus and the symphysis pubis. After insertion, the large prosthesis extends beyond the borders of all potential hernia orifices in the pelvis. The defects are not closed. The mesh envelops the visceral sac and is held in place by intra-abdominal pressure and connective tissue ingrowth.

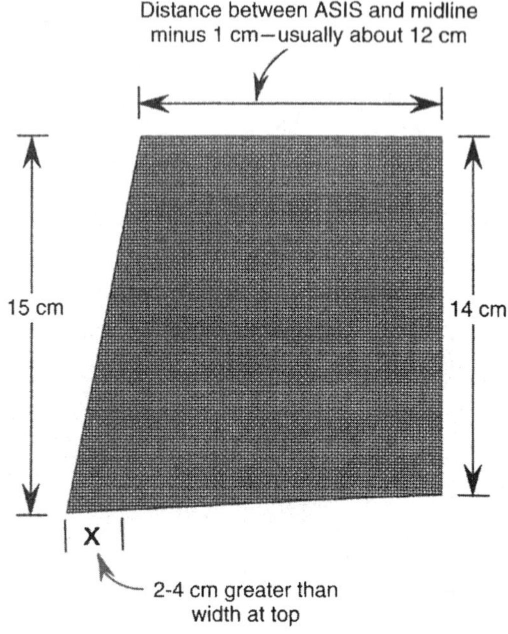

Figure 6-4 Mesh dimensions for unilateral preperitoneal repair.
(From Wantz GE. Atlas of Hernia Surgery. New York: Raven Press, 1991.)

When repairing a unilateral hernia using this technique, a transverse or a lower midline incision can be used. The transverse incision begins just lateral to the midline and two fingerbreadths above the pubic tubercle. The incision is continued in a superior-lateral direction to pass 1 cm cephalad to the location of the internal ring and cephalad to any hernia defects. The incision is approximately 8 cm in length. Importantly, the rectus sheath is incised and the rectus muscle itself is retracted medially, but not divided. The preperitoneal space is entered and hernia sacs reduced under direct vision. Wantz suggested the use of a diamond-shaped mesh for this repair[28] (Figure 6-4). The mesh overlaps the incision by 3 cm in the cephalad direction. Three absorbable sutures are used to secure the upper border of the mesh to the abdominal wall.

Kurzer reviewed his experience with open uni- and bilateral (Stoppa) preperitoneal mesh repairs for recurrent inguinal hernias.[29] A prospective cohort study of 101 consecutive patients with 114 recurrent inguinal hernias was analyzed. He noted no major complications and one infection. There were no testicular complications. His five recurrences (5%) all occurred within the first 6 months, and all occurred among the first 20 patients. He concluded that the open preperitoneal repair is the procedure of choice for complex, multirecurrent inguinal hernias.

Solorzano et al prospectively evaluated the efficacy and safety of GPRVS in patients at high risk for recurrence.[30] Sixty-four patients with 124 inguinal hernias underwent repair according to the method of Stoppa. Of these, 19 patients (30%) were operated on for recurrent or rerecurrent hernias. Factors predicting a high risk for recurrence included large hernia size (greater than 5 cm), failure of one or more previous repairs, and chronic obstructive pulmonary disease. After a mean follow-up of 24 months, the recurrence rate was 1% per inguinal hernia or 2% per patient. Although the majority of repairs in this study were done for primary hernias, the excellent overall results suggest that the repair may yield superior results for the repair of complex, recurrent hernias.

LAPAROSCOPIC PREPERITONEAL REPAIRS FOR RECURRENT HERNIA Previous studies on open repairs of recurrent inguinal hernias noted frequent recurrences, testicular damage or nerve injury. For the recurrent hernia, a second groin exploration via the open technique would necessitate dissecting through scar tissue. In the early phases of the development of minimally invasive surgery, Ger described a method for laparoscopic mesh implantation.[31] The laparoscopic repair is based on the preperitoneal approach and the use of mesh. Significant controversy has arisen regarding the choice of method of repair of inguinal hernias with the addition of laparoscopy to the surgeon's armamentarium. In 2001, the National Institute for Clinical Excellence in the United Kingdom published practice guidelines on the use of laparoscopic surgery for inguinal hernia.[32] They recommended that laparoscopic surgery be considered for recurrent and bilateral hernias only.

Nonetheless, laparoscopic repair of recurrent inguinal hernias is becoming increasingly accepted in surgical practice. Although the learning curve requires some time, once mastered, the laparoscopic approach allows for excellent anatomical definition of the hernia and the surrounding anatomy.

Proponents of the laparoscopic approach for the repair of groin hernias emphasize the advantages of minimal pain, rapid return to work and normal activities, better visualization, decreased wound infection, and cost savings due to more rapid return to work. If such benefits occur for patients undergoing primary inguinal repair, there may be even greater advantages to patients undergoing recurrent repair.

Opponents of the laparoscopic approach emphasize the need for general anesthesia, the duration of the operation, the operative costs, the necessity for advanced laparoscopic skills, and the higher rate of severe complications. Long-term follow-up to track recurrences is also not available. However, many of those who oppose laparoscopy as a primary repair technique agree that the laparoscopic approach is a reasonable approach for the repair of recurrent inguinal hernias that have previously been repaired using a conventional anterior approach. Definitive outcome and cost data will need to be analyzed to determine if the laparoscopic approach will be the procedure of choice in the future.

Due to obvious difficulty in recruiting patients, large randomized trials of recurrent hernia repairs do not exist. Case series, however, have reported low rerecurrence rates after recurrent hernia repair using the laparoscopic method.[33,34]

The European Union Hernia Trialists collaboration evaluated the effects of laparoscopic and open hernia repair on recurrence and persisting pain.[35] The reduction in recurrence was similar after laparoscopic and open mesh placement. The laparoscopic group had less persistent pain and had a more rapid return to normal activities. The laparoscopic repair took longer to perform. Of concern is the finding that the laparoscopic technique may increase the risk of rare but serious complications. The group found that visceral and vascular injuries were more frequent in the laparoscopic group than in the open hernia repair group (combined, 4.7 versus 1.1 per 1000).

Memon et al evaluated the laparoscopic treatment for recurrent hernias after previous open repair.[36] Ninety-six recurrent hernias were repaired in 85 patients. Long-term follow-up was performed by questionnaire, examination, or both in 76 patients. Sixty-five (86%) preferred the laparoscopic repair, 8 (1%) preferred the conventional repair, and 10 (13%) failed to reply. Satisfaction with the laparoscopic repair was noted by 70 (92%) of the patients, and 6 (8%) were either dissatisfied or did not answer. Finally, 72 (95%) of the patients stated that they would recommend laparoscopic surgery to their family and friends.

The techniques for laparoscopic hernia repair include the transabdominal preperitoneal (TAPP) repair and the totally extraperitoneal (TEP) approach. The hernia repair is the same in both techniques, yet the approach to the preperitoneal space differs.

TAPP APPROACH The TAPP technique is less desirable than the TEP technique, because it violates the peritoneal space. The approach to the preperitoneal space is through the abdomen and increases the risk of visceral injury and adhesion formation. Additionally, if mesh is exposed intraperitoneally, adhesion to mesh with subsequent bowel obstruction or fistula can result. In the TAPP repair, the trocars are placed into the abdominal cavity and pneumoperitoneum is established. A peritoneal flap is made over the inguinal region to enter the preperitoneal space. After reduction of the hernia and placement of the mesh, the flap is reapproximated with staples or sutures.

Beets compared the open and laparoscopic (TAPP) preperitoneal mesh repair for recurrent inguinal hernia.[37] Seventy-nine patients with 93 recurrent and 15 concomitant primary inguinal hernias were prospectively randomized between GPRVS (37 patients) and TAPP (42 patients). Mean operating time was 56 minutes with GPRVS versus 79 minutes with TAPP ($p < 0.0001$) Most complications were minor, except for a pulmonary embolus and an ileus, both after GPRVS. Patients had less pain and more rapid return to work with the TAPP, but costs were similar. Recurrence rates at a mean follow-up of 34 months were 1 in 52 (1.9%) for GPRVS versus 7 in 56 (12.5%) for TAPP. The authors concluded that laparoscopic repair of recurrent hernia has lower morbidity than GPRVS. TAPP, however, is a challenging procedure and failure rate is higher. It is unclear to what extent the laparoscopic learning curve contributed to the higher recurrence rate following TAPP.

Mahon et al randomized 120 patients with bilateral, recurrent or bilateral and recurrent hernias to the TAPP or open mesh repair.[38] Although it is clear from the manuscript that 35% of the patients underwent surgery for recurrent hernia, the results as they pertain specifically to this subgroup of patients with recurrent hernias are not described in detail. Following evaluation of all study patients, they found that the TAPP was faster, less painful, and allowed for earlier return to work compared with open mesh repair. Four patients undergoing laparoscopic repair suffered a recurrence compared with one patient in the open group. Overall, there were more complications in the open group; however, there were two bowel injuries in the laparoscopic group. In this study, 13% of patients undergoing open repair had persistent groin pain at 3 months. This number was significantly reduced to 1% in the laparoscopic approach. Of the patients undergoing recurrent hernia repair, more of those undergoing laparoscopic repair thought the overall experience of their second repair was superior to that of their original repair.

TEP APPROACH In the TEP approach, access to the preperitoneal space is gained directly, without entering the abdominal cavity. Blunt dissection can be used to enter the preperitoneal space, but a balloon dissector advanced to the pubis facilitates the approach. The balloon is insufflated, creating a cavity in the preperitoneal space. Reduction of the hernia and placement of the mesh follows. The TEP approach is more difficult to learn. However, it allows the surgeon to remain clear of the abdominal cavity, thereby minimizing adhesions and maintaining the integrity of the peritoneal lining over the mesh. When first performed, surgeons used several staples to secure the mesh to the posterior inguinal wall. Tacks were also placed medial to the inferior epigastric vessels, to the Cooper's ligament, the lacunar ligament, the posterior rectus musculature, and the transversus abdominis aponeurotic arch. Laterally, it was common practice to secure the mesh to the lateral extension of the transversus aponeurotic arch and the superior edge of the iliopubic tract. Many patients developed neurosensory symptoms during the earlier years of the laparoscopic approach, primarily in the lateral femoral cutaneous nerve and genitofemoral nerve distribution (located dorsal to the lateral iliopubic tract). As a consequence, it is now recommended to avoid stapling, particularly in the triangular area inferior to the internal inguinal ring. Bordered by the ductus deferens medially and the spermatic vessels laterally in the male, this triangle contains the external oblique artery and vein and the femoral nerve. The obturator artery lies medial to the triangle of doom over Cooper's ligament. With more experience with the laparoscopic approach, it has become clear that few, if any, tacks are required for fixation of the mesh when using the preperitoneal approach. These tacks should only be placed medially into the pubis or Cooper's ligament. Independent of the use of tacks or staples, adequate overlap over the pubic bone is necessary to prevent medial recurrences. There is no need for a keyhole incision in the mesh for the cord structures, as long as the peritoneum/hernia sac is adequately reduced. Adequate lateral extension of the mesh is crucial: ideally, the mesh should extend at least 3 cm beyond the internal ring. The preperitoneal space must be dissected superiorly to the level of the umbilicus and medially beyond the linea alba. Incomplete dissection with inadequate identification of all landmarks may precipitate recurrence.

Recurrences after the laparoscopic approach often result from the use of a mesh that is too small. I usually use an 11 cm by 14 cm mesh. The mesh must be large enough to overlap the midline and cover all defects. Meticulous hemostasis is of utmost importance, because the mesh may become displaced by hematoma. The mesh can also migrate or fold.

There are few published studies on the results of the TEP technique for recurrent hernia repair. Scheuerlein et al from Germany evaluated the use of TEP in 181 patients with recurrent hernias.[39] Their rerecurrence rate was 0%. They also noted that 12% of the patients undergoing TEP had postoperative pain. This rate can be compared with conventional data on groin pain after hernia repair that varies between 3% and 37%. Scheuerlein et al speculated that the lower postoperative pain is likely due to the fact that they did not secure the mesh and avoided electrocautery.

Van der Hem et al retrospectively reviewed 104 patients with 108 recurrent hernias who underwent TEP repair.[40] The authors determined that median time from primary repair to recurrence was 36 months, and median duration of surgery was 63 minutes. Twelve percent of the patients had a postoperative complication. Only two direct rerecurrences (2%) occurred as a result of inadequate positioning of the mesh.

Complications of Recurrent Herniorrhaphy

Complications of recurrent hernia repairs are, in principle, the same as for primary repairs. Scar tissue, as can be encountered during a recurrent repair, lacks elasticity. Therefore, the incidence of postoperative seromas and hematomas is higher, particularly for the latter, due to impaired contractility of blood vessels. One maneuver that is particularly important to minimize hematoma and seroma formation is avoiding dissection of the distal sac. Nevertheless, the incidence of wound infection is similar to that of primary repairs.

Postoperative neuralgia after a recurrent hernia repair is uncommon, especially if no neuralgia was present after the first repair. Treatment algorithms for these relatively rare cases include local anesthetic and steroid injections, systemic analgesics, anti-inflammatory agents, antidepressants, nerve ligation, and electrical stimulation. Rarely does an additional surgical procedure solve the problem.

Injury to the vasculature, viscera, and testicular structures in a previously operated field can be minimized by use of meticulous dissection techniques and awareness of the anatomy. Needless to say, recurrent hernia can also be complicated by a recurrent hernia.

Conclusion

Recurrent inguinal hernias are a significant burden to patients and to society. In the United States alone, they affect over 70,000 patients per year. The repair of recurrent inguinal hernias has significantly evolved over the past decade. The change in surgical practice is illustrated by the observations of Barrat et al.[41] They evaluated 163 recurrent hernia repairs performed from 1991 to 2000. Over the study period, use of the Shouldice repair for recurrent hernias decreased from 90% to 0%, while the use of mesh for recurrent hernia repairs increased from 10% to 100%. During the same time period, Lichtenstein repairs for recurrent hernias increased to a total of 77% of cases. Recurrent inguinal herniorrhaphies done by a TEP approach increased from 11% to 23% for recurrences after a Lichtenstein procedure, or after conventional repair in working and/or physically active patients without contraindications to general anesthesia. A Stoppa repair has not been used since 1998. If a recurrence follows a TEP or Stoppa technique, the authors preferred to use a Lichtenstein technique.

In my opinion, although controversial for primary repairs, mesh is an excellent option for repair of recurrences. I prefer to place the mesh preperitoneally, unless the primary repair was done by the preperitoneal approach with mesh, or by a conventional myoaponeurotic anterior repair. In the latter situation, I often use the "plug and patch" technique, although this comes at the price of encountering scar tissue during the reoperation.

In patients who previously had a Lichtenstein repair, I prefer to place the mesh preperitoneally via a laparoscopic totally extraperitoneal (TEP) approach. A giant scrotal recurrence or history of previous lower abdominal surgery does not preclude a laparoscopic repair, but increases operative complexity and difficulty. I also offer the laparoscopic approach to patients with a unilateral recurrent and contralateral primary repair, to those with primary bilateral hernias, and to those who specifically request a laparoscopic repair of primary hernias or recurrent hernias after myoaponeurotic repairs. I emphasize to the patients, however, that although the overall complication rate with the laparoscopic repair is similar to that for an open repair, the risk of a serious injury to the bowel, bladder, or vasculature has been reported to be greater with the laparoscopic approach. The open preperitoneal repair is an attractive alternative for nonlaparoscopic surgeons faced with unusual, complex, rerecurrent hernias after anterior repairs, and in cases in which the patient has contraindications to laparoscopic surgery (e.g., significant medical comorbidities).

REFERENCES

1. Memon MA, Fitzgibbons RJ. Assessing risks, costs, and benefits of laparoscopic hernia repair. Annu Rev Med 1998;49:63–77.
2. MacFadyen BV, Mathis CR. Inguinal herniorrhaphy: complications and recurrences. Semin Laparosc Surg 1994;1:128.
3. Wantz GE. Prosthetic repair of groin hernioplasties. In: Atlas of Hernia Surgery. New York: Raven Press, 1991.
4. Schumpelick V, Kupeczyk-Joeris D, Töns C, Pfingsten F. Reparation der Rezidivleistenhernie-Taktik, Technik und Ergebinsse. Chirurg 1990; 61:526–529.
5. Guthy E, Boom H. Multiple recurrence in inguinal hernia. Langenbecks Arch Chir 1983;361:316–318.

6. Lawrence K, McWhinnie D, Goodwin A, et al. Randomized controlled trial of laparoscopic versus open repair of inguinal hernia: early results. Br Med J 1995;311:981–985.
7. Welsh DRJ. The Shouldice inguinal hernia repair. Prob Gen Surg 1995; 12:93–100.
8. Dudda W, Schunk R. Repair of inguinal and femoral hernias by the Lotheissen-McVay technique. Late follow-up in 1202 cases. Langenbecks Arch Chir 1990;372:351–358.
9. Gardener E, Gray D, O'Rahilly R. Blood vessels, lymphatic drainage, and nerves. In: Anatomy: A Regional Study of Human Structure. Philadelphia: WB Saunders, 1975.
10. The EU Hernia Trialists Collaboration. Repair of groin hernia with synthetic mesh. Meta-analysis of randomized controlled trials. Ann Surg 2002;235: 322–332.
11. Zheng H, Si Z, Kasperk R, et al. Recurrent inguinal hernia: disease of the collagen matrix? World J Surg 2002;26:401–408.
12. Read RC. Attenuation of rectus sheath in inguinal herniation. Am J Surg 1970;120:610.
13. Read RC. Collagen synthesis and direct inguinal herniation. In: Inguinal Hernia: Advances or Controversies? Oxford: Radcliff Medical Press, 1994.
14. Bielecki K, Puwaski R. Is cigarette smoking a causative factor in the development of inguinal hernia? Pol Tyg Lek 1998;43:974.
15. Read RC. Blood protease/antiprotease imbalance in patients with acquired herniation. Prob Gen Surg 1995;12:41–46.
16. Abrahamson J. Factors and mechanisms leading to recurrence. In:Prostheses and Abdominal Wall Hernias. Austin: Landes, 1994.
17. Lichtenstein IL. Hernia Repair Without Disability. Saint Louis: Ishiyaku Euroamerica, 1986.
18. Bassini E. Nuovo metodo sulla cura eradicale dell'ernia inguinale. Arch Soc Ital 1887;4:379–382.
19. Lichtenstein IL, Shulman AG, Amid PK. The cause, prevention, and treatment of recurrent groin hernia. Surg Clin North Am 1993;73:529–544.
20. Leber GE, Garb JL, Alexander AI, Reed WP. Long-term complications associated with prosthetic repair of incisional hernias. Arch Surg 1998;133:378–382.
21. Gilbert AI, Grahan MF. Improved sutureless technique: advice to experts. Prob Gen Surg 1995;12:117–119.
22. Rutkow IM, Robbins AW. Open mesh plug hernioplasty. Prob Gen Surg 1995;12:121–127.
23. Amid PK. Routine mesh repair. Crucial Controversies in Surgery 1997; 4B:63–70.
24. Bay-Nielsen M, Nordin P, Nilsson E, Kehlet H. Operative findings in recurrent hernia after a Lichtenstein procedure. Am J Surg 2001;182:134–136.

25. Gianetta E, Cuneo S, Vitale B, et al. Anterior tension-free repair of recurrent inguinal hernia under local anesthesia. A 7-year experience in a teaching hospital. Ann Surg 2000;231:132–136.

26. Haapaniemi S, Gunnarsson U, Nordin P, Nilsson E. Reoperation after recurrent groin hernia repair. Ann Surg 2001;234:122–126.

27. Stoppa RE, Warlaumont CR. The preperitoneal approach and prosthetic repair of groin hernia. In: Hernia. Philadelphia: JB Lippincott, 1989.

28. Wantz G, Fischer E. Recurrent inguinal hernia. In: Current Surgical Therapy. Saint Louis: Mosby, 2001.

29. Kurzer M, Belsham P, Kark A. Prospective study of open preperitoneal mesh repair for recurrent inguinal hernia. Br J Surg 2002;89:90–93.

30. Solorzano CC, Minter RM, Childers TC, et al. Prospective evaluation of the giant prosthetic reinforcement of the visceral sac for recurrent and complex bilateral inguinal hernias. Am J Surg 1999;177:19–22.

31. Ger R, Monroe K, Duvivier R, Mishrick A. Management of indirect inguinal hernias by laparoscopic closure of the neck of the sac. Am J Surg 1990;159: 370–373.

32. National Institute for Clinical Excellence. Guidance on the use of laparoscopic surgery for inguinal hernia. National Institute for Clinical Excellence: London, 2001.

33. Kald A, Anderberg B, Smedh K. Laparoscopic groin hernia repair: results of 200 consecutive herniorrhaphies. Br J Surg 1995;82:618–620.

34. Topal B, Hourlay P. Totally preperitoneal endoscopic inguinal hernia repair. Br J Surg 1997;84:61–63.

35. McCormack K, Scott N, Go P, et al. EU Hernia Trialists Collaboration. Laparoscopic techniques versus open techniques for inguinal hernia repair. Cochrane Database Syst Rev 2003;1:CD001785.

36. Memon M, Feliu X, Sallent E, et al. Laparoscopic repair of recurrent hernias. Sug Endosc 1998;13:807–810.

37. Beets G, Dirksen C, Go P, et al. Open or laparoscopic preperitoneal mesh repair for recurrent inguinal hernia? A randomized controlled trial. Surg Endosc 1999;13:323–327.

38. Mahon D, Decadt B, Rhodes M. Prospective randomized trial of laparoscopic (transabdominal preperitoneal) versus open (mesh) repair for bilateral and recurrent inguinal hernia. Surg Endosc 2003;17:1386–1390.

39. Scheuerlein H, Schiller A, Schneider C, et al. Totally extraperitoneal repair of recurrent inguinal hernia. Results from 179 consecutive patients. Surg Endosc 2003;17:1072–1076.

40. van der Hem JA, Hamming JF, Meeuwis JD, Oostvogel HJ. Totally extraperitoneal endoscopic repair of recurrent inguinal hernia. Br J Surg 2001;88:884–886.

41. Barrat C, Surlin V, Bordea A, Champault G. Management of recurrent inguinal hernias: a prospective study of 163 cases. Hernia 2003;7:125–129.

CHAPTER 7

Reoperative Surgery for Melanoma

Nicholas E. Tawa, Jr., MD, PhD

Précis

Melanoma is a cancer diagnosed with increasing incidence, and patients with recurrent disease will be encountered in daily general surgical practice with some frequency. The use of sentinel lymph node biopsy (SNB) has improved risk stratification for patients with metastasis, and has deepened our understanding of the natural history of melanoma. New imaging technologies have also allowed earlier identification of metastatic lesions amenable to surgical resection. In this brief review, a pragmatic approach to the management of advanced melanoma is described.

Overview

Reoperative procedures for melanoma encompass several clinical scenarios, ranging from completion lymphadenectomy following a microscopically positive sentinel node biopsy to resection of bulky metastatic disease. The tragedy associated with decision-making for patients with distant metastasis is their short expected survival, as balanced against the goal of palliation, and in some cases, a low but real expectation for long-term or even curative benefit. Many melanoma patients are also young, and the physician may feel pressured to intervene even when such efforts are futile. Under such circumstances, denying surgery can be a sad but wiser course.

In this review, a familiarity with the technique and rationale of SNB and the principles governing excision of a primary lesion are assumed, as described in available reviews.[1,2] The newly revised AJCC staging system for cutaneous melanoma is also referenced here, and is fully delineated elsewhere.[3]

RADIOLOGIC EVALUATION

As the resolution of radiological procedures such as FDG-positron emission tomography (PET) scanning and cross-sectional imaging (computed tomography [CT], magnetic resonance imaging [MRI]) continues to improve, clinically occult metastases in patients with a prior history of melanoma are more easily identified.[4] If such lesions are found, early resection may benefit some patients. Conversely, how frequently serial imaging should be used, which modality is superior, and whether nonvisceral body sites (e.g., brain) should be included routinely are unresolved. In addition, whether such aggressive approaches are economically sensible or result in improved overall survival is uncertain. For patients with a prior history of hematogenous metastasis, or for those on systemic therapy protocols, imaging at 3- to 6-month intervals is standard. A special instance is the patient in whom a metastatic lesion is strongly suggested by PET, but is nonpalpable or poorly imaged by modalities such as CT. Under such circumstances, high-resolution ultrasound or experimental hand-held PET probes may be helpful for localization.

PATIENT SELECTION

Several factors appear to predict improved outcome following resection of metastatic disease, or are otherwise important considerations prior to surgery.[5,6]

1. The presence of a solitary lesion, as opposed to multiple lesions in one organ or the simultaneous involvement of multiple organs. For example, resection of a peripheral soft tissue metastasis, e.g., one involving muscle (stage IV A disease), consolidated by postoperative radiotherapy, would be a more attractive procedure than resection of a complex visceral lesion (e.g., patients with stage IV B or C disease).
2. A prolonged disease-free interval from the primary lesion to the initial metastatic event, or elapsing between unrelated metastatic events.[7] However, this parameter is probably not as predictive of benefit for melanoma as in epithelial cancers, such as adenocarcinoma of the colon.
3. Lack of involvement of the central nervous system or lung. For example, it is imperative that, before embarking on any major resection, the brain is imaged to rule out concurrent, asymptomatic metastasis. If hemorrhage into such a lesion occurs perioperatively, the results can be disastrous. Alternatively, following successful treatment for brain metastasis (craniotomy, radiotherapy, or both together), a patient presenting with an isolated visceral lesion may remain an appropriate candidate for resection.
4. An anticipated overall survival of at least 3 to 6 months.
5. An acceptable morbidity for the procedure itself, taking into account the age and physiologic state of the patient. However, advanced age alone should not preclude intervention if other factors are favorable.
6. The patient's overall treatment history, including prior trials of experimental systemic therapy.

RATIONALE FOR RESECTION OF METASTATIC LESIONS

Randomized trials of outcome following aggressive surgical management for metastatic melanoma are not available. However, several retrospective studies suggest that in well-selected patients, relapse-free survival may be extended by several months, or in some cases, years.[5,6] Whether surgery in such cases affects overall survival is less clear. Dramatically favorable outcomes are often anecdotal and must be balanced against the approximate 5% of patients who will experience spontaneous remission of their disease. Some authors have suggested that resection of metastases removes a reservoir of tumor potentially capable of seeding yet additional distant sites, thus protecting the patient from such events, while freeing the immune system to counter smaller residual deposits of melanoma.[8] Unfortunately, there is no good evidence to support this view. Therefore, the best justification for surgery (and the one which should guide decision-making), is palliation of symptoms such as pain, obstruction, or hemorrhage, and the possibility of enhancing the relapse-free interval.

Similarly, the goal of completion lymphadenectomy (see below) remains most clearly to allow accurate staging (for prognosis and to allow selection for systemic therapy) and to prevent the subsequent development of bulky disease.[9] Bulky adenopathy may entail more difficult surgery, incurs a higher incidence of complications such as seroma formation, and may favor increased subsequent local recurrence. Certain subset analyses of previous randomized trials of elective node dissection suggested that relatively thin melanomas showed some overall survival benefit from lymphadenectomy when compared to thicker primary lesions.[10] However, such data are not statistically rigorous. If true, such observations may support the concept that regional lymph nodes can be the sole reservoir of metastatic disease, and that extirpation is of long-term benefit. This latter issue is only now being addressed by well-designed prospective trials, conducted with accurate staging as obtained by SNB, for example in the Sunbelt Melanoma Trial.[11]

Lymphadenectomy

Resection of regional lymph nodes may occur in several different clinical contexts. In each case, attention to the anatomic borders defining the draining nodal basin, with avoidance of lesser procedures (e.g., sampling only clinically obvious lesions) is desirable, both to maximize local control and minimize recurrence, and to ensure accurate staging.

COMPLETION LYMPHADENECTOMY FOLLOWING A POSITIVE SENTINEL NODE BIOPSY

The axillary, superficial groin (inguinal and femoral), and deep pelvic (external iliac and obturator) nodal basins are the most prevalent sites for dissection after a positive SNB performed for primary melanoma of the trunk or extremity. Many general surgeons also possess adequate training to pursue the more common cervical node procedure, i.e., modified radical neck dissection (with sparing of the internal jugular vein and spinal accessory nerve). However, with the advent of sentinel node localization for head and neck primaries, a more refined approach to definitive management at these sites is often preferred. For example, dissection of the superficial parotid gland, with sparing of the facial nerve branches, may be necessary to fully pursue findings upon lymphoscintigraphy.[12] Such procedures are beyond the expertise of most general surgeons if a low rate of complications is desired. This reality advocates for the management of patients with head and neck primaries within specialized referral centers.

In counseling patients preoperatively, sufficient experience has been gained to predict the expected yield of involved nodes at the time of the initial sentinel node localization and at definitive lymphadenectomy.[13,14] Thus, for T1b lesions (less than 1 mm and Clark level IV or ulcerated), which is the minimal invasive melanoma warranting SNB (see below), up to 7% of patients will have a positive node. For T2 lesions (1 to 2 mm) these rates are approximately 10% (nonulcerated) versus 25% (ulcerated); for T3 lesions (2 to 4 mm), they are 24% (nonulcerated) versus 37% (ulcerated); and for T4 lesions (more than 4 mm), the incidence rises dramatically to 30% (nonulcerated), and as high as 58% for ulcerated primaries. Tumor thickness also has predictive power for the anticipated results from completion lymphadenectomy. For example, for lesions less than 2 mm (T1 or T2), it is unlikely that an additional positive node will be found in addition to the already resected sentinel node (less than 5%), whereas for thicker lesions (more than 2 mm) the incidence rises to 25% to 30%. Similarly, the number of nodes harboring metastasis and recovered at the time of the initial SNB procedure is also predictive. In the majority of patients (70%), if only one microscopically involved sentinel node is recovered, all others will prove negative. Under such circumstances, 20% of individuals will have one additional positive node found, 7% will have two additional, and a small number (2%) three more nodes. From such data, one concludes that in the majority of cases the sentinel node is a solitary metastasis, although a large nodal focus or the presence of extracapsular invasion may increase the likelihood of residual disease.

TECHNIQUE OF RESECTION

Certain technical caveats are worthy of mention for these otherwise standard operative procedures. Excision of the previous nodal biopsy incision as a narrow skin ellipse probably lessens the chance of local recurrence. Similarly, unlike other neoplasms, such as breast cancer, extranodal extension of disease, or the presence of tumor deposits in the surrounding adipose tissue (presumably due to seeding of the feeding lymphatic channels), is common in melanoma. Therefore, skin flaps should be raised well away from the incision, with the goal of an honest en bloc resection of all soft tissue within the nodal basin. Skeletonization of the relevant muscles defining each basin (for the axilla, the latissimus, serratus, and pectoralis; and for the groin, the adductor longus and sartorius) should be achieved. Although the superior margin of the axilla and what constitutes a level III dissection are variably defined, skeletonization of the inferior surface of the axillary vein and extraction of tissue along its extreme medial extent, requiring elevation of the pectoralis minor, should be adequate. More aggressive efforts give an unacceptable incidence of extremity lymphedema and risk injury to the brachial plexus. In the axilla, the two major motor nerves (thoracodorsal and long thoracic) should be identified and skeletonized, if a thorough resection has been achieved. There seems to be no rule regarding how the caudal border of the axilla is defined anatomically.

Resection of the nodal basin in the groin carries a much higher incidence of local wound complications (persistent seromas, flap necrosis, wound dehiscence or infection) than at other sites, and carries a higher risk for lymphedema.[15] Therefore, patients should be counseled appropriately prior to operation. Excision of the fascia lata bordered by the sartorius and adductor longus should be performed, with resection of all underlying soft tissue within the femoral triangle and skeletonization of the femoral vessels, except for the lymphatic investment of the femoral vein. The more superficial subcutaneous tissue, which may also harbor nodes, should be excised en bloc within thin flaps, reaching a superior margin 3 to 6 cm above the inguinal ligament (to encompass the inguinal nodes, particularly if the primary is truncal), with the medial margin the external ring. Medial transposition of the sartorius to cover the exposed vessels is mandatory in all cases. Although some authors favor essentially a vertical incision, with a transverse J-extension distally to cover the femoral triangle,[16] this approach does not allow full access to the groin. The rationales for this technique are a possible lesser incidence of lymphedema (by avoiding the transaction of feeding superficial lymphatics incurred by a transverse upper thigh incision) and to accommodate the practice of splitting the inguinal ligament if deep pelvic nodes are pursued. However, this latter approach to the pelvis is ill-advised due to the difficult problem of managing the fascial defect that will inevitably result, with the potential for future herniation. Furthermore, if faced with such a defect, the use of prosthetic material for repair (e.g., a polypropylene mesh plug) is to be discouraged, given the high incidence of local wound complications following groin dissection (particularly infection).

As an alternative, a transverse upper thigh "S" incision is recommended, 2 cm below the inguinal ligament, extending from the pubic tubercle to the anterior superior iliac spine. If dissection of the external iliac nodes is desired, a new oblique counter-incision is made in the inguinal region. The oblique musculature and transverse abdominis are divided, usually just lateral to the internal ring, and the peritoneum reflected superiorly, giving excellent exposure of the deep vessels. If deep access to the proximal femoral canal is required, the superficial epigastric vessels can be divided. The soft tissue surrounding the external iliac artery and vein is removed, with attention to any clinically evident lesions, including extension to the common iliac bifurcation and the obturator foramen. Complete vascular control is usually easy to achieve at the outset and seems advisable and safer for the patient, particularly if bulky disease is present.

The finding of a positive sentinel node at unusual sites, specifically the popliteal, epitrochlear, or supraclavicular regions, occurs rarely.[17] In these cases, it is unclear if a formal node dissection can be conceived or should be carried out, and the potential for nerve injury is fairly high (particularly the brachial plexus for supraclavicular pathology). Although the deep lymphatics course with the popliteal vessels, in the other sites mentioned, there is no anatomically organized nodal grouping.

Furthermore, in general, if a sentinel node is found, e.g., at the elbow or knee, it will often be superficial and not beneath the muscle fascia or associated with the major vessels. Such decisions must be made on an individual basis. A similar issue arises with the finding of a so-called "in transit" sentinel node upon lymphoscintigraphy, i.e., a positive node arising outside of an established nodal basin, for example in the trunk. Such in transit nodes have been shown to have similar prognostic significance to positive nodes found elsewhere and therefore are important to pursue.[18] Whether wide re-excision of such an area after disease is found is necessary to prevent local recurrence is unclear. If only microscopic disease was present and the surgeon feels that an appropriate quantity of surrounding soft tissue was recovered at the time of the initial biopsy, re-excision may not be required.

APPROACH TO DEEP PELVIC NODE DISSECTION

The technical approach to deep pelvic node dissection was discussed earlier. Which patients benefit from the procedure is uncertain,[9,16] and morbidity from lymphedema appears higher when coupled with superficial groin dissection. It seems unlikely that surgery always clears the lymphatic tissue of metastatic disease in the pelvis, given the diffuse pattern of ductal branching beginning superior to the inguinal ligament. As an extreme example, sentinel node biopsy can be applied to primary anal melanomas, with a high incidence of (at times bilateral) occult inguinal node metastasis.[19] Some workers have even described a potential prolongation of the disease-free interval by an aggressive approach to nodal dissection in such cases.[20] However, when these patients recur locally, the pattern of late lymphatic spread is often diffuse, involving the rectovaginal septum and other poorly accessible retroperitoneal structures. A prior iliac lymphadenectomy would retrospectively prove futile in that instance. Therefore, the management of deep pelvic nodes is to some extent predicated on whether disease in this location is considered only a local-regional issue, or a manifestation of true metastatic disease, without consensus. In some cases, a limited approach to resection of an isolated iliac nodal recurrence, potentially using minimally invasive technique (laparoscopy), may be justified in a patient for whom the value of a more aggressive procedure is dubious.

In selecting patients for deep pelvic node dissection, certain prognostic variables help predict iliac nodal involvement. These include a positive Cloquet's (femoral canal) node, the involvement of more than three nodes in the superficial compartment, or the presence of bulky disease.[21] However, in many patients, there will be no obvious node at the anticipated location of the femoral canal. Furthermore, as deep iliac dissection is essentially a separate procedure from superficial femoral lymphadenectomy, it can easily be delayed, allowing time for permanent histopathology, possible additional imaging of the pelvis, and a separate surgical consent. Overall, in the absence of a clear survival value for resection of even microscopically positive superficial nodes, as opposed to pelvic nodes, it is difficult to recommend iliac node dissection universally. In uncertain cases, or if the patient is considered at increased risk, radiologic imaging can be helpful to identify suspicious iliac lesions and to facilitate preoperative diagnostic fine needle aspiration cytology.

MANAGEMENT OF BULKY LYMPHATIC METASTASIS

Persons prone to bulky metastasis include those with metastatic melanoma of unknown primary, patients with a nodal recurrence (often after an otherwise "successful" SNB performed in the same basin earlier), or in unfortunate patients with high-risk primaries who have palpable nodal disease at initial diagnosis. For these, all of the principles of surgical technique described earlier are helpful. It is common practice to offer postoperative radiotherapy if matted nodes, extracapsular extension, or tumor deposits in the soft tissue are present, although prospective evidence favoring efficacy of this modality is available only for central nervous system metastases.[22] In the axilla, the metastatic process can extend along the subclavian vein to the mediastinum, undermining the pectoralis minor and potentially enveloping the brachial plexus. The anatomic approach for excision may require division of the pectoralis minor tendon, partial claviculectomy, or limited chest wall resection. An increased potential for local recurrence, attributable to incomplete margins, and occult extension into adjoined but unrelated nodal compartments such as the neck or mediastinum, may also be anticipated. In these rare cases, it is often hard to conceive lasting benefit, given the surgical morbidity and the high incidence of short-term distant metastasis.

APPLICATION OF SENTINEL NODE BIOPSY FOR IN-TRANSIT DISEASE

One application of SNB which is uniquely "reoperative" is for identifying occult nodal metastases in patients presenting with newly recurrent regional melanoma, despite an earlier apparently successful operation. Little is known about the difference in incidence of nodal metastasis between patients lacking an initial SNB who have a newly identified in transit recurrence, when compared to asymptomatic patients with similar stage primary lesions. The relevant hypothesis predicts that an in-transit lesion defines a "vector" of lymphatic spread from the original primary to the relevant nodal basin. Therefore, the in-transit lesion can be used as the injection site for preoperative scintigraphy, to define its drainage pattern and allow exploration of the relevant regional nodes. For example, in a study by Morton et al, nearly half of all in-transit patients had at least one positive node when managed in this way, and relapse-free survival appeared better in patients demonstrated to be node-negative.[23]

DELAYED SENTINEL NODE MAPPING FOLLOWING DEFINITIVE WIDE LOCAL EXCISION

In certain cases, patients will present whose original pathology warrants a sentinel node procedure for staging, but who have undergone wide excision regardless, without node sampling. In many cases, these are patients with stage IB disease, i.e., those with T1b lesions (less than 1 mm thickness but a discordantly deep Clark level of IV, or with ulceration present). However, it is increasingly recognized that T1b patients can present with lymphatic metastasis, often after an unusually prolonged interval (3 to 5 years), and that sentinel node mapping in such patients yields a 5% to 7% incidence of positivity. Therefore, pursuing a delayed SNB may seem desirable under various circumstances. A common assumption is that a prior wide excision, by disrupting the original pattern of lymphatic drainage, renders SN mapping less accurate, and therefore less predictive, than in a virginal setting. However, when studied, such concerns seem unjustified, particularly as the incidence of nodal recurrence and overall survival appear to be similar in patients staged by immediate versus delayed SNB and then followed for prolonged periods.[24,25] A more practical issue is the fairly frequent inability in this setting to obtain transmittal of the tracer beyond the injection site at the time of lymphoscintigraphy, presumably due to scarring or lymphatic transaction induced by prior surgery.

MANAGEMENT OF WOUND COMPLICATIONS

Liberal use of closed suction drains, with strict criteria for removal (less than 20 to 30 mL/day for at least 2 to 3 days) helps to reduce seromas in most patients. These devices can be maintained for up to 3 to 4 weeks. However, it is well known that no drain works perfectly, and persistent seromas are best treated by open drainage and packing, including use of an immobilizing VAC suction dressing to initiate healing if the soft tissue defect is large. Lesser measures (repeated aspiration, Penrose drainage, or percutaneous ultrasound-guided drainage) are often short-lived, may induce infection, and by failing to resolve the problem may delay subsequent systemic chemotherapy and radiotherapy. Persistent cellulitis following node dissection can also be a difficult problem, and at times may benefit from prolonged (e.g., 2 to 6 months) suppressive oral antibiotic therapy.

Management of Metastatic or Locally Recurrent Melanoma

Some primary lesions can be difficult to clear microscopically. Desmoplastic melanoma (a locally infiltrative spindle cell variant) can spread extensively through the dermis, as can the much less threatening lesion of melanoma in situ, occasionally giving a surprisingly positive margin after wide excision. In such cases, multiple 2- to 3-mm punch biopsies can be harvested at 1 and 2 cm from the recent scar to give a rough predictive map of the distribution of residual disease. A more modern approach for the evaluation of close margins, particularly in the head and neck, is laser confocal microscopy. For desmoplastic lesions, or if extensive "micro-satellitosis" (e.g., IIIC disease) was present in the initial specimen, margins of excision (from studies of primary melanoma) should be 2 to 3 cm. Consolidative postoperative radiotherapy may be useful in this setting to lower local recurrence. However, if a large skin graft was applied or there was early graft loss with extensive scar formation, radiotherapy may promote only formation of a chronic wound, with no discernible benefit.

RECURRENCE IN SCAR OR IN SOFT TISSUE

A limited local recurrence, or a nodular subcutaneous metastasis, is generally managed by excision to a microscopically negative margin. How much of a formal margin is required is unclear, and will be balanced by the perceived operative morbidity. Some metastases can be quite large, and in certain cases (e.g., a gluteal recurrence with extension into the sciatic notch), margin clearance can be difficult. A related question influencing the extent of operation is whether patients with even a straightforward scar recurrence have the same prognosis as before, or if this situation heralds an increased short-term incidence of subsequent metastatic events.

EXCISION OF IN-TRANSIT METASTASES

Limited in-transit lesions of the extremities can be approached by periodic excision until this approach becomes impractical due to an excessive burden of recurrent sites. The role of isolated or hyperthermic limb perfusion continues to be evaluated for these unfortunate patients. Although early responses can be dramatic, there is no clear overall survival benefit,[26] and to add to the frustration, new in-transit lesions will frequently arise de novo following perfusion. This latter phenomenon presumably reflects nests of dermal lymphatic metastases that were dormant and thus resistant to this otherwise toxic therapy. For islands of locally persistent, but anatomically limited in-transit disease (e.g., at the ankle), radiation may be helpful to control recurrences. Aside from its use as a means of primary control of disease at the time of initial operation, limb amputation has no role in managing in-transit disease. However, in unusual cases, such as for the relief of intractable pain or for improved toilet in the face of extensive tumor necrosis, amputation may sometimes be indicated.

GASTROINTESTINAL TRACT

Survival rates decrease progressively for involvement of skin and subcutaneous tissue, distant nodes, the gastrointestinal (GI) tract, lung, bone, liver, and brain, with median survival ranging from 4 to 15 months.[6] Therefore, GI tract metastases are usually associated with disseminated disease and short survival, although as for other sites, some very long-term responses to surgery have been described. The classic indications for palliative resection are obstruction, bleeding, or perforation. If the metastatic process involves the pancreas or duodenum, definitive resection will be impossible. When gastric outlet obstruction is the primary issue and a draining gastrojejunostomy is impractical (either because of the overall condition of the patient or concurrent carcinomatosis), a percutaneous radiologically guided gastrostomy can vent the stomach and prevent the need for a nasogastric tube. During resection for extensive mesenteric metastasis, injury to the feeding or anatomically important vessels should be avoided, even if a positive margin will result. Certainly, dramatic interventions such as use of an interposition jump graft for vascular reconstruction should never be pursued in this setting. If resection for relief of bowel obstruction is impossible, a draining enteroenterostomy or a skin stoma may be wiser options. In the liver, some series have emphasized aggressive resection for metastatic ocular melanomas, although there is probably nothing unique about the metastases themselves. Overall, outcomes are poor, particularly if multiple lesions are present, and the role of newer modalities (e.g., cryo- or radiofrequency ablation) in lieu of surgical resection is undefined. For anal or vaginal primaries, the consensus choice for initial resection is usually wide excision. If these patients recur locally, a larger salvage procedure, e.g., abdominoperineal resection or even pelvic exenteration, may initially seem attractive. Unfortunately, the vast majority of these individuals will show distant metastasis soon after local recurrence becomes an issue, and this reality will supersede the earlier surgical concern and obviate aggressive local therapy.

RETROPERITONEUM

Not infrequently, isolated metastasis to the kidney, adrenal gland, bladder, or retroperitoneal soft tissue will occur. The preferred approach to such lesions is extraperitoneal, either by a true retroperitoneal tenth or eleventh rib lateral incision, or if necessary, a higher thoracoabdominal incision, with division of the costal margin and violation of the diaphragm. These patients usually recover quickly and show little morbidity from surgery, even if nephrectomy is required.

IS "INDUCTION" THERAPY WITH SURGICAL SALVAGE A VIABLE CONCEPT?

As discussed earlier, Morton and coworkers have proposed that in some patients with metastasis, aggressive debulking may render them more responsive to subsequent immunological therapies,[6,8] which is an area of controversy. Along the same lines, in centers treating patients with interleukin-2 or with related forms of biochemotherapy for distant metastasis, initial response rates can be quite high (50% to 60%). In some of these, only a few residual lesions may persist, and they may prove stable on subsequent imaging. Whether an aggressive approach to surgical salvage makes more sense in this than in other settings is unknown. Such surgery is also often propelled by the desire to render the patient "without evidence of disease," in order to facilitate enrollment in additional protocol-based therapies. This practice seems of dubious benefit, given the prevalence of associated occult distant metastases in these high-risk patients.

REFERENCES

1. Gershenwald JE, Thompson W, Mansfield PF, et al. Multi-institutional melanoma lymphatic mapping experience: the prognostic value of sentinel lymph node status in 612 stage I or II melanoma patients. J Clin Oncol 1999;17:976–983.

2. Heaton KM, Sussman JJ, Gershenwald JE, et al. Surgical margins and prognostic factors in patients with thick (>4 mm) primary melanoma. Ann Surg Oncol 1998; 5:322–328.

3. Balch CM, Soong SJ, Gershenwald JE, et al. Prognostic factors analysis of 17,600 melanoma patients: validation of the American Joint Committee on Cancer melanoma staging system. J Clin Oncol 2001;19:3622–3634.

4. Prichard RS, Hill ADK, Skehan SJ, et al. Positron emission tomography for staging and management of malignant melanoma. Br J Surg 2002;89: 389–396.

5. Allen PJ, Coit DG. The surgical management of metastatic melanoma. Ann Surg Oncol 2002;9:762–770.
6. Essner R. Surgical treatment of malignant melanoma. Surg Clin North Am 2003;83:109–156.
7. Crowley NJ, Seigler HF. Relationship between disease-free interval and survival in patients with recurrent melanoma. Arch Surg 1992;127:1303–1308.
8. Ollila DW, Hsueh EC, Stern SL, et al. Metastasectomy for recurrent stage IV melanoma. J Surg Oncol 1999;71:209–213.
9. Mann GB, Coit DG. Does the extent of operation influence the prognosis in patients with melanoma metastatic to inguinal nodes? Ann Surg Oncol 1999;6:263–271.
10. Balch CM, Soong S, Ross MI, et al. Long-term results of a multi-institutional randomized trial comparing prognostic factors and surgical results for intermediate thickness melanomas (1.0 to 4.0 mm). Intergroup Melanoma Surgical Trial. Ann Surg Oncol 2000;7:87–97.
11. McMasters KM. The Sunbelt Melanoma Trial. Ann Surg Oncol 2001;8: 41S–43S.
12. Eicher SA, Clayman GL, Myers JN, et al. A prospective study of intraoperative lymphatic mapping for head and neck cutaneous melanoma. Arch Otolaryngol Head Neck Surgery 2002;128:241.
13. McMasters KM, Wong SL, Edwards MJ, et al. Factors that predict the presence of sentinel lymph node metastasis in patients with melanoma. Surgery 2001;130: 151–156.
14. McMasters KM, Wong SL, Edwards MJ, et al. Frequency of nonsentinel lymph node metastasis in melanoma. Ann Surg Oncol 2002;9:137–141.
15. Shaw JH, Rumball EM. Complications and local recurrence following lymphadenectomy. Br J Surg 1990;77:760–764.
16. Karakousis CP, Emrich LJ, Driscoll DL, et al. Survival after groin dissection for malignant melanoma. Surgery 1991;109:119–126.
17. Thompson JF, Hunt JA, Culjak G, et al. Popliteal lymph node metastasis from primary cutaneous melanoma. Eur J Surg Oncol 2000;26:172–176.
18. McMasters KM, Chao C, Wong SL, et al. Interval sentinel lymph nodes in melanoma. Arch Surg 2002;137:543–549.
19. Tien HY, McMasters KM, Edwards MJ, et al. Sentinel lymph node metastasis in anal melanoma: a case report. Int J Gastrointest Cancer 2002;32:53–56.
20. Kadison AS, Essner R, Bleicher RJ, et al. Primary mucosal melanoma: the role of lymphatic mapping. Proceedings of ASCO 2002;21:1365.
21. Shen P, Conforti AM, Essner R, et al. Is the node of Cloquet the sentinel node for the iliac/obturator node group? Cancer J 2000;6:93–97.
22. Stevens G, Thompson JF, Firth I, et al. Locally advanced melanoma: results of postoperative hypofractionated radiation therapy. Cancer 2000;88: 88–94.

23. Yao KA, Hsueh EC, Essner R, et al. Is sentinel lymph node mapping indicated for isolated local and in-transit recurrent melanoma? Ann Surg 2003;238:743–747.

24. Leong WL, Ghazarian DM, McCready DR. Previous wide local excision of primary melanoma is not a contraindication for sentinel lymph node biopsy of the trunk and extremity. J Surg Oncol 2003;82:143–146.

25. McCready DR, Ghazarian DM, Hershkop MS, et al. Sentinel lymph-node biopsy after previous wide local excision for melanoma. Can J Surg 2001;44: 432–434.

26. Thompson JF, Kam PC, Waugh RC, et al. Isolated limb infusion with cytotoxic agents: a simple alternative to isolated limb perfusion. Semin Surg Oncol 1998; 14:238–247.

CHAPTER 8

Reopertive Pancreaticoduodenal Surgery

Shimul A. Shah, MD; Charles M. Vollmer, Jr., MD;
Mark P. Callery, MD, FACS

Introduction

The pancreas can be a formidable adversary to surgeons even when a primary operation is undertaken. For most pancreatic diseases, reoperations are usually a result of an inadequate initial procedure and, due to the complexity of these conditions, treatment goals are often not met. This review will analyze primary treatment goals and causes of failure for specific pancreatic conditions. The surgical management of complications following both primary operations and reoperations is also discussed.

Management of Complications from Pancreatic Surgery

COMPLICATIONS OF PANCREATIC RESECTION

Despite the complexity of pancreatic surgery, there has been a dramatic improvement in morbidity and mortality rates after pancreatic surgery over the last 25 years. A number of complications have been identified following pancreatic resection that may require surgical intervention. The reoperative rate following pancreatic resection is usually less than 10%, but can be as high as 46%.[1–5]

A pancreatic leak is usually defined as an amylase-rich drain output that is three to five times that of the serum concentration. This is usually evident 3 to 7 days after surgery. These leaks, which once occurred 7% to 19% of the time, are associated with significant increases in hospital stays and morbidity. However, these rates have recently declined to less than 5% in most specialists' hands.[1,4,6] The most common presentation is a fever associated with leukocystosis, abdominal pain, and ileus. Computed tomography (CT) scan may show a fluid collection or abscess in about 20% of these patients. This situation rarely requires reoperation and can be conservatively managed with bowel rest, total parenteral nutrition (TPN), and percutaneous drainage. Minor leaks will resolve in almost all patients. For persistent pancreatic fistulas, octreotide may be a useful adjunct by decreasing the volume of pancreatic secretion, and therefore permitting a more rapid closure of the fistula.

If the patient becomes septic, and a localized cause is not radiographically identified, then a laparotomy should be performed as a last-ditch effort to save the patient. Early intervention can prevent death. Upon reexploration for sepsis, no source may be identified. The pancreas is often presumed to be the cause in this setting, and the area around the pancreas is rarely explored thoroughly, to prevent disruption of a possible intact anastomosis. If there is any question of a pancreatic leak, a completion pancreatectomy should be performed. This may be the only means of containing and controlling infection. Ductal obliteration may be an option to preserve endocrine function. The surgical management is driven by the amount of retroperitoneal inflammation, and rarely is there a role for taking down and revising the pancreatic anastomosis in this setting.[5]

Delayed gastric emptying is defined by the need for a nasogastric tube for more than 14 days postoperatively. This can occur with both a pylorus-preserving operation and a standard Whipple. Most patients respond to bowel rest and gastric decompression. Although this complication can occur in up to one-third of patients, few require reoperation.[1,7]

PANCREATIC FISTULA

Pancreatic fistula is a serious complication that most commonly occurs with operations involving the pancreas or adjacent organs such as the stomach, spleen, colon, adrenal gland, or kidney. Fistulas are best evaluated by fistulogram or endoscopic retrograde cholangiopancreatography (ERCP). Initial management consists of resting the pancreas and gastrointestinal (GI) tract by nasogastric suction and limitation of oral intake. In some instances, TPN may be used as an adjunct to provide nutritional support. Adequate drainage of the fistula is necessary to prevent sepsis. The value of octreotide in the management and prevention of pancreatic fistulae remains controversial. Octreotide has been used to decrease the volume of output, but has not been shown to accelerate fistula closure nor to improve survival in patients with a pancreatic fistula.[8] Yeo and colleagues found that prophylactic octreotide after pancreaticoduodenectomy did not decrease the rates of postoperative fistulae, mortality, or length of hospital stay.[9] This study suggests that octreotide is probably warranted only in the scenario of a small duct in conjunction with a soft-textured gland.

A fistula that is kept open by an anatomic problem will not heal with a pharmacological approach. If pancreatic duct obstruction is present proximal to the fistula, due to malignancy, stricture, calculus, or the fibrosis of chronic pancreatitis, an attempt must be made to address the underlying problem. Reoperation is therefore necessary. When possible, resection of a dominant mass or complete internal drainage of the pancreatic duct including the fistula will successfully correct the problem when these approaches are possible. Fistulas located in the body or tail of the pancreas may be treated by distal pancreatectomy. The simplest maneuver for

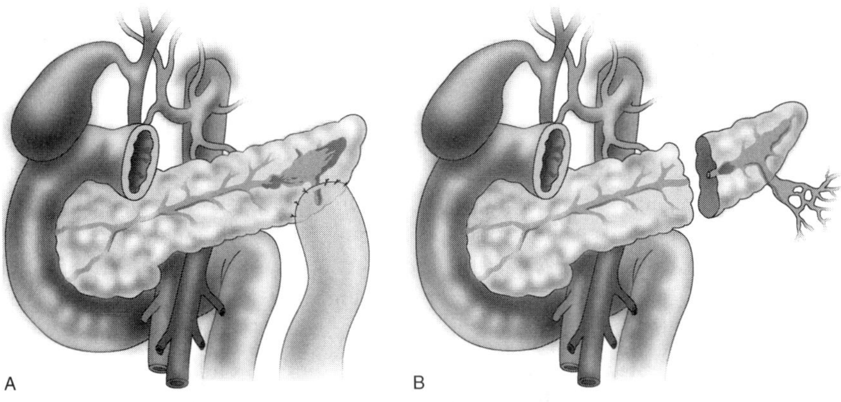

Figure 8-1 (A) Persistent pancreatic fistulas arising at any point along the pancreatic duct may be drained internally into a Roux-en-Y loop of jejunum. (B) For fistulas arising along the body or tail, distal pancreatectomy including the fistula is the procedure of choice.

(Modified from Aranha GV, Prinz RA, Greenlee HB. Reoperations for pancreatitis and pancreatic cancer. In: McQuarrie DG, Humphrey EW, Lee JT, eds. Reoperative General Surgery. St. Louis, MO: Mosby, 1997.)

fistulas in association with benign disease involves dissection of the fistula tract and drainage into a Roux-en-Y loop of jejunum (Figure 8-1).

PANCREATIC ABSCESS

Localized abscesses of the pancreas can usually be successfully treated by conventional open or percutaneous drainage techniques. The major problem lies in the differentiation from a sterile pancreatic phlegmon and infected pancreatic necrosis. Aggressive drainage and even debridement is often necessary in the cases of infected necrosis. Pancreatic phase CT scans are valuable in distinguishing the difference between sterile and infected necrosis, the presence of gas and the potential for drainage.[10–12] CT-guided fine-needle aspiration for smear and culture is the most accurate tool in determining the presence of pancreatic necrosis, but is not itself sufficient as a treatment modality, with recurrence rates approaching 70%.[13,14] Direct catheter drainage is associated with a much lower recurrence when drainage outputs are followed with sinography to assess for adequacy of drainage and presence of retained debris.[15]

Widespread pancreatic and peripancreatic infected necrosis often requires repeated open drainages with necrosectomy and placement of large-bore sump drains. Repeated debridements and drainages, sometimes coupled with open packing of the abdomen, are sometimes necessary. In this scenario, it is often prudent to be less, rather than more, aggressive when debriding, taking care not to injure major vascular structures. The mortality rate for infected pancreatic necrosis has decreased to almost 10% in most studies, although it must be noted that these represent "highly" selected patients.[16–18]

PANCREATIC ASCITES

Pancreatic ascites is usually the result of a disruption of the main pancreatic duct or, alternatively, a leaking pseudocyst that leads to massive ascites. Acute peritonitis does not develop, because the pancreatic enzymes have not been activated by the proteolytic duodenal enzymes. Treatment consists of bowel rest, TPN, and repeated paracenteses. Octreotide may have some benefit, but the role is not yet clear. Conservative therapy avoids surgery in approximately 50% of patients.

Surgery is indicated if nonoperative therapy is unsuccessful over a period of 3 to 4 weeks.[19,20] ERCP can be used to identify a ductal leak. The surgical failure rate is as low as 12% to 18% if a point of leakage is found on ERCP before surgery, but it can be as high as 50% if a discrete source is not found on ERCP.[21] Because disruptions in the pancreatic duct are thought to be caused by an increased pressure within the pseudocyst or the pancreatic duct, endoscopic therapy by sphincterotomy or by insertion of a transpapillary stent may reduce intraductal pressure.[22] If a pseudocyst is present, internal drainage into the appropriate adjacent viscus, either endoscopically or surgically, is the preferred treatment. If a direct leak from the pancreatic duct is identified, an anastomosis between the site of ductal rupture and a Roux limb of jejunum achieves controlled drainage. Fistulas and pseudocysts located in the body or tail of the pancreas can be treated by distal pancreatectomy.

Reoperations for Benign Conditions

RECURRENT PANCREATITIS

Chronic pancreatitis is primarily a nonsurgical disease and should be managed medically. Relief of chronic pain from pancreatitis is a difficult problem. However, this has long been recognized as the primary indication for surgical intervention. Surgery is also necessary in cases complicated by pseudocyst, pancreatic abscess, fistula, biliary obstruction, splenic vein thrombosis leading to hemorrhage, and ductal fibrosis.[23,24]

Although many operations have been devised to relieve pain from pancreatitis, only pancreatic duct drainage and pancreatic resection have proven to be beneficial.[25–30] Pancreatic duct drainage is the procedure of choice in patients with a dilated duct, because it relieves pain and preserves both exocrine and endocrine function. The success rates for abolishing pain using a lateral pancreaticojejunostomy range from 77% to 93%.[23,31–40] A dilated pancreatic duct (larger than 5 mm) confirmed by ERCP allows for a relatively straightforward side-to-side pancreaticojejunal anastomosis. For the daunting problem of an underlying cancer masked in diffuse fibrosis from chronic pancreatitis, multiple biopsies should be performed at the time of initial operation if there is any concern for malignancy.

A pancreaticoduodenectomy or distal pancreatectomy is favored, depending on the location of the scarring or mass.

Resection is preferred over decompression techniques in the absence of ductal dilation, the presence of a dominant mass, or a suspected malignancy. When inflammatory changes are confined to a specific area of the pancreas, it is tempting to assume that resection of this area will relieve the pain. This assumption is often incorrect. These problems can be further magnified by noncompliance and continued alcohol and narcotic abuse commonly seen in these patients, thus reinforcing the importance of proper patient selection. Resection is associated with a high incidence of metabolic problems related to pancreatic function including insulin-dependent diabetes and steatorrhea.[31–33]

Patients who develop or continue to have pain after pancreaticojejunostomy or pancreatic resection should undergo a complete reevaluation. All potential causes of pain, including peptic ulcer disease, biliary disease, and colitis should be considered equally with recurrent pancreatitis. Once these other causes of pain have been ruled out, the effectiveness and technique of the initial operation must be reevaluated.

ERCP provides the best assessment of the patency of the pancreaticojejunostomy and the completeness of drainage. It also identifies areas of undrained pancreatic duct within the head or uncinate process after resections and limited drainage procedures. If there is incomplete drainage of the pancreatic ductal system or any undrained segments after resection, redrainage of the pancreatic duct is the preferred approach, since completion pancreatectomy is the alternative.[41–43] Redrainage is a less formidable operation than resection and is more effective in achieving pain relief without sacrificing endocrine and exocrine function of the pancreas. Prinz et al. achieved an overall 71% relief of pain in 14 (10%) of 138 patients who underwent redrainage after initial pancreaticojejunostomy.[42] From seven patients who had undergone a pancreatic resection after unsuccessful drainage procedure, none were rendered pain-free, and furthermore, three died from complications of diabetes management. This excellent rate of pain relief after redrainage compares favorably with the quoted 80% success rate after initial pancreaticojejunostomy.[41]

The most important objective of pancreaticojejunostomy is the complete drainage of the pancreatic ductal system and not the length of the anastomosis created. During redrainage procedures, the anterior surface of the pancreas should be completely exposed from duodenum to tail. The duct can be palpated and confirmed with needle aspiration of water-clear exocrine fluid. In difficult circumstances, intraoperative ultrasound will facilitate identification of the duct in a fibrotic pancreas (Figure 8-2). Once identified, the duct should be opened widely from one end of the pancreas to the side of the previous pancreaticojejunostomy or transection level of distal pancreatectomy. Both the duct of Wirsung and the duct of Santorini should be drained from the splenic hilum to as close as possible to the duodenum (Figure 8-3). After inadequate drainage procedures, the redundancy of the original Roux limb of jejunum almost always permits it to be used for the new wider drained anastomosis. If a distal resection was the original procedure, a new jejunal Roux limb will need to be crafted if none was used in the

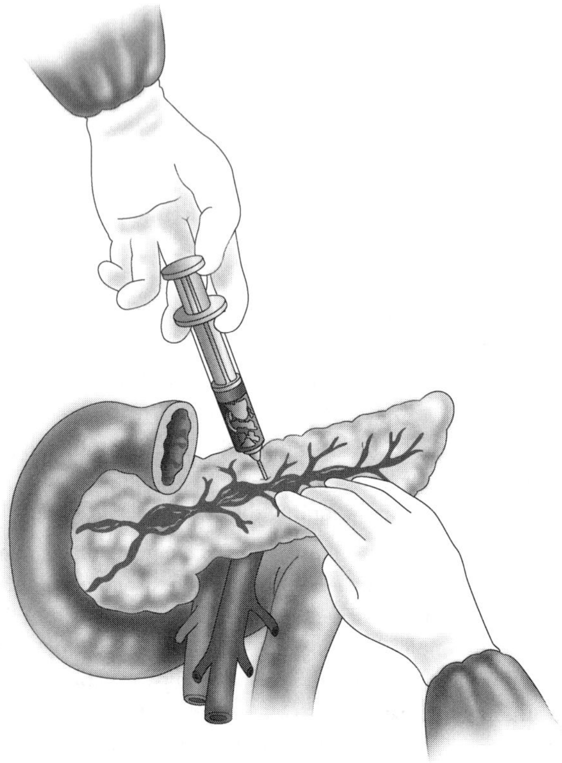

Figure 8-2 Identification of a dilated pancreatic duct and confirmation with needle aspiration of water-clear exocrine fluid.

(Modified from Prinz RA, Deiziel DJ, Bransky AS. Roux-en-Y pancreaticojejunostomy for chronic pancreatitis. In: Baker RJ, Fischer JE, eds. Mastery of Surgery. Philadelphia: Lippincott, Williams, and Wilkins, 2001.)

initial operation. A one-layer anastomosis with monofilament suture between the fibrous capsule of the pancreas and the seromuscular layer of the opened jejunum can be created with either an interrupted or a continuous technique.

The poor results of distal pancreatectomy after unsuccessful pancreatic drainage are due to the frequent occurrence of undrained segments of the pancreatic duct in the head and uncinate process of the gland. These segments of dilated duct must be addressed to achieve satisfactory pain relief. If an area of obstructed pancreatic duct remains in the rim of pancreas adjacent to the duodenum after a distal or near-total pancreatectomy, continued pain can be expected. This supports performing a pancreaticoduodenectomy to relieve pain from recurrent pancreatitis.[25,44] Various modifications of pancreatic resection techniques have been offered in hopes of both preserving pancreatic parenchyma and preventing the need for resection of adjacent organs such as the duodenum, bile duct, or spleen.[45–47] Pancreaticoduodenectomy,

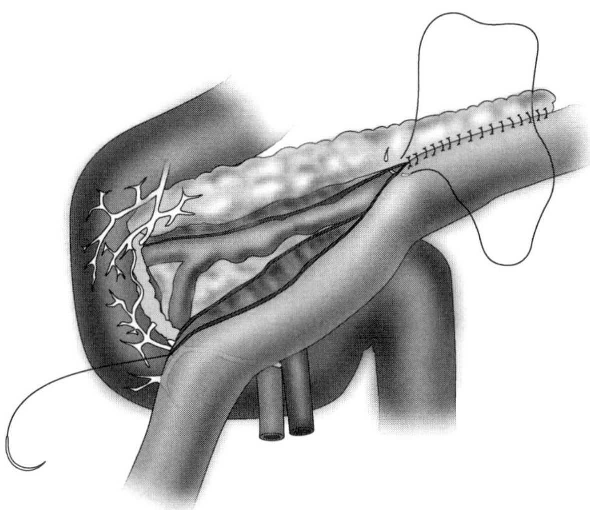

Figure 8-3 Complete drainage of the pancreatic ductal system with the duct of Wirsung and the duct of Santorini drained from the splenic hilum to as close as possible to the duodenum. In the head of the gland, the anterior superior and inferior pancreaticoduodenal arteries should be suture-ligated to prevent bleeding.

(Modified from Prinz RA, Deiziel DJ, Bransky AS. Roux-en-Y pancreaticojejunostomy for chronic pancreatitis. In: Baker RJ, Fischer JE, eds. Mastery of Surgery. Philadelphia: Lippincott, Williams, and Wilkins, 2001.)

performed in high-volume centers, safely warrants consideration, since it is more complete for pain relief.

PANCREATIC PSEUDOCYST

Reoperation for pancreatic pseudocysts is required in 15% to 20% of patients. Recurrent or persistent pseudocyst, bleeding, error in diagnosis, and residual pancreatic disease are all potential causes for initial operative failure. The most common cause for reoperation is a missed pseudocyst, but this occurrence should be waning now that CT scan and ultrasound provide a more accurate delineation of the presence of multiple cysts prior to the initial endeavor. One must be certain intraoperatively that no cysts are missed. Fine-needle aspiration of any suspicious area can be employed to prevent this.

Continued or recurrent abdominal and back pain after pseudocyst drainage is another reason for reoperation. This is usually a manifestation of underlying chronic pancreatitis. An ERCP should be obtained in any patient who develops a pseudocyst in the setting of chronic pancreatitis to determine if the pancreatic duct is dilated. ERCP also distinguishes communication between the duct and cyst. Drainage from the unroofed pancreatic duct and pseudocyst can be achieved in the

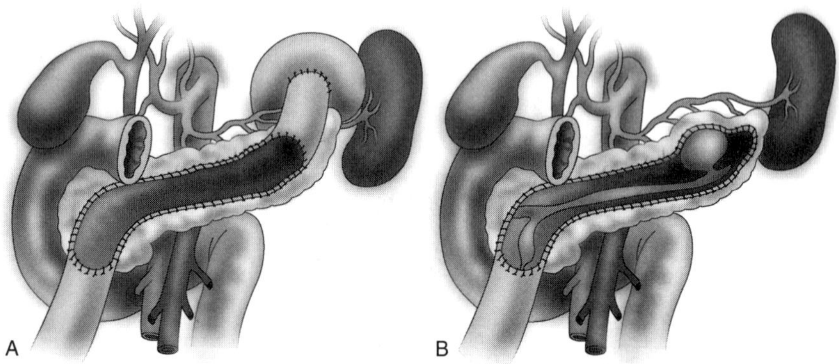

Figure 8-4 Simultaneous drainage of the pseudocyst and the pancreatic duct can be performed. As shown here, the same Roux-en-Y limb is used to drain both the pseudocyst and the dilated pancreatic duct where the pseudocyst is in the tail of the pancreas (A) and the midbody of the pancreas (B).

(Modified from Aranha GV, Prinz RA, Greenlee HB. Reoperations for pancreatitis and pancreatic cancer. In: McQuarrie DG, Humphrey EW, Lee JT, eds. Reoperative General Surgery. St. Louis, MO: Mosby, 1997.)

same setting using the same Roux-en-Y jejunal loop, and can usually be performed with no increase in morbidity[48,49] (Figure 8-4). Alternatively, Nealon and colleagues have recently reported that ductal drainage alone in chronic pancreatitis with pseudocysts is sufficient and effective in completely resolving associated pseudocysts. In their series, pancreaticojejunostomy alone without drainage of the cyst led to decreased operative time, less dissection, and most importantly, no pseudocyst recurrence in 47 patients.[50]

Lateral pancreaticojejunostomy should be performed if the duct is dilated. In patients with continued or recurrent pain after pseudocyst drainage, the pancreatic duct is first evaluated by ERCP. If cystogastrostomy had previously been performed, this is taken down and the entire pancreatic duct, including the previous site of drainage into the stomach, is incorporated into a side-to-side pancreaticojejunostomy. This usually represents failure to recognize and treat chronic pancreatitis simultaneously during the first procedure employed to drain the pseudocyst. The defect in the posterior wall of the stomach is closed primarily. If the initial operation was a cyst-jejunostomy (Figure 8-5), the same Roux loop can be used to drain the adjacent opened pancreatic duct.[50]

CYSTIC NEOPLASMS OF THE PANCREAS

The most common cystic lesions of the pancreas are pseudocysts. However, cystadenomas represent about 10% of the nonmalignant cystic lesions of the pancreas, and the even more rare cystadenocarcinoma represents only 1% of primary pancreatic malignant lesions.[51,52] These cystic lesions typically present with symptoms of abdominal pain, weight loss and, less frequently, nausea, vomiting, and weakness.

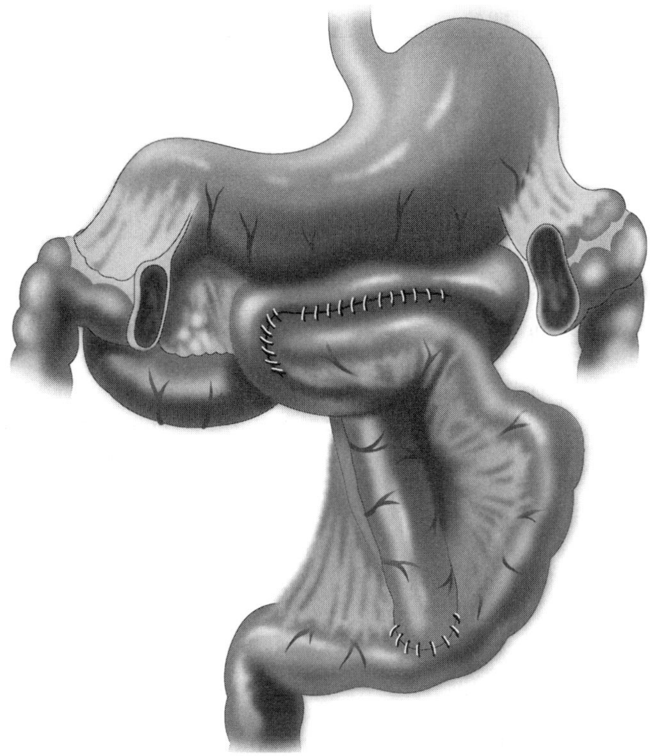

Figure 8-5 Roux-en-Y cystojejunostomy.

(Modified from Bradley EL. In: Baker RJ, Fischer JE, eds. Mastery of Surgery. Philadelphia: Lippincott, Williams, and Wilkins, 2001.)

Jaundice, pancreatitis, or steatorrhea are infrequent presentations; however, cystadenocarcinomas present more often with jaundice than do cystadenomas (28% versus 6%). Two variants are recognized—serous and mucinous. Most serous lesions are identified by imaging, and since they are benign they can be safely observed. Total excision of mucinous cystic lesions is the preferred method of treatment because of their higher propensity toward malignancy. Upon exploration, differentiation from a pseudocyst is usually made by the smooth, rounded appearance of a defined capsule present with a pseudocyst. Cystadenomas are more lobulated and septated and can have local inflammatory effects.

Failure to distinguish a pseudocyst from these true cystic lesions at the initial operation results in the persistence of symptoms and failure of resolution of the cyst. This emphasizes the need for a cyst wall biopsy at the initial procedure. Internal drainage is not adequate, even for cystadenomas, because of the viscosity of the cyst contents and its multiloculated nature. Percutaneous aspiration alone will fail and may delay the correct diagnosis. A Roux limb placed on a suspected pseudocyst will often initially need to be removed or, alternatively, the stomach will be involved with tumor and will require resection. A left subtotal pancreatectomy is the preferred treatment for symptomatic cysts in the tail or body of the pancreas. Some lesions in the head require a pancreaticoduodenectomy or even total pancreatectomy if they are large.[51,52]

Special Problems in Reoperation for Malignancy

REOPERATIVE PANCREATICODUODENECTOMY

Selected patients thought to have unresectable disease at an initial laparotomy may benefit from restaging and reexploration at pancreatic specialty centers. Single institution experiences have shown that reoperations for periampullary carcinoma have resectability, morbidity, mortality, and long-term survival rates similar to initial resections[53–58] (Table 8-1). In the absence of extrapancreatic disease, local resectability is most commonly due to extension of tumor in the retroperitoneum along the proximal 4 cm of the superior mesenteric artery, or portal vein encasement. Pancreatic phase CT scan is still the diagnostic test of choice to assess resectabilty upon referral after exploration at another institution. Tyler and Evans found that CT scan accurately predicted resectability in 14 (74%) of 19 patients.[57] Patients with previous enteric and biliary bypass can still undergo standard Whipple operation (Figure 8-6). Prolonged surgical exploration to assess local-regional resectability, while attempting to preserve the previous biliary or gastric anastomosis is inappropriate, and the previous anastomoses should be taken down to facilitate exploration based on favorable assessment on the preoperative CT scan (Figure 8-7). This maneuver is required to evaluate the superior porta hepatitis. The Johns Hopkins group found improved survival in the reoperative group at 1 and 5 years, but this was attributed due to a trend of less-advanced tumors in the reoperative group.[56] An aggressive approach to reexploration by a pancreatic specialist should be advocated, because surgery remains the only option for cure in patients with periampullary cancer.

Table 8-1 Reoperative Pancreaticoduodenectomy

Author	Surgically Treated (n)	Successfully Resected (n)	Early Morbidity (%)	Perioperative Mortality (%)
Moosa 1979[53]	17	11	NR	NR
Jones 1985[54]	NR	50	NR	NR
Hashimi 1989[55]	18	11	NR	9
McGuire 1991[41]	46	33	38	2
Tyler 1994[57]	23	14	21	0
Robinson 1996[58]	NR	29	28	0
Sohn 1999[56]	78	52	32	3.8

NR, not reported.

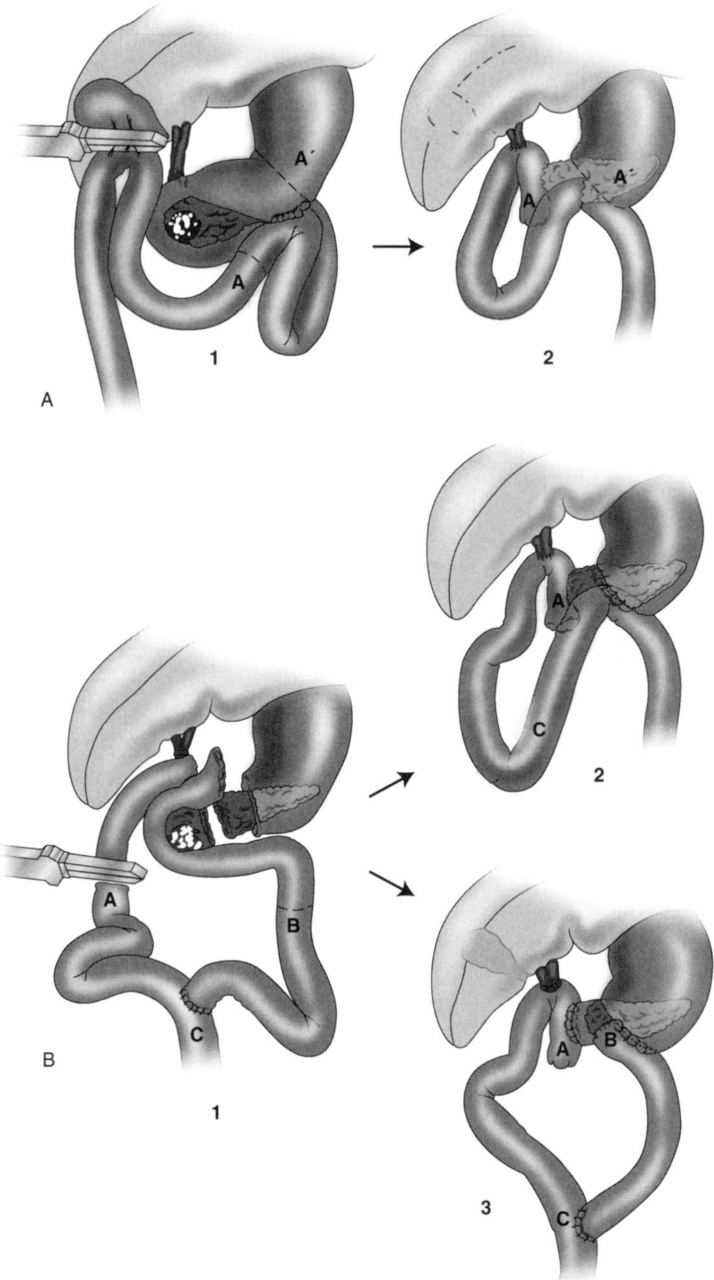

Figure 8-6 Options for reconstruction of the gastrointestinal tract in patients who undergo reoperative pancreaticoduodenectomy after palliative biliary and gastric bypass procedures. (A) Loop gastrojejunostomy and cholecystojejunostomy, (B) Roux-en-Y choledochojejunostomy.

(Modified from Tayler DS, Evans DB. Reoperative pancreaticoduodenectomy. Ann Surg 1994; 219:215.)

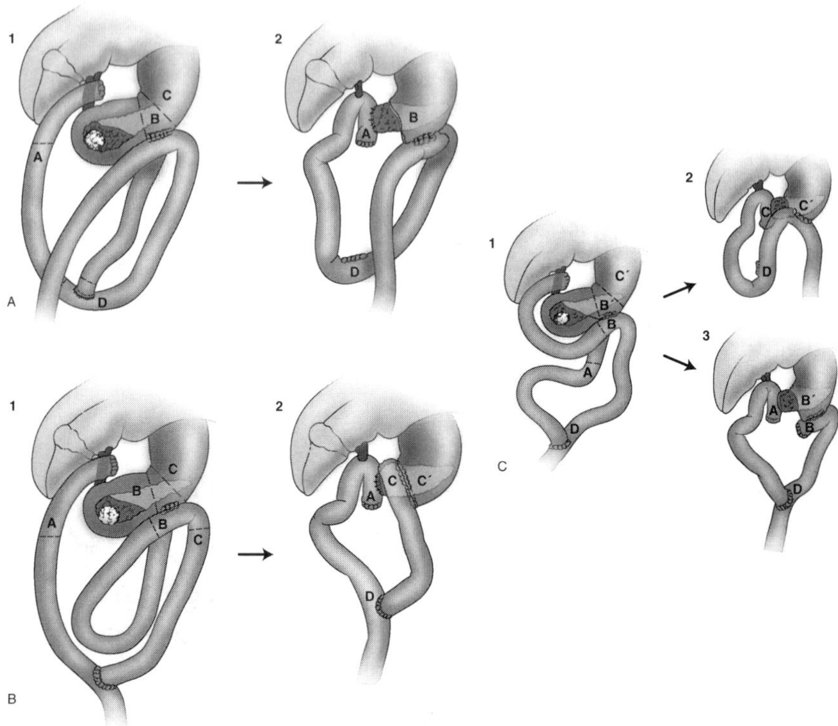

Figure 8-7 Options for reconstruction of the GI tract in patients who undergo reoperative pancreaticoduodenectomy after palliative biliary and gastric bypass procedures. (A) Roux-en-Y choledochojejunostomy with the gastrojejunostomy placed distal to the jejunostomy. During pancreaticoduodenectomy, the gastrojejunostomy was preserved in this illustration. (B) Roux-en-Y choledochojejunostomy with a loop gastrojejunostomy placed proximal to the jejunostomy. During pancreaticoduodenectomy, the gastrojejunostomy was resected in this illustration. (C) Roux-en-Y choledochojejunostomy and gastrojejunostomy. During pancreaticoduodenectomy, the gastrojejunostomy was preserved in C-3; if resected, the final reconstruction would be similar to B-2.

(Modified from Tayler DS, Evans DB. Reoperative pancreaticoduodenectomy. Ann Surg 1994;219:216.)

COMPLETION PANCREATECTOMY

Problems related to the pancreatic enteric anastomosis continue to be the most important cause of postoperative morbidity and mortality. Completion pancreatectomy is rarely necessary, but if surgical complications of the pancreaticoduodenectomy occur and persist, then early surgical intervention maximizes survival. Meticulous surgical technique in creation of the pancreaticoenterostomy is treatment when operating for malignant neoplasms of the pancreas, and especially the ampulla and duodenum. Chronic pancreatitis induces a fibrous reaction that results in a firm gland that holds sutures well, allowing for a pancreaticoenterostomy with greater integrity.

The neoplasm-bearing pancreas has a soft consistency and has been shown to have a higher rate of breakdown, leading to completion pancreatectomy.[59] In a review of the Mayo Clinic experience, Smith et al found that all patients who underwent Whipple resection for chronic pancreatitis avoided a completion pancreatectomy, while 6% who underwent pancreatoduodenectomy for cancer underwent total gland resection.[60] Ampullary tumors result in complete pancreatectomy in 6.0% to 8.3% of patients compared to 3.0% to 3.5% for ductal lesions in these two series. This is attributed to the infrequency of pancreatitis with ampullary tumors, whereas it is commonly associated with pancreatic ductal adenocarcinoma.[59,60] Pancreaticoduodenectomy with external drainage of the pancreatic duct may be an option in patients with small unobstructed ducts or a soft, friable pancreas.[61,62]

Because of the variety of available medications, interventional techniques, parental nutrition, and antibiotics, most complications of pancreaticoduodenectomy can be treated without operation. However, sometimes these approaches are inadequate, and completion pancreatectomy is usually undertaken as the only hope to save the life of a patient. The surgeon is faced with a pancreatic anastomotic dehiscence in a critically ill patient and no hope of repair or diversion. The decision to operate is often difficult, but should be made early, before systemic manifestations of the complication begin to appear. Technically the procedure can be demanding, but the main challenge lies in the patient's ability to tolerate the major postoperative challenges including fluid shifts, large blood loss, endocrine and exocrine insufficiency, and malnutrition.[59,60]

INTRADUCTAL PAPILLARY MUCINOUS TUMORS

Intraductal papillary mucinous tumors (IPMTs) are being recognized more frequently in patients with abdominal pain due to ductal obstruction from mucin or papillary growth in the pancreatic duct. Recurrent pancreatitis with hyperamylasemia is the most common presentation. The disease is most common in the pancreatic head, and usually represents an indolent, relapsing pattern of pancreatitis over 2 years.[63] The prognosis of IPMT is obviously better than that of ductal adenocarcinoma of the pancreas, as not all tumors show evidence of invasive malignancy. It has a slow growth rate and a late tendency toward metastasis. The exact biology of IMPT is unclear, but it does have malignant potential.[64,65]

Complete resection of diseased pancreas is the treatment of choice for IPMT. Since the prognosis is favorable, we prefer to preserve pancreatic function when possible at the initial resection and elect to perform a pylorus-preserving pancreatectomy for tumors in the head of the pancreas, segmental resection for tumors in the body, and distal pancreatectomy for tumors in the tail. The diffuse type of IPMT usually warrants a total pancreatectomy. Frozen section should be performed to ensure margins free of dysplasia and to rule out panductal extension. Patients should be followed with MRCP or ERCP and EUS.

Recurrent IPMT usually behaves aggressively. The disease-free interval is usually long and patients should be followed closely for at least 4 years.[66] CEA and CA 19-9 may have some benefit, but their exact roles are unclear. The site of recurrence is almost always the remnant pancreas. In these cases, the biology of IPMT is likely a multicentric or diffuse pattern. The treatment is therefore total pancreatectomy.[66]

Reoperative Surgery for Neuroendocrine Disease

INSULINOMA

Organic hyperinsulinism is a rare disease that accounts for about 90% of endocrine pancreatic tumors. The trouble stems from beta-cell hyperfunction causing the potentially life-threatening sequelae of insulin hypersecretion and neutroglycopenia. Solitary adenomas are the most frequent presentation and they are equally distributed throughout the pancreas. Other rare causes include multiple adenomas (often in association with MEN-1), malignant insulinoma, adenomatosis, and diffuse hyperplasia. The prognosis of hyperinsulism is good, and the chance of reversal of that state is high when treated at high-volume centers.[67] The four criteria to establish the diagnosis of insulinoma include a blood glucose of 40 to 50 mg/dL, a concomitant insulin level of 6 μU/mL, a C-peptide level of greater than 0.2 nmol, and an absence of sulfonylurea on plasma screening. Close to 90% of these small tumors can be localized through the use of preoperative studies like angiography and CT, in conjunction with intraoperative ultrasound and manual palpation.[68–71] Two large studies that have reviewed reoperative therapy for persistent hyperinsulism have shown the reoperative rate to be 13% to 16%.[67,68]

Patients with multiple tumors or diffuse hyperplasia are at high risk of developing recurrent disease. In addition to family history, thorough operative exploration with routine use of IOUS is mandatory. IOUS increases the intraoperative detection rate, but still may miss multiple tumors in up to one-third of patients.[69] Some series report that about half of these patients with multiple tumors will indeed have MEN-1.[70] Routine genetic testing is now available to identify unknown familial disease in such patients and may aid in ensuring adequate resection. Concomitant hypoglycemia and hyperinsulinemia, coupled with elevated C-peptide levels and negative plasma sulfonylurea screen, should rule out factitious hypoglycemia.

Insensitive preoperative imaging modalities in the 1960s and 1970s led to poor tumor localization. Extensive and blind resections were more commonplace and naturally led to many failures. Selective angiography has now become the gold standard for preoperative localization, but the combination of CT, transabdominal ultrasound, intraoperative ultrasound, or angiography will currently localize the tumors in close to 75% of patients. Surgical experience in mobilization and palpation of the pancreas also aids in localizing the tumor.[71] Portal venous sampling (PVS),[72] selective arterial injection of calcium,[73] and endoscopic ultrasound[74] have also been advocated for tumor localization. In patients requiring reexploration, we favor PVS or arterial injection of calcium. However, the major determinant of a successful resection is not preoperative localization, but rather intraoperative identification.

Reexploration for recurrent hyperinsulinism will usually lead to an extensive resection, or, less likely, a solitary adenoma is identified and an enucleation can be performed. Cure of one problem, unfortunately, can be replaced with a new morbid diagnosis. Diabetes is more common after reoperation, even with repeated enucleations. Better localization studies have now led to many more enucleations and rarely, if ever, blind resections. Distal resection from tail to superior mesenteric vein with sequential intraoperative glucose monitoring is acceptable if all diagnostic moves fail. The majority of MEN-1 patients have been found to have multiple tumors, and therefore, we favor subtotal distal pancreatectomy with enucleation of tumors from the head of the pancreas. Fistulas are a common complication following enucleation of larger lesions. Intraoperative secretin for diagnosis, fibrin glue, and octreotide[75] are modalities that have each been used to resolve this problem. The cure rate for insulinomas is high, even in the reoperative setting.

GASTRINOMA

Gastrinomas are rare endocrine tumors of the pancreas and duodenum, which are usually less than 2 cm in diameter, and that cause Zollinger-Ellison syndrome. The diagnosis is established by the gastrin radioimmunoassay. The secretin stimulation test confirms the presence of this neuroendocrine tumor if the clinical presentation is confusing.[76] Since gastrinomas are small, preoperative localization procedures often fail. Ultrasound, CT, magnetic resonance imaging (MRI), angiography, octreotide scan, and EUS are all modalities used to attempt localization of gastrinomas. A standardized surgical exploration of the pancreas with intraoperative ultrasound and duodenal exploration should result in detection and excision of gastrinomas in almost all cases.[77,78]

Patients referred after operative failure are either hypergastrinemic after a previous negative exploration or hypergastrinemic after a partial resection. Options include medical management, total gastrectomy, or a wide aggressive resection. Of patients with the diagnosis of gastrinoma, 50% will have no gross tumor found at the first exploration.[79–81] These patients have often had previous operations or complications of ulcer disease or morbid obesity, making the exploration difficult. In these patients, the diagnosis and operative strategy should be reinvestigated. All excised tissue should be histologically reexamined and the preoperative localization studies repeated with the addition of PVS, if not already performed. PVS has been shown to localize gastrinomas in 80% of cases.[82] Angiography is highly specific for disease not metastatic to the liver. CT may not be helpful if there is no liver involvement. Selected patients with MEN may benefit from surgical resection to debulk gross disease.

Upon exploration, the pancreas should be exposed thoroughly and a Kocher procedure performed to expose duodenum. The gastrinoma should be excised by enucleation if possible. In the reoperative setting, pancreaticoduodenectomy or distal pancreatectomy is not rewarding if performed blindly. The most likely patient to benefit will have ectopic gastrinoma missed at first exploration. Intraoperative modalities such as ultrasound, manual palpation, and thorough investigation of the gastrinoma triangle will aid in the search for the tumor. If all preoperative studies are negative, the tumor can still be found intraoperatively over 85% of the time in experienced hands.[83,84] The ideal treatment of gastrinoma would be complete excision of the primary tumor. Norton and colleagues advocate aggressive resections even in patients with likely recurrence in the future.[85]

REFERENCES

1. Cameron JL, Pitt HA, Yeo CJ, et al. One hundred and forty-five consecutive pancreaticoduodenectomies without mortality. Ann Surg 1993;217:430–438.
2. Pellegrini CA, Heck CF, Raper S, et al. An analysis of the reduced morbidity and mortality rates after pancreaticoduodenectomy. Arch Surg 1989;124: 778–781.
3. Fernandez-del Castillo C, Rattner DW, Warshaw AL. Standards for pancreatic resection in the 1990s. Arch Surg 1995;130:295–300.
4. Trede M, Schwall G. The complications of pancreatectomy. Ann Surg 1998;207:39–47.
5. Cunningham JD, Weyant MT, Levitt M, et al. Complications requiring reoperation following pancreatectomy. Int J Pancreatol 1998;24:23–29.
6. Cullen JJ, Sarr MG, Ilstrup DM. Pancreatic anastomotic leak after pancreaticoduodenectomy: incidence, significance, and management. Am J Surg 1994;168:295–298.
7. Yeo CJ. Management of complications following pancreaticoduodenectomy. Surg Clin North Am 1995;75:913–924.
8. Prinz RA, Pickelman JR, Hoffman JP. Treatment of pancreatic cutaneous fistulas with a somatostatin analog. Am J Surg 1988;155:36–42.
9. Yeo CJ, Cameron JL, Lillemoe KD, et al. Does prophylactic octreotide decrease the rates of pancreatic fistula and other complications after pancreaticoduodenectomy? Ann Surg 2000;232:419–429.
10. vanSonnenberg E, Wittich GR, Chon KS, et al. Percutaneous radiologic drainage of pancreatic abscesses. Am J Roentgenol 1997;168:979–984.
11. Ashley SW, Perez A, Pierce EA, et al. Necrotizing pancreatitis: contemporary analysis of 99 consecutive cases. Ann Surg 2001;234:572–580.
12. Men S, Akhan O, Koroglu M. Percutaneous drainage of abdominal abscess. Euro J Rad 2002;43:204–218.
13. Mithofer K, Mueller K, Warshaw AL. Interventional and surgical treatment of pancreatic abscess. World J Surg 1997;21:162–168.
14. Grosso M, Gandini G, Cassinis MC, et al. Percutaneous treatment (including pseudocystogastrostomy) of 74 pancreatic pseudocysts. Radiology 1989;173: 493–497.
15. Neff R. Pancreatic pseudocysts and fluid collections: percutaneous approaches. Surg Clin North Am 2001;81:399–403.
16. Beger HG. Operative management of necrotizing pancreatitis-necrosectomy and continuous closed post operative lavage of the lesser sac. Hepatogastroenterology 1991;38:129–133.

17. Bradley EL III. Management of infected pancreatic necrosis by open drainage. Ann Surg 1987;206:542–550.

18. Bradley EL III. A fifteen year experience with open drainage for infected pancreatic necrosis. Surg Gynecol Obstet 1993;177:215–222.

19. Munshi IA, Haworth R, Barie PS. Resolution of refractory pancreatic ascites after continuous infusion of octreotide acetate. Int J Pancreatol 1995;17: 203–206.

20. Ohge H, Yokoyama T, Kodama T, et al. Surgical approaches for pancreatic ascites: Report of three cases. Surg Today 1999;29:458–461.

21. Da Cunha TE, Machado M, Bacchella T, et al. Surgical treatment of pancreatic ascites and pancreatic pleural effusions. Hepatogastroenterology 1995;42: 748–751.

22. Neoptolemus JP, Winslett MC. Pancreatic ascites. In: Chronic Pancreatitis. Berlin: Springer, 1990:262–279.

23. Warshaw AL, Banks PA, Fernandez-del Castillo C. AGA technical review: treatment of pain in chronic pancreatitis. Gastroenterology 1998;115:765–776.

24. Steer ML, Waxman I, Freedman S. Chronic pancreatitis. N Engl J Med 1995;332:1482–1490.

25. Aranha GV, Prinz RA, Greenlee HB. Reoperative General Surgery. St. Louis: Mosby Publishers, 1997:597–620.

26. Warshaw AL, Popp JW, RH Schapiro Jr, et al. Long-term patency, pancreatic function and pain relief after lateral pancreaticojejunostomy for chronic pancreatitis. Gastroenterology 1980;79:289–293.

27. Prinz RA, Greenlee HB. Pancreatic duct drainage in 100 patients with chronic pancreatitis. Ann Surg 1981;194:313–320.

28. Bradley EL III. Long-term results of pancreaticojejunostomy in patients with chronic pancreatitis. Am J Surg 1987;153:207–213.

29. Eckhauser FE, Strodel WE, Krol JA, et al. Near total pancreatectomy for chronic pancreatitis. Surgery 1984;96:599–607.

30. Traverso LW, Kozarek RA. The Whipple procedure for severe complications of chronic pancreatitis. Arch Surg 1993;128:1047–1053.

31. Rattner DW, Fernandez-del Castillo C, Warshaw AL. Pitfalls of distal pancreatectomy for relief of pain in chronic pancreatitis. Am J Surg 1996;171:142–146.

32. Keith RG, Sabil FG, Sheppard RH. Treatment of chronic alcoholic pancreatitis by pancreatic resection. Am J Surg 1989;157:156–160.

33. Hakain AG, Brougham TA, Vogt DP, et al. Long term results of the surgical management of chronic pancreatitis. Am Surg 1994;60:306–308.

34. Izbicki JR, Bloechle C, Knoefel WT, et al. Surgical treatment of chronic pancreatitis and quality of life after operation. Surg Clin North Am 1999;79:913–944.

35. Sohn TA, Campbell KA, Pitt HA, et al. Quality of life and long-term survival after surgery for chronic pancreatitis. J Gastrointest Surg 2000;4: 355–365.

36. Lucas CE, McIntosh B, Paley D, et al. Surgical decompression of ductal obstruction in patients with chronic pancreatitis. Surgery 1999;126: 790–795.

37. Greenlee HB, Prinz RA, Aranha GV. Long-term results of side-to-side pancreaticojejunostomy. World J Surg 1990;14:70–76.

38. Adams DB, Ford MC, Anderson MC. Outcome after lateral pancreaticojejunostomy for chronic pancreatitis. Ann Surg 1994;219:481–487.

39. Nealon WH, Thompson JC. Progressive loss of pancreatic function in chronic pancreatitis is delayed by main pancreatic duct decompression. A longitudinal prospective analysis of the modified Puestow procedure. Ann Surg 1993;217: 458–466.

40. Nealon WH, Townsend CM Jr, Thompson JC. Operative drainage of the pancreatic duct delays functional impairment in patients with chronic pancreatitis. A prospective analysis. Ann Surg 1988;208:321–329.

41. McGuire GE, Pitt HA, Lillemoe KD, et al. Reoperative surgery for periampullary adenocarcinoma. Arch Surg 1991;126:1205–1212.

42. Prinz RA, Aranha GV, Greenlee HB. Redrainage of the pancreatic duct in chronic pancreatitis. Am J Surg 1986;151:150–156.

43. Markowitz TS, Rattner DW, Warshaw AL. Failure of symptomatic relief after pancreaticojejunal decompression for chronic pancreatitis: Strategies for salvage. Arch Surg 1994;129:374–379.

44. Cohen JR, Kuchta N, Geller N, et al. Pancreaticoduodenectomy for benign disease. Ann Surg 1983;197:68–71.

45. Beger HG, Krautzberger W, Bittner R, et al. Duodenum-preserving resection of the head of the pancreas in patients with severe chronic pancreatitis. Surgery 1985;98:467–474.

46. Frey CF, Schmith GJ. Description and rationale of a new operation for chronic pancreatitis. Pancreas 1987;2:701–707.

47. Warshaw AL, Rattner DW, Fernandez-del Castillo C, et al. Middle segment pancreatectomy: a novel technique for conserving pancreatic tissue. Arch Surg 1998;133:327–331.

48. Munn JS, Aranha GV, Greenlee HB, et al. Simultaneous treatment of chronic pancreatitis and pancreatic pseudocyst. Arch Surg 1987;122:662–667.

49. Prinz RA, Aranha GV, et al. Combined pancreatic duct and upper gastrointestinal tract and biliary tract drainage in chronic pancreatitis. Arch Surg 1985;120:361–366.

50. Nealon WH, Walser E. Duct drainage alone is sufficient in the operative management of pancreatic pseudocyst in patients with chronic pancreatitis. Ann Surg 2003;237:614–622.

51. Von Segresser L, Rohner A. Pancreatic cystadenoma and cystadenocarcinoma. Br J Surg 1984;71:449–451.

52. Corbally MT, McAnena OJ, Urmacher C, et al. Pancreatic cyst adenoma—a clinicopathologic study. Arch Surg 1989;124:1271–1274.

53. Moosa AR. Reoperation for pancreatic cancer. Arch Surg 1979;114:502–504.
54. Jones BA, Langer B, Taylor BR, et al. Periampullary tumors: which ones should be resected? Am J Surg 1985;149:46–52.
55. Hashimi H, Sabanatham S. Second look operation in managing carcinoma of the pancreas and periampullary region. Surg Gynecol Obstet 1989;168: 224–226.
56. Sohn TA, Lillemoe KD, Cameron JL, et al. Reexploration for periampullary carcinoma: resectability, perioperative results, pathology, and long-term outcome. Ann Surg 1999;229:393–400.
57. Tyler DS, Evan DB. Reoperative pancreaticoduodenectomy. Ann Surg 1994;219: 211–221.
58. Robinson EK, Lee JE, Lowy AM, et al. Reoperative pancreaticoduodenectomy for periampullary carcinoma. Am J Surg 1996;172:432–438.
59. Farley DR, Schwall G, Trede M. Completion pancreatectomy for surgical complications of pancreaticoduodenectomy. Br J Surg 1996;83:176–179.
60. Smith CD, Sarr MG, vanHeerden JA. Completion pancreatectomy following pancreaticoduodenectomy: clincal experience. World J Surg 1992;16:521–524.
61. Katsaragakis S, Antonakis P, Konstadoulakis MM, et al. Reconstruction of the pancreatic duct after pancreaticoduodenectomy: a modification of the Whipple procedure. J Surg Onc 2001;77:26–29.
62. Marcus SG, Cohen H, Ranson JHC. Optimal management of the pancreatic remnant after pancreaticoduodenectomy. Ann Surg 1995;221:635–648.
63. Traverso LW, Peralta EA, Ryan JA, et al. Intraductal neoplasms of the pancreas. Am J Surg 1998;175:426–431.
64. Milchgrub S, Campuzano M, Casillas J, et al. Intraductal carcinoma of the pancreas. Cancer 1992; 69:651.
65. Sugiyama M, Izumisato Y, Abe N, et al. Predictive factors for malignancy in intraductal papillary-mucinous tumours of the pancreas. Br J Surg 2003;90: 1244–1249.
66. Sho M, Nakajima Y, Kanehiro H, et al. Pattern of recurrence after resection for intraductal papillary mucinous tumors of the pancreas. World J Surg 1998;22: 874–878.
67. Thompson GB, Service J, van Heerden JA, et al. Reoperative insulinomas, 1927 to 1992: an institutional experience. Surgery 1993;114:1196–1206.
68. Simon D, Starke A, Goretzki PE, et al. Reoperative surgery for organic hyperinsulinism: indications and operative strategy. World J Surg 1998;22: 666–672.
69. Grant CS, van Heeerden JA, Charboneau JW, et al. Insulinoma: the value of intraoperative ultrasonography. Arch Surg 1988;123:843–848.
70. Van Heerden JA, Edis AJ, Service FJ. The surgical aspects of insulinomas. Ann Surg 1979;189:677–682.
71. Norton JA, Shawker TH, Doppman JL, et al. Localization and surgical treatment of occult insulinomas. Ann Surg 1990;212:615–620.

72. Vinik AL, Delbridge L, Moattari R, et al. Transhepatic portal vein catheterization for localization of insulinomas: a ten-year experience. Surgery 1991;109:1–11.

73. Doppman JL, Miller DL, Chang R, et al. Insulinomas: localization with selective intra-arterial injection of calcium. Radiology 1991;178:237–241.

74. Rosch T, Lightdale CJ, Botet JF, et al. Localization of pancreatic endocrine tumors by endoscopic ultrasonography. N Engl J Med 1992;326:1721–1726.

75. Buchler M, Friess H, Klempa I, et al. Role of octreotide in the prevention of postoperative complications following pancreatic resection. Am J Surg 1992; 163:125–130.

76. McGuigan JE, Wolfe MM. Secretin injection test in the diagnosis of gastrinoma. Gastroenterology 1980;79:1324–1331.

77. Kisker O, Bastian D, Bartsch D, et al. Localization, malignant potential, and surgical management of gastrinomas. World J Surg 1998;22:651–658.

78. Merrell RC, Mitchell BK. Reoperative General Surgery. St. Louis: Mosby Publishers, 1997;792–798.

79. Norton JA, Collen MJ, Gardner JD, et al. Prospective study of gastrinoma localization and resection in patients with Zollinger-Ellison syndrome. Ann Surg 1986;204:468–479.

80. Thompson JC, Lewis BG, Wiener I, et al. The role of surgery in the Zollinger-Ellison syndrome. Ann Surg 1983;197:594–607.

81. Deveney CW, Deveney KE, Stark D, et al. Resection of gastrinomas. Ann Surg 1983;198:546–553.

82. Roche A, Raisonnier A, Gillon-Savouret MC. Pancreatic venous sampling and arteriography in localizing insulinomas and gastrinomas: Procedure and results in 55 cases. Radiology 1982;145:621–627.

83. McArthur KE, Richardson CT, Barnett CC. Laparotomy and proximal gastrin vagotomy in Zollinger-Ellison syndrome: results of a sixteen-year prospective study. Am J Gastroenterol 1996;91:1104–1111.

84. Ellison EC. Forty-year appraisal of gastrinoma. Ann Surg 1995;22:511–521.

85. Norton JA, Kivlen M, Li M, et al. Morbidity and mortality of aggressive resection in patients with advanced neuroendocrine tumors. Arch Surg 2003;138:859–866.

CHAPTER 9

Reoperative Endocrine Surgery

Rebecca S. Sippel, MD; Herbert Chen, MD

Précis

Reoperative thyroid and parathyroid operations are technically demanding. Several preoperative and intraoperative adjuncts are available to assist the surgeon in the management of these patients. When done by an experienced surgeon, these operations are associated with minimal morbidity and mortality.

Reoperative Thyroid Surgery

Thyroid surgery is the twentieth most common operation performed by general surgeons.[1] The majority of primary operations are done to identify and treat thyroid malignancies. Thyroid reoperations account for only about 5% of all thyroid operations each year.[2] These reoperations can be technically demanding and are associated with a significant risk of complications.

INDICATIONS FOR REOPERATION

Emergent Reexploration—Thyroid reoperation may be indicated in the immediate postoperative period. Bleeding that leads to airway obstruction is the most common indication for emergent reexploration. Although major bleeding that causes airway compromise is a rare complication, the outcome of this complication can be deadly. In a series of 918 patients, Abbas and colleagues found an incidence of major bleeding requiring exploration of 0.7%.[3] The time interval between surgery and the reoperation is usually less than 48 hours, although bleeding has been reported as far out as 5 days postoperatively.[4] If impending airway obstruction is present, the wound should be opened at the bedside and the patient should be taken emergently to the operating room. The majority of hematomas that become symptomatic are deep to the strap muscles. The source of bleeding is identified in most cases, with a mixture of causes including superior thyroid artery, inferior thyroid artery, venous, thyroid, and soft tissues.[4]

Reoperation for Malignancy—Thyroid reoperations for malignancy can occur either in the first few weeks after the primary resection or occur several years after the initial exploration. The current limitations of fine needle aspiration and frozen section in the evaluation of some thyroid nodules (especially follicular thyroid lesions) often leads to the need for an initial diagnostic thyroid lobectomy.[5–7] The management of well-differentiated thyroid cancer is debated, but many surgeons believe that a total thyroidectomy is the treatment of choice for malignant disease. Thus, patients who have a thyroid malignancy on permanent histology after a diagnostic lobectomy usually require a completion thyroidectomy. Removal of all of the thyroid tissue allows the use of I-131 to detect and treat metastatic disease. Furthermore, thyroglobulin can be used as a marker of disease recurrence after I-131 ablation. Interestingly, despite the fact that a full lobectomy was performed at the initial procedure, a significant number of patients are found to have cancer within their remnant lobe. In a review of 116 thyroid reoperations, Levin and associates found a 64% incidence of malignancy in the remaining lobe.[8]

The complication rate in reoperation for malignancy is approximately 8%.[8] Injuries tend to occur when scar tissue is present due to a previous dissection. The highest complication rates are seen in patients who are being treated with a delayed recurrence of tumor after a bilateral resection, or when only a subtotal thyroidectomy was performed and the remaining tissue needs to be resected for cure.

The timing of a reoperation for malignancy is debated. Most advocate returning to the operating room as soon as the diagnosis is made and preferably within 10 days of the primary resection. If this is not possible, some advocate waiting several months before attempting surgery, because the friability of tissues making exploration too dangerous at that time.[2] The timing of completion thyroidectomy has been examined by several groups. They found no significant difference in the complication rate, regardless of the timing of the second thyroid operation.[9,10] If only one side of the neck was dissected during the primary surgery, as with a standard lobectomy, then the risk of resecting the other side should be no greater than that seen at the initial exploration, potentially making exploration safe at any time frame.

Reoperation for Benign Disease (Thyroid Goiters)—Up to one-half of thyroid reoperations are for benign disease.[11] Patients with thyroid nodules and benign goiters are often managed with either a thyroid lobectomy or a subtotal thyroidectomy for diagnostic or symptomatic reasons. Unfortunately, up to 26% of patients will have a recurrence after goiter surgery.[12] Other treatment options, such as radioactive iodine, can be considered before proceeding with reoperation.[13] The most common indication for reoperating on a patient with a benign thyroid disease is compressive symptoms. The risks of reoperation for benign disease are just as high as reoperation for malignancy and approach 22%.[11] In a review of reoperations for substernal goiters, Hsu found a 15% incidence of postoperative complications, with temporary hypocalcemia and vocal cord dysfunction being the most common.[13] Interestingly, in reviewing the pathologic specimens, they found that 8% of recurrent substernal goiters contained a malignancy, which is two to three times higher than the incidence seen with primary thyroid resections.[13]

PREOPERATIVE ASSESSMENT

Reoperative thyroid surgery can be performed in the immediate postoperative period to correct surgical complications such as bleeding, within a few weeks of surgery to complete the management of a thyroid malignancy, or several years later to address a recurrent disease or a second disease process within the neck. Although the preparation for each of these scenarios is somewhat different, some basic principles remain the same regardless of the indication or timing of the procedure.

The first step is to perform a careful review of earlier procedures. The operative notes should be reviewed to identify whether or not the parathyroids or the recurrent laryngeal nerves were identified and preserved. Unfortunately, the previous reports are often difficult to obtain and frequently do not include the pertinent information. Probably more indicative of parathyroid function after the initial surgery are the calcium and parathyroid hormone (PTH) levels from the postoperative period. Low levels may indicate that the parathyroid glands have been devascularized during the first operation, placing them at high risk during a subsequent exploration.

Preoperative laboratory studies may vary based on the indication for the thyroid reexploration. In most cases, thyroid function tests, a thyroid-stimulating hormone (TSH) level, and a serum calcium should be obtained. Serum thyroglobulin may be very helpful for patients with recurrent well-differentiated thyroid cancer, as the thyroglobulin levels tend to correlate with the extent of disease. This lab value is most helpful when the TSH level is elevated (over 60 μIU/mL) after thyroid hormone withdrawal. In patients with recurrent medullary thyroid cancer, the measurement of serum calcitonin and carcinoembryonic antigen are useful markers to follow disease recurrence.

Preoperative evaluation of recurrent laryngeal nerve function is essential. Evaluation of nerve function can be performed in the clinic preoperatively using either direct or indirect laryngoscopy. With a unilateral recurrent laryngeal nerve injury, patients typically present with hoarseness. Some patients are able to compensate for a unilateral nerve injury and remain asymptomatic. A bilateral recurrent nerve injury leads to the disastrous complication of vocal cord paralysis and the potential need for a tracheostomy. The incidence of preexisting recurrent laryngeal nerve injury in patients undergoing reoperation has been shown to be between 2.4% and 4.9%.[2] This information is important in preoperative and intraoperative management. If a patient has a unilateral recurrent laryngeal nerve injury, one could employ additional adjuncts to maintain the integrity of the remaining contralateral recurrent nerve.

LOCALIZATION STUDIES

Imaging studies can play an important role in defining anatomy prior to reoperation. A radionuclide thyroid scan can define the extent of remaining thyroid tissue within the neck and may also localize recurrent disease outside of the thyroid bed. Neck ultrasound (U/S) is also an informative preoperative imaging study. Ultrasound is most effective in identifying disease recurrence in and around the thyroid. If recurrent disease is fixed within the neck or there is concern of tracheal involvement then a computed tomography (CT) or magnetic resonance imaging (MRI) can define the extent of the tumor and determine if invasion of surrounding structures is present. In these cases, endoscopic evaluation of the trachea can determine if the tumor is invading through the larynx or trachea. Intraoperative adjuncts such as ultrasonography can also aid in tumor localization. Although this technique is operator dependent, U/S has been shown to be more sensitive than palpation for identifying tumor nodules.[14]

OPERATIVE APPROACH

The anatomy of the neck and the planes of dissection are often obscured in reoperative thyroid surgery. The landmarks disappear, putting the parathyroids and the recurrent laryngeal nerve at much higher risk for injury. Because of the distortion of tissue planes, most surgeons advocate approaching the thyroid from normal, undisturbed tissue planes. One approach involves extending the previous incision to allow the operation to start laterally and move medially. The dissection is often initiated anterior to the sternocleidomastoid muscle and lateral to the sternohyoid muscles. The sternothyroid and sternohyoid muscles are often densely adherent to the underlying thyroid bed, especially in the case of malignancy. These muscles remain attached to and are dissected with the thyroid gland. If the posterior capsule of the thyroid was not dissected during the previous exploration, then the technique of "capsular dissection" may be utilized to protect the parathyroids and the nerves. After the middle thyroid vein is divided, dissection of the inferior thyroid lobe proceeds; care must be taken to stay right on the thyroid capsule to preserve the nerve and the blood supply to the parathyroids. This technique of capsular dissection for recurrent thyroid surgery has been shown in large series to have a major complication rate of less than 3%.[2]

In patients who already had a posterior dissection, it is often safest to start inferior to the scar tissue and to dissect out the recurrent laryngeal nerve as it emerges from the superior mediastinum.[15] Resecting a fibrosed thyroid upper pole before identifying the ipsilateral recurrent nerve is extremely dangerous. The recurrent laryngeal nerve is at greatest risk for injury as it courses through the ligament of Berry at the cricothyroid articulation. Often the thyroid will be densely adherent to the nerve at this location. If thyroid cancer is invading the recurrent nerve, then the nerve may need to be sacrificed. However, this potential scenario should be discussed with the patient before surgery. In the case of benign disease, it is frequently appropriate to leave a small remnant of adherent thyroid tissue on the recurrent nerve to preserve vocal cord function. Electrical stimulation intraoperatively has been used to aid in the identification and preservation of the recurrent laryngeal nerve. Without the aid of electrical stimulation, the recurrent laryngeal nerve can be identified in about 75% of cases.[12,16]

In most cases, identification of all parathyroid tissue during thyroid reoperation is not possible. If parathyroid tissue is identified, great care should be taken to preserve the blood supply. If the parathyroid glands are unintentionally removed or there is a question of devascularization, then parathyroid autotransplantation should be considered. Prior to reimplantation, a frozen section biopsy should be performed, especially in reoperation for thyroid cancer, to ensure that the transplanted tissue is parathyroid as opposed to a lymph node containing malignant cells. We generally autotransplant parathyroid tissue in 1 mm by 3 mm pieces to the ipsilateral sternocleidomastoid muscle. It is important to mark the location of the autotransplanted tissue with nonabsorbable suture and/or surgical clips, should these parathyroid fragments become hyperplastic.

COMPLICATIONS

Reoperative thyroid surgery can be challenging in several situations. First of all, after a subtotal resection, there is extensive scar tissue. Often the only remaining thyroid tissue is located directly over the recurrent laryngeal nerve and the parathyroid glands. The second issue that can make the reoperation more difficult is the presence of invasive recurrent tumor and involved lymph nodes. Finally if several parathyroid glands have already been removed or if there is a known recurrent laryngeal nerve injury, the chance of long-term complications is high.

The more common complications after thyroid surgery are bleeding, hypoparathyroidism, and recurrent nerve injury. In the reoperative setting, there is a high incidence of all of these complications. The risk of a bleeding complication is higher during reoperative surgery. The incidence of hematomas requiring evacuation is over three times higher in the reoperative setting (2.5% versus 0.7%).[17] Notably, the use of drains has not been shown in any study to prevent the formation of cervical hematomas or to facilitate their early diagnosis.[4] Bleeding leading to postoperative reexploration also increases the risk of other complications. A study by Burkey and associates found a significant increase in the overall complication rate in patients undergoing reoperation for bleeding when compared to those undergoing initial exploration.[4] Of 42 patients in the reexploration for bleeding group, 17% suffered from one or more complications postoperatively.

Prior surgery not only distorts the tissue planes but can also compromise the blood supply to the parathyroids or the recurrent laryngeal nerve. Extensive dissection around these structures can lead to temporary or permanent nonfunctioning, even though the structure itself remains intact. The risk of permanent hypoparathyroidism has been shown to be increased by up to five-fold in patients after thyroid reoperations in comparison to those undergoing initial surgery.[2] If parathyroid tissue is identified at the time of reoperation, it should be treated as if it is the only remaining functioning tissue. Extreme care should be taken to preserve the blood supply in situ. However, if the blood supply to the parathyroid tissue is questionable, the tissue needs to be reimplanted either into the sternocleidomastoid or into the nondominant forearm (brachioradialis muscle). The location of reimplantation is based on the extent of dissection within the neck and the likelihood of requiring further neck exploration in the future. If there is any chance of the patient requiring future neck dissection, the safest alternative is to make a separate incision away from the neck for reimplantation.

Recurrent laryngeal nerve injury manifests as hoarseness or loss of voice quality postoperatively. This can be documented by indirect laryngoscopy. The injury may be temporary (lasting less than 6 months) or permanent. The risk of recurrent laryngeal nerve injury varies by the institution and the experience of the surgeon. Several studies have shown that the risk of injury in the reoperative setting is at least double that seen in primary exploration, with injury rates as high as 14%.[17] Careful dissection and knowledge of the anatomy are key to minimizing the risk of nerve injury. Multiple devices exist that can aid in the identification of the nerves of the neck. Electromyographic monitoring of the recurrent laryngeal nerve can be performed via several different routes. Monitoring electrodes can be on the surface or integrated into the endotracheal tube.[18] The recurrent laryngeal nerve can be successfully identified in the majority of patients by these techniques. However, no studies have demonstrated a reduction in recurrent nerve injury utilizing these technologies.[19] Because of the need for special equipment and monitoring devices, some have opted for other means of monitoring recurrent laryngeal nerve function. The use of laryngeal masked anesthesia (LMA) with visualization of the cords using a fiberoptic scope has been advocated by some as a less expensive alternative, as it uses equipment already available within the operating room. The success of this technique is slightly less due to the inability to use LMA in all patients.[20,21]

In experienced hands the complication rate of reoperative surgery can be minimized. However, the risks of reoperative thyroid surgery are still greater than with a primary exploration, which emphasizes the importance of performing the appropriate procedure at the initial operation.

Reoperative Parathyroid Surgery

Operations for primary hyperparathyroidism have been shown to be successful in 95% to 98% of cases, when performed by an experienced surgeon.[22] The success rate of primary explorations is not matched in the reoperative setting, which has a success rate of only 85% to 95%.[23,24] Reoperation is challenging not only due to the scarring that obliterates landmarks, but also the increase likelihood that these patients have aberrant anatomy, which led to a failed initial exploration. There are several reasons that a primary exploration may fail, including multiple hyperplastic parathyroid glands, ectopically located glands, supernumerary glands, incomplete resection of hyperplastic glands, surgeon inexperience, and inadequate exploration of the neck and upper mediastinum.[25] The most common cause of failure during primary exploration is still a missed adenoma, which occurs in over 50% of cases.[26] The most common location for the missed adenoma is a missed inferior adenoma contained within the thymus.[27] The second most common reason for failure is a missed diagnosis of hyperplasia, which occurs in approximately one-third of patients. It is important to remember that supernumerary parathyroids occur in approximately 13% of the population.

PREOPERATIVE ASSESSMENT

The first step is to confirm the diagnosis of recurrent or persistent hyperparathyroidism. A careful history needs to be taken, focusing especially on a family history

Box 9-1 NIH 2002 Guidelines for Operative Treatment of Asymptomatic Primary Hyperparathyroidism[9]*

1. Serum calcium over 1.0 mg/dL above the upper limit of normal
2. 24-h urinary calcium more than 400 mg
3. Creatinine clearance reduced by 30%
4. Bone mineral density t-score less than –2.5 at any site
5. Age under 50

*Patients with clear symptoms of primary hyperparathyroidism should undergo surgery. These guidelines are for asymptomatic patients.

of endocrine disorders as well as their disease-related symptoms. Serum calcium and PTH levels should be verified. A urinary calcium should also be obtained in all patients, as up to 10% of patients with a failed primary exploration have been found to have familial hypercalcemic hypocalciuria, a disease that is not cured by parathyroidectomy.[28] It is also important to reassess the indications for operative intervention, especially in the asymptomatic and the elderly. There has been a re-evaluation of the NIH recommendations for surgical treatment of patients with primary hyperparathyroidism (Box 9-1).[29] The risks of reoperative parathyroid surgery are significantly greater than those of primary exploration, including recurrent laryngeal nerve injury, permanent hypoparathyroidism, and persistent hyperparathyroidism. The benefits of surgery must outweigh the risks for any given patient. Hasse and colleagues evaluated the quality of life of patients after reoperative parathyroid surgery and found that 20% of patients were so unhappy with the results of their surgery that they wished that they had not consented to the surgery.[30]

Review of the operative records and available histopathology can provide information about which parathyroid glands were identified, the extent of the dissection, and the presence of aberrant anatomy. Despite the fact that many reports lack sufficient detail, Rotstein and colleagues found that careful review of operative notes and pathology allowed them to predict the correct side of the pathology in 75% of cases.[23]

LOCALIZATION STUDIES

Preoperative localization is essential in reoperative parathyroid surgery. Noninvasive studies of both the neck and mediastinum can be very beneficial. The most informative study is a Tc-99m sestamibi scan, which can localize the lesion in over half of patients.[31] However, sestamibi can be negative and has a false positive rate of 17%.[24] Thallium subtraction is another nuclear medicine study, which can be used to localize parathyroids (Figure 9-1). While many have abandoned the use of this test in favor of Tc-99m sestamibi scans, we have found that it can be beneficial in half of patients who do not localize on a Tc-99m sestamibi scan.[32] The next most commonly obtained test is a U/S. The usefulness of ultrasound varies greatly because

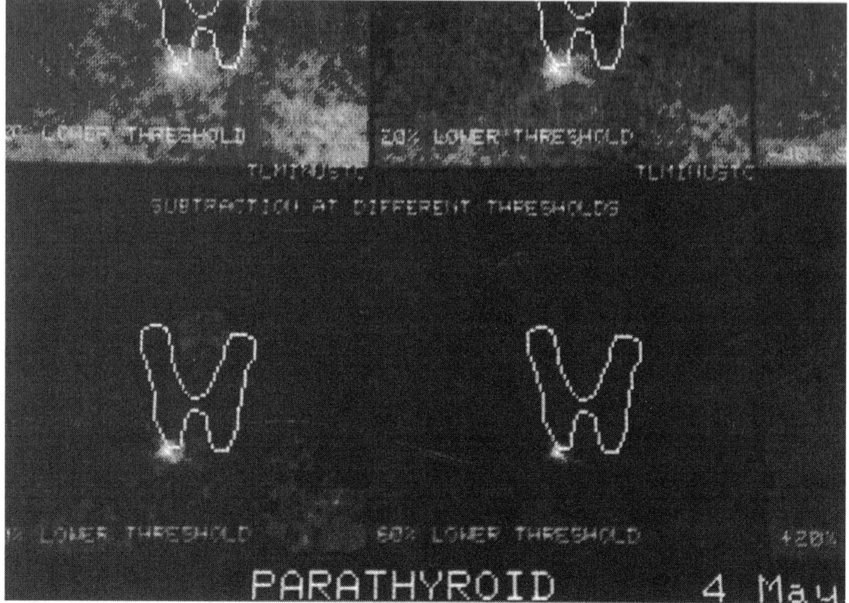

Figure 9-1 A thallium-201/Tc-99m sestamibi subtraction scan showing a right lower parathyroid adenoma.

it is very operator-dependent. However, most studies show that U/S, like sestamibi, is beneficial in over half of patients. The combination of U/S and sestamibi scan has been shown to successfully identify 94% of adenomas.[33] MRI scans can also be used for localization. MRI appears to be the most beneficial when glands are located in ectopic locations, especially the mediastinum. CT scans have been shown to localize lesions in only about a third of patients and appear to be most beneficial when glands are located in the tracheoesophageal groove.[26] Given the incidence of false positives with each of these tests, most authors would advocate having at least two positive studies before proceeding with repeat exploration. A combination of U/S, sestamibi, and MRI has been shown to have a diagnostic precision of nearly 90%.[34]

When noninvasive studies are not in agreement, invasive studies may provide additional localizing information. If questionable lesions are located in the neck, then fine-needle aspiration can be used to confirm the presence or absence of parathyroid tissue within the lesion. Selective venous sampling (SVS) can also be of great benefit. While it does not define the anatomy, SVS can help to guide the surgeon to the region of the abnormality. Jones and colleagues evaluated the utility of SVS when noninvasive studies were conflicting and they found it was useful in 75% of cases.[24]

The costs of preoperative localization can be high, but when successfully utilized, it decreases the operative time by 50%. When all the operative and preoperative costs are combined, it is actually 28% less expensive to perform the needed preoperative localization studies than it is to take a patient directly to the operating room.[35]

OPERATIVE APPROACH

In patients undergoing an initial parathyroid exploration in the absence of a localization scan, an experienced endocrine surgeon can successfully locate and resect the parathyroid abnormality more than 95% of the time with a bilateral neck exploration.[22] In sharp contrast, a parathyroid reexploration should generally not be performed without a positive localization study. The operative strategy must be tailored to the side and location of the predicted lesion. If the preoperative localization study reveals an abnormal parathyroid in the superior position, an incision along the anterior border of the sternocleidomastoid allows a posterior approach to the gland (lateral to the strap muscles). These glands can be located retroesophageally, in the posterior mediastinum, or in the carotid sheath. Occasionally an undescended parathyroid gland can be just inferior or in the submandibular gland.[36] If the preoperative localization study reveals an abnormal parathyroid gland in the lower position, a medial approach through the old incision is often preferred. In these cases, the parathyroid can be in the thymus or intrathyroid.[27] If an intrathyroidal parathyroid adenoma is identified, a thyroid lobectomy should be performed.

Preoperative localization studies may be suggestive of a mediastinal location. Any suspicion of a mediastinal adenoma by sestamibi should be confirmed with either CT or MRI. With clear localization in the mediastinum (Figure 9-2), a repeat neck exploration can be eliminated and the patient can be taken directly to the operating room for resection of the mediastinal lesion. The technique of radioguided parathyroidectomy via video-assisted thoracoscopic surgery (VATS) combined with intraoperative PTH testing is an effective approach for patients with primary hyperparathyroidism and mediastinal parathyroid lesions.[37]

There are special considerations for patients undergoing a reexploration for either secondary or tertiary hyperparathyroidism. If the patient has disease recurrence after undergoing a subtotal parathyroidectomy, the abnormal tissue may either be an enlarged remnant or a fifth gland that is located in an ectopic location. Sestamibi localization should help to identify the location of the abnormal tissue. The abnormal tissue should be resected, with a portion of it being cryopreserved and a portion of it being autotransplanted into the forearm. When the recurrence occurs after a total parathyroidectomy with a forearm implant, it may be either due to graft hyperplasia in the arm or due to a fifth gland. Sestamibi scans can be performed on both the arm and the neck.[38] Bilateral venous sampling should also be performed to look for a PTH gradient, which can help localize the abnormality. Again, any tissue that is removed should be cryopreserved in case the patient becomes hypoparathyroid postoperatively.

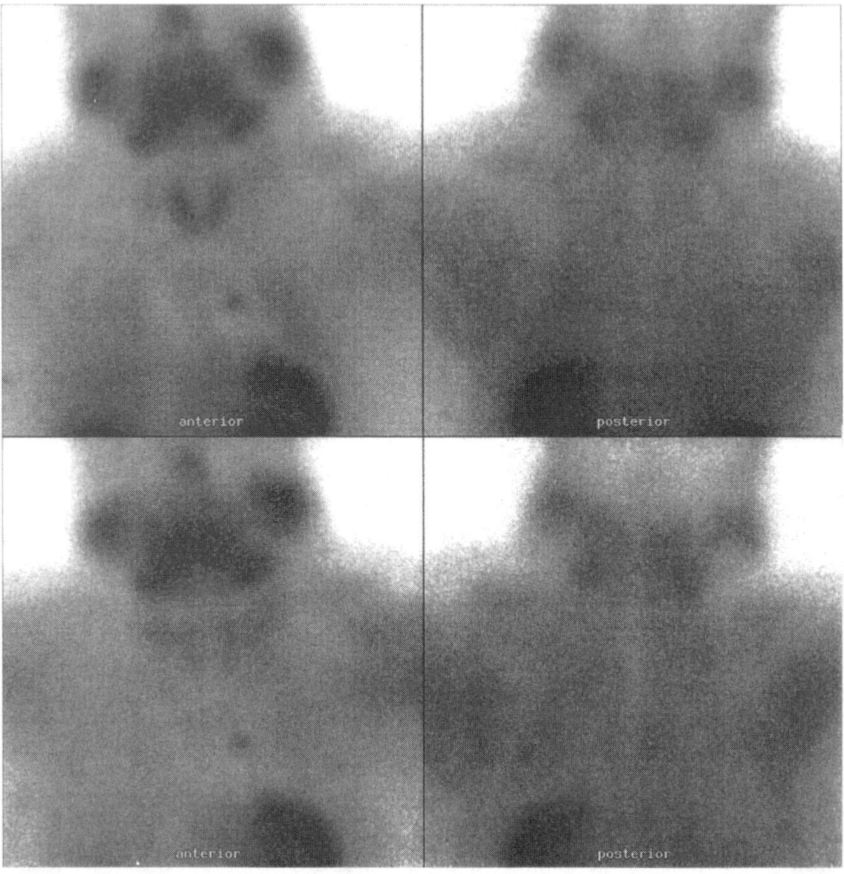

Figure 9-2 A Tc-99m sestamibi of the neck and mediastinum revealing a parathyroid adenoma in the anterior mediastinum.

INTRAOPERATIVE ADJUNCTS

Several intraoperative adjuncts can be applied to aid in the intraoperative identification of parathyroid tissue at reoperation (Box 9-2). Radioguided surgery has been shown to be very effective for intraoperative localization in patients with recurrent primary hyperparathyroidism as well as secondary/tertiary hyperparathyroidism.[38–41] Preoperative injection of 10 mCi of Tc-99m sestamibi is performed 1 to 2 hours prior to surgery. Background counts are obtained using a collimated gamma probe, and the glands are identified by their elevated counts (Figure 9-3). Hyperplastic glands have been shown to have ex-vivo counts over 20% of background.[42] Intraoperative ultrasound has also been applied with some success. The detection rate of intraoperative ultrasound can be double that seen with preoperative ultrasound.[43] However, the use of intraoperative ultrasound requires technical expertise, and the efficacy is very operator-dependent. The development of the

Box 9-2 Intraoperative Adjuncts for Reoperative Parathyroidectomy

1. Radioguided surgery
2. Intraoperative ultrasound
3. Intraoperative PTH monitoring
4. Recurrent laryngeal nerve monitoring

intraoperative PTH assay has proven very effective in primary explorations, but also can play an essential role in reoperative surgery (Figure 9-4). The intraoperative assay can be used to confirm that all of the hyperfunctioning tissue has been removed, with a 98% accuracy rate.[44,45] It can also be utilized to help localize the abnormal glands intraoperatively. Differential venous sampling from the jugulars can be performed intraoperatively to identify the side of the abnormality. Another technique that has been utilized is manual massage of the tissue, which can lead to a spike in blood PTH levels.[44]

Recurrent laryngeal nerve monitoring can also be used in parathyroid explorations to aid in the identification and preservation of the recurrent nerves (discussed in Reoperative Thyroid Surgery, above).

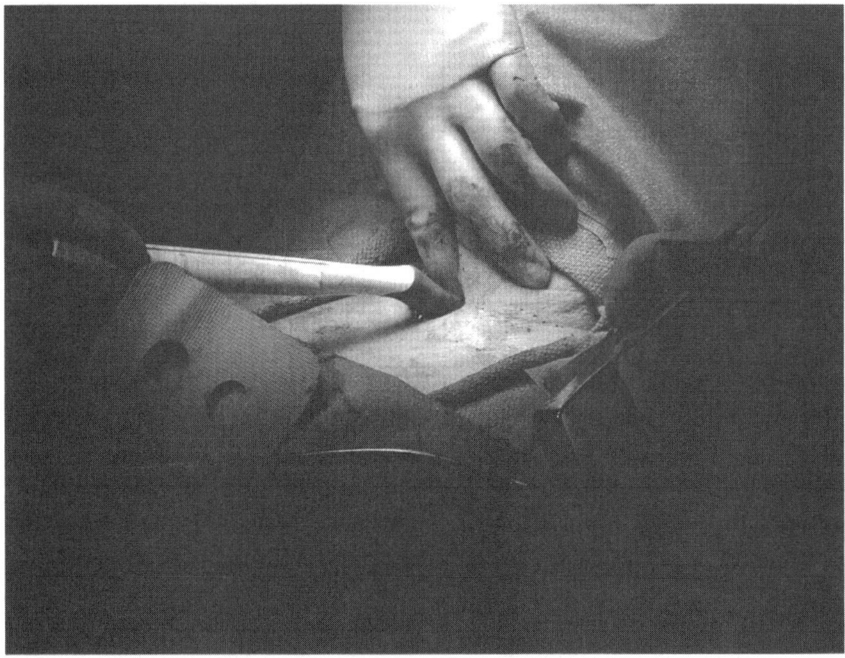

Figure 9-3 Intraoperative use of a radioprobe guides the dissection aids in the identification of the abnormal parathyroid glands.

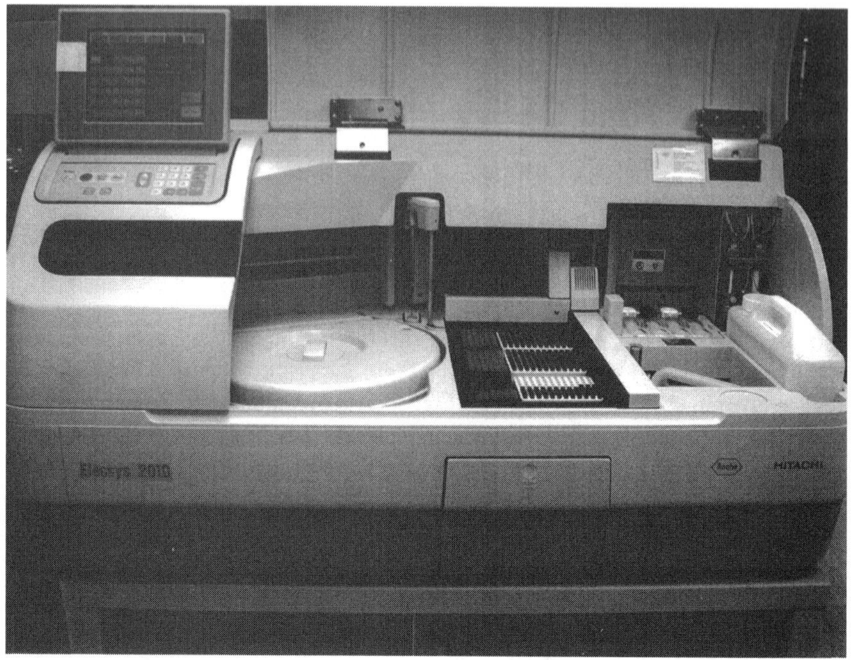

Figure 9-4 The Elecsys 2010 system can be used to perform the intraoperative PTH assay.

If the patient has had multiple glands removed previously or an extensive bilateral neck exploration, care must be taken to preserve the remaining parathyroid tissue. If viable parathyroid tissue in the neck cannot be confirmed, then any parathyroid tissue that has been removed should be cryopreserved for future autotransplantation.

COMPLICATIONS

Compared with first neck explorations, repeat operations are associated with a significantly greater morbidity. Transient hypocalcemia is a common complication after reoperative parathyroid surgery, occurring in up to 25% of patients.[31] The incidence of permanent hypoparathyroidism is between 5% and 10%.[46] In a series of 228 patients reported by Jaskowiak and associates, 5.3% of patients ultimately required a parathyroid autograft for management of their hypoparathyroidism. These numbers help to emphasize the importance of cryopreserving parathyroid tissue any time there is a question regarding the amount of remaining viable parathyroid tissue. The incidence of recurrent laryngeal nerve injury has ranged from 1.2% to 4%.[46] Unfortunately, much of the data reported in the literature are from major academic institutions with extensive experience in reoperative parathyroid surgery, and their data are likely not representative of the results in general practice.

Conclusion

Reoperative thyroid and parathyroid surgery accounts for a small percentage of the endocrine surgeries done each year. These procedures can be technically demanding and require an extensive knowledge of the anatomy of the neck as well as the anatomic variations that can exist. When done by an experienced surgeon, these procedures can be safely performed with minimal morbidity and mortality.

REFERENCES

1. Rutkow IM. Surgical operations in the United States: 1979 to 1984. Surgery 1987;101:192–200.
2. Reeve TS, Delbridge L, Brady P, et al. Secondary thyroidectomy: a twenty-year experience. World J Surg 1988;12:449–453.
3. Abbas G, Dubner S, Heller KS. Re-operation for bleeding after thyroidectomy and parathyroidectomy. Head Neck 2001;23:544–546.
4. Burkey SH, van Heerden JA, Thompson GB, et al. Reexploration for symptomatic hematomas after cervical exploration. Surgery 2001;130:914–920.
5. Chen H, Zeiger MA, Clark DP, et al. Papillary carcinoma of the thyroid: can operative management be based solely on fine-needle aspiration? J Am Coll Surg 1997;184:605–610.
6. Chen H, Nicol TL, Zeiger MA, et al. Hurthle cell neoplasms of the thyroid: are there factors predictive of malignancy? Ann Surg 1998;227:542–546.
7. Callcut R, Selvaggi S, Mack E, et al. The utility of frozen section evaluation for follicular thyroid lesions. Ann Surg Oncol 2003;10:S21–S22.
8. Levin KE, Clark AH, Duh QY, et al. Reoperative thyroid surgery. Surgery 1992;111:604–609.
9. Tan MP, Agarwal G, Reeve TS, et al. Impact of timing on completion thyroidectomy for thyroid cancer. Br J Surg 2002;89:802–804.
10. Chao TC, Jeng LB, Lin JD, Chen MF. Reoperative thyroid surgery. World J Surg 1997;21:644–647.
11. Wilson DB, Staren ED, Prinz RA. Thyroid reoperations: indications and risks. Am Surg 1998;64:674–678.
12. Muller PE, Jakoby R, Heinert G, Spelsberg F. Surgery for recurrent goitre: its complications and their risk factors. Eur J Surg 2001;167:816–821.
13. Hsu B, Reeve TS, Guinea AI, et al. Recurrent substernal nodular goiter: incidence and management. Surgery 1996;120:1072–1075.
14. Desai D, Jeffrey RB, McDougall IR, Weigel RJ. Intraoperative ultrasonography for localization of recurrent thyroid cancer. Surgery 2001;129:498–500.
15. Thomas CG Jr. Reoperative thyroid surgery. In: McQuarrie D, Humphrey E, Lee J, eds. Reoperative General Surgery. St. Louis: Mosby-Year Book; 1997:771–779.
16. Dackiw AP, Rotstein LE, Clark OH. Computer-assisted evoked electromyography with stimulating surgical instruments for recurrent/external laryngeal nerve identification and preservation in thyroid and parathyroid operation. Surgery 2002;132:1100–1106.

17. Menegaux F, Turpin G, Dahman M, et al. Secondary thyroidectomy in patients with prior thyroid surgery for benign disease: a study of 203 cases. Surgery 1999;126:479–483.

18. Tschopp KP, Gottardo C. Comparison of various methods of electromyographic monitoring of the recurrent laryngeal nerve in thyroid surgery. Ann Otol Rhinol Laryngol 2002;111:811–816.

19. Marcus B, Edwards B, Yoo S, et al. Recurrent laryngeal nerve monitoring in thyroid and parathyroid surgery: the University of Michigan experience. Laryngoscope 2003;113:356–361.

20. Eltzschig HK, Posner M, Moore FD Jr. The use of readily available equipment in a simple method for intraoperative monitoring of recurrent laryngeal nerve function during thyroid surgery: initial experience with more than 300 cases. Arch Surg 2002;137:452–456.

21. Scheuller MC, Ellison D. Laryngeal mask anesthesia with intraoperative laryngoscopy for identification of the recurrent laryngeal nerve during thyroidectomy. Laryngoscope 2002;112:1594–1597.

22. Chen H, Zeiger MA, Gordon TA, Udelsman R. Parathyroidectomy in Maryland: effects of an endocrine center. Surgery 1996;120:948–952.

23. Rotstein L, Irish J, Gullane P, et al. Reoperative parathyroidectomy in the era of localization technology. Head Neck 1998;20:535–539.

24. Jones JJ, Brunaud L, Dowd CF, et al. Accuracy of selective venous sampling for intact parathyroid hormone in difficult patients with recurrent or persistent hyperparathyroidism. Surgery 2002;132:944–950.

25. Levin KE, Clark OH. The reasons for failure in parathyroid operations. Arch Surg 1989;124:911–914.

26. Brennan MF, Norton JA. Reoperation for persistent and recurrent hyperparathyroidism. Ann Surg 1985;201:40–44.

27. Wadstrom C, Zedenius J, Guinea A, et al. Re-operative surgery for recurrent or persistent primary hyperparathyroidism. Aust NZ J Surg 1998;68:103–107.

28. Marx SJ, Stock JL, Attie MF, et al. Familial hypocalciuric hypercalcemia: recognition among patients referred after unsuccessful parathyroid exploration. Ann Intern Med 1980;92:351–356.

29. Bilezikian JP, Potts JT Jr, Fuleihan G, et al. Summary statement from a workshop on asymptomatic primary hyperparathyroidism: a perspective for the 21st century. J Bone Miner Res 2002;17(supp2):N2–N11.

30. Hasse C, Sitter H, Brune M, et al. Quality of life and patient satisfaction after reoperation for primary hyperparathyroidism: analysis of long-term results. World J Surg 2002;26:1029–1036.

31. Jaskowiak N, Norton JA, Alexander HR, et al. A prospective trial evaluating a standard approach to reoperation for missed parathyroid adenoma. Ann Surg 1996;224:308–320.

32. Sippel R, Bianco J, Wilson M, et al. Can thallium subtraction scanning play a role in the preoperative imaging for minimally invasive parathyroidectomy? Clin Nucl Med 2004;29:21–26.

33. Feingold DL, Alexander HR, Chen CC, et al. Ultrasound and sestamibi scan as the only preoperative imaging tests in reoperation for parathyroid adenomas. Surgery 2000;128:1103–1109.

34. Rodriquez JM, Tezelman S, Siperstein AE, et al. Localization procedures in patients with persistent or recurrent hyperparathyroidism. Arch Surg 1994;129: 870–875.

35. Nilsson B, Fjalling M, Klingenstierna H, et al. Effects of preoperative parathyroid localisation studies on the cost of operations for persistent hyperparathyroidism. Eur J Surg 2001;167:587–591.

36. Axelrod D, Sisson JC, Cho K, et al. Appearance of ectopic undescended inferior parathyroid adenomas on technetium Tc 99m Sestamibi scintigraphy—A lesson from reoperative parathyroidectomy. Arch Surg 2003;138:1214–1218.

37. O'Herrin JK, Weigel T, Wilson M, Chen H. Radioguided parathyroidectomy via VATS combined with intraoperative parathyroid hormone testing: the surgical approach of choice for patients with mediastinal parathyroid adenomas? J Bone Miner Res 2002;17:1368–1371.

38. Sippel R, Bianco J, Chen H. Radioguided parathyroidectomy for recurrent hyperparathyroidism caused by forearm graft hyperplasia. J Bone Miner Res 2003;18:939–942.

39. Chen H, Mack E, Starling JR. Radioguided parathyroidectomy is equally effective for both adenomatous and hyperplastic glands. Ann Surg 2003;238: 332–337.

40. Nichol PF, Starling JR, Mack E, et al. Long-term follow-up of patients with tertiary hyperparathyroidism treated by resection of a single or double adenoma. Ann Surg 2002;235:673–678.

41. Norman J, Denham D. Minimally invasive radioguided parathyroidectomy in the reoperative neck. Surgery 1998;124:1088–1092.

42. Chen H, Mack E, Starling JR. Radioguided parathyroidectomy is equally effective for both adenomatous and hyperplastic glands. Ann Surg 2003;238: 332–337.

43. Rossi HL, Ali A, Prinz RA. Intraoperative sestamibi scanning in reoperative parathyroidectomy. Surgery 2000;128:744–750.

44. Irvin GL III, Molinari AS, Figueroa C, Carneiro DM. Improved success rate in reoperative parathyroidectomy with intraoperative PTH assay. Ann Surg 1999;229:874–878.

45. Bergenfelz A, Isaksson A, Lindblom P, et al. Measurement of parathyroid hormone in patients with primary hyperparathyroidism undergoing first and reoperative surgery. Br J Surg 1998;85:1129–1132.

46. Wells SA Jr, Debenedetti MK, Doherty GM. Recurrent or persistent hyperparathyroidism. J Bone Miner Res 2002;17(suppl 2):N158–N162.

CHAPTER 10

Reoperative Gastroesophageal Surgery

Mercedeh Baghai, MD; Kent R. VanSickle, MD;
C. Daniel Smith, MD

Reoperation After Antireflux Surgery

Antireflux surgery (ARS) is appropriate and effective management for patients with gastroesophageal reflux disease (GERD) refractory to medical management, on life-long acid suppression, or suffering from side effects of the medical management.[1] Over the past two decades, the operations have evolved from predominantly open thoracic approaches to, now, a predominantly laparoscopic abdominal approach, with similar, if not better outcomes.[2,3] As the procedures have evolved, and patterns of failure and complications have been better characterized, the morbidity and mortality has decreased (2.1% and 0.3% respectively) with long-term symptomatic success rates of over 90%.[4,5]

Despite these excellent outcomes, there remain a small subset of patients who, after ARS, continue to suffer from persistent or recurrent GERD or develop new symptoms such as dysphagia or chest pain. Although many of these patients respond to nonoperative medical and endoscopic therapies, a small percentage (2% to 16%) ultimately undergo revisional antireflux surgery.[4,6]

Reoperation after antireflux surgery, like most reoperative surgery, is technically challenging and fraught with potential complications.[7–9] Additionally, success rates are typically lower than with the primary procedure. Therefore, an understanding of the potential early and late complications following ARS, the patterns of ARS failures and the necessary preoperative workup, and appropriate patient selection are critical in maintaining low morbidity while achieving reasonable success with redo ARS.

IMMEDIATE PERIOPERATIVE ISSUES

Major surgical complications immediately after primary ARS occur in 2% to 3% of patients.[4,6] These include leaks from esophageal or gastric perforations (1%), acute wrap herniation (0.5%), and bleeding (0.2%). The most important predictors of favorable outcome with these complications are early diagnosis and timely operative intervention.

Leaks

ETIOLOGY The most clinically significant immediate postoperative complication is a perforation leading to a leak. This can result from a delayed perforation caused by inadvertent electrocautery injury to the esophagus or stomach, or from ischemia of the gastric wall due to close cauterization of a short gastric vessel. Additional causes may include unrecognized perforation due to difficult dissection during mobilization of the cardia or esophageal hiatus while passing an instrument around the esophagus or while passing the esophageal dilator into the stomach.[4,10]

DIAGNOSIS AND WORKUP An unrecognized leak can be life-threatening. We commonly perform intraoperative endoscopy if dissection is particularly difficult or a leak is suspected. The esophagus and stomach are distended with air while submerged under water, and air bubbles are sought. Some advocate injecting methylene blue through a nasogastric tube in the distal esophagus; however, we have cases in which this technique failed to identify a perforation that was subsequently found with endoscopic insufflation as described. Postoperatively, signs of sepsis such as fever, leukocytosis, oliguria, and tachycardia should not be dismissed and must be thoroughly evaluated. An early gastrograffin swallow may help establish the diagnosis when otherwise clinically equivocal. If a leak is suspected, there is no role for diagnostic or therapeutic endoscopy in the early postoperative setting.

MANAGEMENT If a leak is found or suspected, early reoperation is essential. This can be achieved laparoscopically with a relatively low conversion rate.[4,6,11,12] If minimal or no contamination is found, a primary repair covered by a fundoplication, periesophageal fat patch, or fibrin glue is reasonable. In this setting, a deep drain and gastrostomy tube are also necessary to control the esophagogastric secretions. If excessive inflammation or contamination is encountered, surgical drainage with diversion and a venting/feeding gastrojejunostomy tube may be the safest immediate solution.

Acute Wrap Herniation

ETIOLOGY Another technical complication, usually requiring immediate reoperation is acute transdiaphragmatic wrap herniation (0.5% to 1.3%).[4,6] The cause of an acute wrap herniation is usually mechanical or technical in nature. Issues such as incomplete crural closure, closure under tension, or suture disruption may be etiologic. Most commonly, the acute herniation is preceded by a sudden increase in intra-abdominal pressure secondary to coughing or postoperative nausea and vomiting.[13–15]

DIAGNOSIS AND WORKUP Acute wrap herniation may present as a sudden, severe, unrelenting midepigastric pain associated with nausea, vomiting, and dysphagia. It can also present more subtly, as new dysphagia following an episode of retching. Workup should include a gastrograffin swallow, which would be diagnostic. Again, an upper endoscopy is rarely indicated in this acute setting.

MANAGEMENT The best management of this problem is prevention, with careful hiatal reconstruction and aggressive use of perioperative antiemetics. If patients retch in the immediate postoperative period, they should immediately undergo a contrast swallow. If wrap herniation is detected early (within 7 days), reoperation is indicated. Here, the hernia is reduced and the esophageal hiatus reconstructed. However, if wrap herniation is identified more than 7 days postoperatively, it is usually best to avoid redo ARS for at least 6 weeks because of the potential for dense adhesions and a very difficult repair. Reports have been made of tension-free crural repairs for both primary and reoperative paraesophageal herniation using different prosthetic biomaterial;[16,17] however, this remains controversial, mostly because of lack of long-term data pertaining to the risks of esophageal erosion and/or obstruction.

Bleeding

ETIOLOGY Postoperative hemorrhage is unusual (0.2% to 0.75%) and most often results from an iatrogenic injury to the spleen or the short gastric vessels.[4,6] Upper GI bleeding from missed peptic ulcer, severe esophagitis, or acute gastritis has been described but is very rare.[18]

DIAGNOSIS AND WORKUP Diagnosis of the acute intra-abdominal hemorrhage is predominantly a clinical diagnosis based on the patient's hemodynamics and serial hematocrits.

If the presenting problem is an acute upper GI bleed, the initial evaluation should include an upper endoscopy to localize and possibly address the lesion therapeutically. If bleeding is not localized endoscopically, one should consider the source to be inside the fundal wrap.

MANAGEMENT If the patient is returned to the operating room, one can start with a laparoscopic exploration only if the patient is stable and the surgeon is skilled in advanced laparoscopy.

In case of the unremitting upper GI bleed that is not controlled by endoscopic measures, reoperation may also be warranted. In this setting, one can undo the fundoplication and perform intraoperative endoscopy to manage a bleeding site within the wrap.

Once the patient is beyond the immediate perioperative period and discharged to home, the subsequent complications are usually divided into the categories of early problems (less than 6 weeks) and late problems (beyond 6 weeks).

EARLY POSTOPERATIVE PROBLEMS

The early morbidity associated with antireflux surgery can range from benign gas bloating to dysphagia and food impaction.[19] It is important to recognize that more than half of the patients develop some degree of new "transient" symptom that will resolve with time. Reoperation in this early postoperative period is extremely rare.

Dysphagia and Food Impaction

PRESENTATION The most common of the early complications is transient dysphagia, seen in over half of the patients and most commonly due to postoperative edema or a tight wrap. The onset is typically about the tenth postoperative day and should resolve by 3 weeks. Most patients will complain of difficulty swallowing solids, and in severe cases, intolerance of liquids. This postoperative edema, accompanied by dietary indiscretions and consumption of solid foods (patients should not consume solids for 1 month after surgery), can lead to food impaction.

DIAGNOSIS AND WORKUP The diagnosis in this setting is primarily based on clinical presentation alone. Contrast swallow will document the narrowing of the distal esophagus or the slow transit of contrast into the stomach. In most cases, an upper endoscopy is not indicated for diagnostic purposes. However, if the symptoms do not resolve with conservative treatment, an endoscopic evaluation may be useful to ensure that the wrap is not severely twisted, causing obstruction, or that an ulcer had not developed within the wrap.

MANAGEMENT Reassurance and continuation of a soft food/liquid diet is the primary management. Early dilation is rarely indicated and risks early wrap disruption and recurrent GERD. We reserve this for the small subgroup of patients with dysphagia persisting more than 6 weeks or high-grade food impaction. If dilation becomes necessary, serial dilation with Savory or Maloney dilators are preferred over balloon dilatation, because the sudden inflation pressures of the balloon dilators can lead to acute wrap disruption.

Gas Bloating or Aerophagia

PRESENTATION Other symptoms such as early bloating or aerophagia ("air swallowing") with postprandial discomfort can also occur. This is most commonly seen with a tight wrap or excessive edema in a patient who preoperatively had symptoms of bloating or delayed gastric emptying (DGE).

DIAGNOSIS AND WORKUP The most important element of the workup here is documenting a preoperative gastric emptying study. Patients who initially present with bloating associated with their GERD symptoms are more likely to have bloating complications postoperatively.[20] These patients should undergo a gastric emptying study as part of their preoperative evaluation. If DGE is identified prior to surgery, a concurrent pyloroplasty or venting gastrostomy may help avoid the postoperative symptoms.[13]

MANAGEMENT The majority of the symptoms of gas bloating, pain, and aerophagia will resolve without specific intervention.[19] However, if the symptoms persist and the gastric emptying study suggests DGE, the intervention will depend on the degree of DGE. If the $T^{1/2}$ of the study is abnormally long, but less than twice the upper limit of normal, we have shown in a recent comparative study that a temporizing venting PEG can successfully relieve the symptoms without the need for a surgical pyloroplasty.[21,22] However if the $T^{1/2}$ is prolonged by more than twice the upper limit of normal, the patient will likely need a pyloroplasty, which often times can be performed laparoscopically.

LATE POSTOPERATIVE PROBLEMS

Antireflux operations are performed to eliminate pathologic gastroesophageal reflux. Late failure in this setting is defined as either unsuccessful control of the reflux or new problems resulting from the anatomic alterations of the surgery. Despite the variability in the primary antireflux operations performed in the United States, such as the Nissen fundoplication, the Hill posterior gastropexy, or the Belsey Mark IV repair, all repairs seem to have a similar long-term failure rate of 5% to 15%.[23]

In our earlier series of 1000 consecutive patients undergoing laparoscopic antireflux surgery for GERD and paraesophageal hernias, we found a 3.6% reoperation rate at 7 years' follow-up.[4] This rate was similar between the GERD and the paraesophageal hernia subgroups. However, the patients with more severe reflux, as evidenced by esophageal stricture and Barrett's esophagus, had a higher rate of revisional surgery than those with uncomplicated GERD (8% versus 3.6%, respectively). Over 90% of the revisional operations after laparoscopic fundoplication were performed within the first 2 years of follow-up.[24]

ETIOLOGIES OR PATTERNS OF FAILURE Patterns of failure for laparoscopic ARS differ from open ARS. Nonetheless, they can all be classified in one of the categories of anatomic or physiologic failure (Box 10-1). Over the years, as the patterns of failure have been better defined, many authors have identified important intraoperative technical factors that may contribute to failures (Box 10-2).[13,14,19,25] Careful attention to these critical steps of the procedure may help reduce this failure rate and may, in fact, explain some of the differences between failure rates at different institutions.[26,27]

The reason to emphasize these mechanisms of failure is that prevention of failure in these patients is a vastly more effective and reliable measure of long-term success than any subsequent attempt at medical, endoscopic, or surgical intervention.

Box 10-1 Anatomic and Physiologic Patterns of Failure of Antireflux Surgery

ANATOMIC PATTERNS OF FAILURE (FIGURES 10-1 AND 10-2)

1. Complete or partial wrap disruption
2. Misplaced or slipped wrap
3. Transdiaphragmatic wrap herniation
4. Wrap too tight or too long
5. Twisted wrap
6. Tight crural closure

PHYSIOLOGIC PATTERNS OF FAILURE

1. Incorrect initial diagnosis (e.g., achalasia)
2. Unrecognized associated foregut problem (e.g., delayed gastric emptying, esophageal body dysfunction, peptic ulcer disease

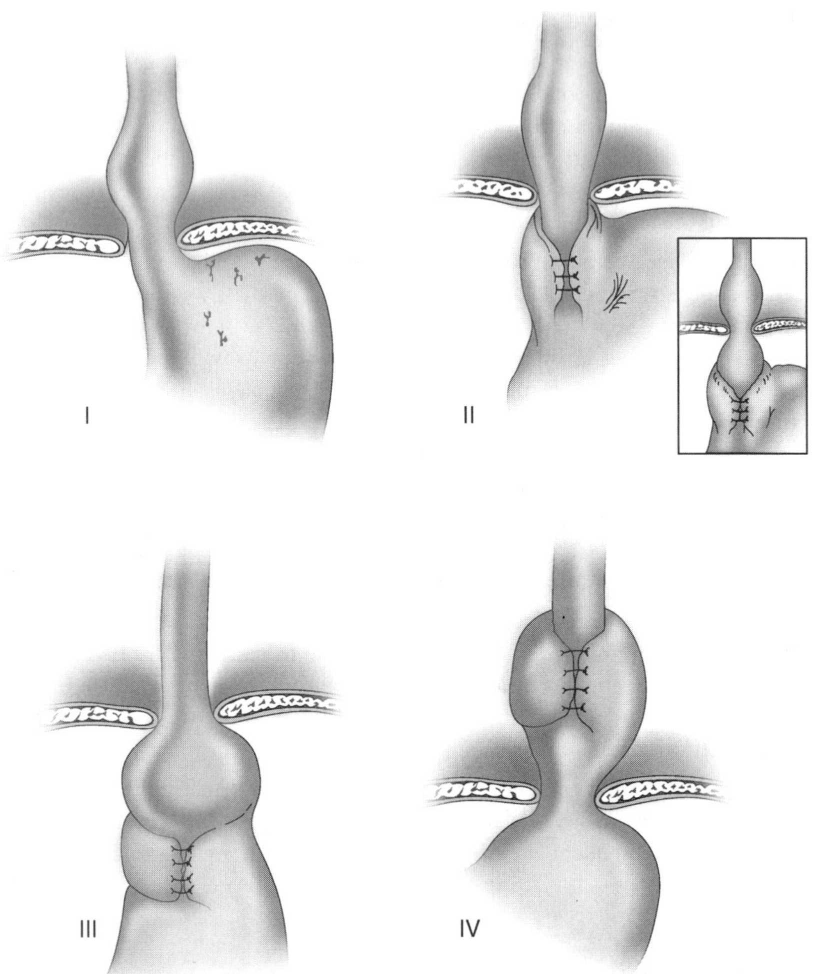

Figure 10-1 Four types of surgical failure of Nissen fundoplication: (I) Wrap disruption, (II) Gastric herniation above the wrap, (III) "Slipped" Nissen, and (IV) Wrap herniation.

(From Hinder RA. Gastroesophageal reflux disease. In: Bell RH Jr, Rikkers LF, Mulholland MW, eds. Digestive Tract Surgery: A Text and Atlas. Philadelphia: Lippincott-Raven Publishers, 1996:19.)

WORKUP Before undertaking revisional ARS, a thorough evaluation is essential. This should include a complete history and physical; and adjunct studies of barium swallow, upper endoscopy, esophageal physiologic studies of manometry, pH testing, and a gastric emptying study. The history should specifically seek and document symptoms of heartburn, regurgitation, and dysphagia, and compare these with the patient's preoperative symptomatology. Specifically, asking about early

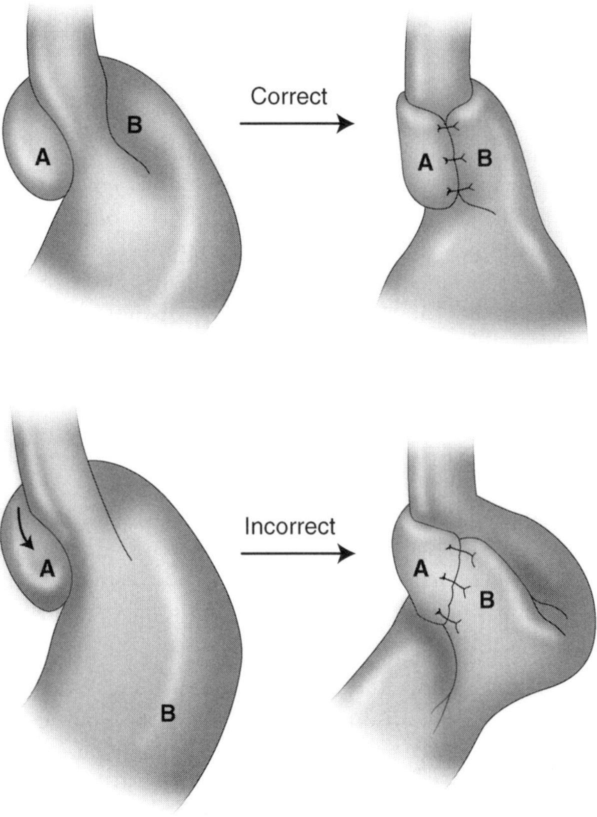

Figure 10-2 Another failure mechanism, "twisted" wrap: Using gastric body instead of fundus to perform fundoplication.

Box 10-2 Intraoperative Technical Errors Leading to Late Surgical Failure

1. Inadequate esophageal mobilization
2. Misplacement of the fundic wrap too low onto the stomach or choice of the body of the stomach for the wrap
3. Inadequate fixation of the fundic wrap
4. Inadequate takedown of the short gastric attachments (Rossetti-Nissen fundoplication), leading to a twisted wrap
5. Inadequate closure of the crura or primary suture closure under tension
6. Inadequate hiatal dissection with or without incomplete reduction of paraesophageal hernia and hernia sac[28]

postprandial bloating will help identify those most likely to have delayed gastric emptying. A copy of the previous operative report may help delineate any potential problems in the first operation that may have led to an anatomic failure and serve as a roadmap in the reoperation.

An upper endoscopy is the single most useful test for identifying and characterizing anatomic failure, especially wrap twisting, misplacement, or transdiaphragmatic herniation. Barium swallow is often only confirmatory. Esophageal function tests with pH monitoring and manometry are also necessary to assess recurrent GERD or motility problems. Manometry is critical in assessing esophageal clearance, both to ensure that the proper operation was performed previously and to base the type of reoperative fundoplication on the status of esophageal motility, sphincter pressures, and clearance.

MEDICAL AND ENDOSCOPIC MANAGEMENT

RECURRENT REFLUX If the failure is secondary to recurrent reflux symptoms, a trial of medical management with proton pump inhibitors (PPIs) is indicated. However, both the patient and the physician should realize that success of medical management is lower in operated than nonoperated patients.[29,30] At the least, this can allow for esophagitis, ulcerations, and edema to resolve prior to further intervention. Furthermore, symptom control with PPIs may also predict favorable response to revisional ARS.[31]

If the workup does not reveal an obvious anatomic or technical etiology for the recurrence of symptoms, but documents pathologic gastroesophageal reflux, endoscopic antireflux procedures may be considered.[32] Radiofrequency ablation of the lower esophageal sphincter (STRETTA, Curon Medical) has been shown to be effective in 70% to 85% of patients with primary GERD,[33–35] although this has not yet been studied in those who have failed ARS. In a recent animal model, we demonstrated that this technique can be performed with reasonable accuracy and efficacy after previously failed ARS, using fluoroscopic guidance.[36] The clinical experience in this setting is extremely limited; however, in our recent study of STRETTA in eight patients after failed fundoplication, seven documented improvement in GERD symptoms at a 1-year mean follow-up.[37]

Other endoscopic techniques, such as the submucosal injection of an expanding biopolymer or the endoscopic suturing device,[38] may also be an alternative to reoperation for a loose wrap or hypotensive lower esophageal sphincter. All such endoscopic therapies are currently approved as primary therapy for GERD, and none have any significant data from use in revisional ARS.[32,39,40]

DYSPHAGIA If failure is secondary to new or progressive dysphagia, an intact but misaligned, misplaced, or herniated wrap is usually the etiology. With dysphagia in the absence of a paraesophageal hernia or a slipped, misplaced, or twisted fundoplication, a nonoperative trial of dilatation can be attempted. Balloon dilatation is usually not recommended because the sudden inflation pressures can potentially disrupt the wrap. However, serial dilations with Savory or Maloney dilators may be successful in resolving the problem of an otherwise uncomplicated tight or long wrap.

REOPERATIVE MANAGEMENT As mentioned earlier, the key predictors of positive surgical outcomes are patient selection and operative technique. Regarding patient selection, those patients who present with recurrent or new symptoms of reflux or dysphagia, and have a corresponding anatomic abnormality, experience the best results with revisional ARS.[7,19,41]

Regarding operative technique, the experience of the surgeon with reoperative ARS is key in determining the outcome of these operations. Revisional ARS is technically challenging, and experience and skill with reoperative abdominal surgery along with understanding of the esophagogastroduodenal physiology and anatomy is imperative in achieving the best functional result. Historically, reoperative antireflux surgery has been approached through an open laparotomy or thoracotomy, which was determined largely by whether the primary procedure was abdominal or thoracic. With increasing skill and experience in laparoscopic techniques, laparoscopic revisional ARS has been shown to be safe and efficacious.[11] However, if the patient has had multiple open foregut procedures, laparoscopic reoperation may not be feasible, and a thoracotomy may then be the safest alternative. In particular, reconstruction of the hiatus in case of recurrent paraesophageal hernia or esophageal shortening may best be managed through a thoracic approach. Irrespective of the approach, the operation should be crafted to the pathophysiology and anatomy identified in the preoperative workup. For example, if the manometry documents a severe motility disorder, then the wrap should be taken down and redone with a 270° (Toupet or Dor) fundoplication. Or in the case of esophageal shortening, an esophageal lengthening procedure like a Collis gastroplasty may be needed.[42–44]

Regardless of the reason for failure, some general principles apply to all revisional ARS, as listed in Box 10-3.

Results of Reoperative Antireflux Surgery—Most series report acceptable results for revisional ARS. Success rates usually range from 70% to 85%,[24] as opposed to

Box 10-3 General Principles in the Conduct of Revisional Antireflux Surgery

1. Dissect hiatus completely and mobilize esophagus well into the mediastinum
2. Specifically ensure adequate fundic mobilization and take down additional short gastric vessels if necessary[45]
3. Always take apart the previous fundoplication
4. Use intraoperative endoscopy to assess esophageal length and integrity of esophagus and stomach (identify perforations)
5. Calibrate wrap over esophageal dilator
6. Use gastrostomy tube liberally if concerned about potential esophagus or stomach injury, prolonged return of GI function, or ability to eat
7. Aggressively prevent postoperative nausea and retching with prophylactic antiemetics on all patients[25]

the success rates of 85% to 95% for primary operations. A decade ago, Jamieson reported a 79% success rate in a meta-analysis of 564 redo patients from 14 series.[46] This success rate falls to 66% and 50%, respectively, with third and fourth reoperations.[47] The morbidity and mortality are also higher in this reoperative group. Morbidity rates range from 2% to 46%,[8,9] and mortality rates are reported to range anywhere between 0.5% to17%.[48] In our own series of 251 reoperative cases, overall morbidity and mortality were 14% and 0.4%, respectively.[49]

As mentioned earlier, these redo patients can be highly complex and technically challenging, and the operations inherently carry a high complication rate and lower success rates. Therefore, before considering a patient for reoperative antireflux surgery, one must carefully determine the cause of failure, assess the severity of their symptoms, and ultimately weigh these factors against the risks of a redo operation, in order to determine the necessity for intervention and the likelihood of its success.

Reoperation After Surgery for Achalasia

The pathophysiology of achalasia—a hypertensive lower esophageal sphincter (LES) that fails to relax completely, and abnormal esophageal body peristalsis—is an irreversible process, and as such, esophageal body function will always be abnormal.[50] Treatment is primarily directed toward alleviating the obstructed distal esophagus, and the current treatment of choice for most patients with achalasia is an esophagomyotomy. First described by Heller in 1914,[51] this procedure is now generally performed laparoscopically and has gained acceptance both in the surgical and medical communities as the gold standard for treatment. The management of patients who have failed primary surgical treatment of achalasia is challenging and difficult. This chapter will focus on two issues for patients requiring reoperations for previous achalasia therapy: (1) those presenting with immediate perioperative problems (i.e., perforation), and (2) those with persistent or recurrent symptoms (i.e., treatment failures).

REOPERATION FOR ESOPHAGEAL PERFORATION

Esophageal perforation during Heller myotomy for achalasia is a well-recognized problem, and is reported to occur in 4% to 15% of patients.[50,52–54] This problem is managed by suture closure of the mucosal laceration, and in many cases this is feasible laparoscopically. Fortunately, a perforation that is unrecognized intraoperatively and discovered as a postoperative esophageal leak is an unusual complication, occurring in less than 1% of patients.[50] Early recognition and treatment are critical in order to avoid the significant associated morbidity and mortality.

ETIOLOGIES Most esophageal mucosal injuries occur in patients whom have undergone previous therapy for achalasia, particularly endoscopic treatments such as dilation or botulinum toxin (Botox) injection.[53,55] Scarring from previous therapy obscures normal anatomy, and dissection in this area can lead to immediate or delayed mucosal injury. An early report suggested previous pneumatic dilatation as an independent risk factor for mucosal perforation,[56] and Sharp et al reported five of eight perforations occurring in patients with a previous therapeutic procedure (Botox, dilation, or myotomy).[54] Other etiologies include electrocautery thermal injury and instrumentation.

CLINICAL PRESENTATION The early identification of esophageal leak after Heller myotomy requires a high index of suspicion and appropriate immediate attention. Many surgeons performing this procedure routinely obtain contrast studies of the esophagus on postoperative day 1 to rule out unrecognized leaks. Any patient with worsening abdominal pain, tenderness or guarding, fever, tachycardia, or oliguria is highly suggestive of a perforation, and should be investigated immediately.

WORKUP Esophageal perforation is a true surgical emergency, and a high index of suspicion and prompt evaluation is the key to successful management. Any patient with a suspected perforation should undergo a thorough evaluation. A water-soluble contrast (i.e., gastrograffin) swallowing study is indicated to secure the diagnosis, and a barium swallow may be added if the gastrograffin study is negative.

MANAGEMENT Therapy should be directed toward both repairing the leak and establishing adequate control of upper GI tract secretions. Leaks that are detected early postoperatively (on routine day 1 contrast swallow or within 24 hours) can usually be managed laparoscopically. If the tissue is viable, primary repair with an absorbable suture and reinforcement of the repair with tissue glue or a tissue patch (e.g., repositioning or creating a fundoplication over the repair) is appropriate. Placing a drain in the abdominal cavity near the repair along with a nasogastric tube in the esophagus proximal to the repair and a gastrostomy tube is important for control of GI secretions while the repair heals. Patients are maintained on parenteral nutrition for 7 to 10 days before restudying the esophagus.

If the presentation of esophageal perforation is delayed (over 24 hours) or if the tissue around the perforation is not viable, placement of drains and intestinal tubes may be all that can be accomplished. In ill patients with large perforations, esophageal and gastric exclusion may be a useful temporizing procedure with future plans for delayed resection and reconstruction. Rarely should resection be attempted as initial management.

CONCLUSION Reoperation for esophageal perforation after achalasia therapy is fortunately a rare event. Most mucosal injuries are recognized at the time of myotomy, either directly or with intraoperative endoscopy, and can be repaired primarily. Because of the high morbidity and mortality associated with an esophageal perforation, a high index of suspicion and prompt treatment are key to successful management. Primary reinforced repair is preferable, unless significant scarring and/or contamination are present.

REOPERATION FOR TREATMENT FAILURE

ETIOLOGY Most patients who have failed operative management present with recurrent (or persistent) dysphagia (Box 10-4). Incomplete or inadequate myotomy is the most common cause, and has typically been more common after a thoracic esophagomyotomy, as performing a complete myotomy onto the proximal 2 to 3 cm

Box 10-4 Causes of Recurrent Symptoms

1. Incomplete/inadequate myotomy
2. Gastroesophageal reflux (with or without stricture)
3. Scarring and fibrosis from previous treatment
4. Esophageal carcinoma
5. Fundoplication
6. End-stage achalasia

of stomach is more difficult using the transthoracic approach.[57] An inadequate myotomy is also certainly possible with an abdominal approach, and is usually seen early in a surgeon's experience with the laparoscopic Heller myotomy.[52]

Gastroesophageal reflux and stricture is another cause of failure, particularly in those patients in whom an antireflux procedure was not a part of their esophagomyotomy. Fortunately, with the acceptance of the Heller myotomy and partial fundoplication (either Dor or Toupet) as the treatment of choice in most patients, the incidence of symptomatic reflux and subsequent stricture is low.[52,53] However, the issue of adding an antireflux procedure remains controversial, and some surgeons routinely perform the Heller myotomy without fundoplication.

Although most often associated with gastroesophageal reflux, the presence of a stricture must always alert the surgeon to the possibility of esophageal carcinoma, particularly due to the known increased incidence of squamous cell carcinoma in patients with long-standing achalasia.[50] Also, scarring and fibrosis from a previous myotomy, pneumatic dilatations, or intersphincteric botulinum toxin injection may contribute to stricture at the LES, and this has been reported in several studies.[55,58]

For patients in whom an antireflux procedure was added, recurrent dysphagia may be related to technical error in the fundoplication. Current recommendations in the literature support the use of either the partial posterior (Toupet) or the partial anterior (Dor) fundoplication.[52,53,55,59,60] The symptoms are usually due to esophageal distortion from a malpositioned partial fundoplication.[53,57] A 360° fundoplication should never accompany an esophagomyotomy for achalasia.

Finally, patients with long-standing achalasia and significant esophageal dilation (more than 7 cm) preoperatively have a higher rate of failure with esophagomyotomy.[61] This is most likely due to the loss of the conduit function of the atonic esophagus and now more sacular esophagus. Relieving esophageal outlet obstruction with the myotomy only partly corrects for the dilated and tortuous esophagus that does not empty well.

MANAGEMENT Treatment should be tailored to the underlying problem. If an incomplete or inadequate myotomy is the cause, attempts at pneumatic dilatation should be the initial choice of therapy. Zaninotto et al were able to successfully treat seven of nine patients with recurrent dysphagia from incomplete myotomies with repeated "gentle" dilatations.[60] Generally, lower balloon pressures, shorter dilation times, and more frequent attempts are recommended in order to reduce the risk of perforation in the area of a previous cardiomyotomy. For patients in whom repeat pneumatic dilatations fail, a laparoscopic redo Heller myotomy can be performed, using endoscopic guidance to ensure a completed cardiomyotomy and to assess the possibility of a perforation.

The approach to a redo myotomy is similar to a primary procedure. Careful attention must be paid to the area of the previous myotomy, however, and under no circumstances should an effort be made to redo the myotomy in this area, as only mucosa with overlying scar tissue remains and a perforation is highly likely. It is recommended that the new myotomy be performed 180° away from the previous site (typically posterior),[57] but with adequate visualization a successful anterior cardiomyotomy can be performed safely.

Conclusion

With widespread acceptance and improvement in techniques of the laparoscopic Heller myotomy, reoperations for patients with achalasia should gradually decrease. Before embarking on any therapy for an achalasia recurrence, a careful and thorough evaluation is imperative to secure the diagnosis and to direct treatment at the underlying cause for primary failure. Conservative measures (i.e., medical, endoscopic) should be employed initially, reserving redo myotomy or esophagectomy for refractory failures.

REFERENCES

1. Hinder RA, Filipi CJ, Wetscher G, et al. Laparoscopic Nissen fundoplication is an effective treatment for gastroesophageal reflux disease. Ann Surg 1994; 220:472–481.
2. Fuchs KH, Feussner H, Bonavina L, et al. Current status and trends in laparoscopic antireflux surgery: results of a consensus meeting. The European Study Group for Antireflux Surgery (ESGARS). Endoscopy 1997;29:298–308.
3. Stein HJ, Feussner H, Siewert JR. Antireflux surgery: a current comparison of open and laparoscopic approaches. Hepatogastroenterology 1998;45:1328–1337.
4. Terry M, Smith CD, Branum GD, et al. Outcomes of laparoscopic fundoplication for gastroesophageal reflux disease and paraesophageal hernia. Surg Endosc 2001;15:691–699.
5. Hinder RA, Perdikis G, Klinger PJ, DeVault KR. The surgical option for gastroesophageal reflux disease. Am J Surg 1997;103(5A):144S–148S.
6. Carlson MA, Frantzides CT. Complications and results of primary minimally invasive antireflux procedures: a review of 10,735 reported cases. J Am Coll Surg 2001;193:428–439.
7. Awad ZT, Anderson PI, Sato K, et al. Laparoscopic reoperative antireflux surgery. Surg Endosc 2001;15:1401–1407.
8. Pointner R, Bammer T, Then P, Kamolz T. Laparoscopic refundoplications after failed antireflux surgery. Am J Surg 1999;178:541–543.

9. Neuhauser B, Hinder RA. Laparoscopic reoperation after failed antireflux surgery. Semin Lap Surg 2001;8:281–286.
10. Schauer PR, Meyers WC, Eubanks S, et al. Mechanisms of gastric and esophageal perforations during laparoscopic Nissen fundoplication. Ann Surg 1996;223:43–52.
11. Floch NR, Hinder RA, Klingler PJ, et al. Is laparoscopic reoperation for failed antireflux surgery feasible? Arch Surg 1999;134:733–737.
12. Curet M, Josloff RK, Schoeb O, Zucker KA. Laparoscopic reoperation for failed antireflux procedures. Arch Surg 1999;134:559–563.
13. Hunter JG. Approach and management of patients with recurrent gastroesophageal reflux disease. J Gastrointest Surg 2001;5:451–457.
14. Horgan S, Pohl D, Bogetti D, et al. Failed antireflux surgery: what have we learned from reoperations? Arch Surg 1999;134:809–817.
15. Idani H, Narusue M, Kin H, et al. Acute intrathoracic incarceration of the stomach after laparoscopic Nissen fundoplication. Surg Laparosc Endosc Perc Tech 2000;10:99–102.
16. Frantzides CT, Madan AK, Carlson MA, Stavropoulos GP. A prospective randomized trial of laparoscopic polytetrafluoroethylene (PTFE) patch repair vs simple cruroplasty for large hiatal hernia. Arch Surg 2002;137:649–652.
17. Granderath FA, Kamolz T, Schweiger UM, Pointner R. Laparoscopic refundoplication with prosthetic hiatal closure for recurrent hiatal hernia after primary failed antireflux surgery. Arch Surg 2003;138:902–907.
18. Laws H, McKernan, J. Endoscopic management of peptic ulcer disease. Ann Surg 1993;217:548–555.
19. Hinder RA, Klingler PJ, Perdikis G, Smith SL. Management of the failed antireflux operation. Surg Clin North Am 1997;77:1083–1098.
20. Kamolz T, Bammer T, Granderath FA, Pointner R. Comorbidity of aerophagia in GERD patients: outcome of laparoscopic antireflux surgery. Scand J Gast 2002;37:138–143.
21. Farrell TM, Richardson WS, Halkar R, et al. Nissen fundoplication improves gastric motility in patients with delayed gastric emptying. Surg Endosc 2001;15:271–274.
22. Van Sickle K, et al. Delayed gastric emptying in patients undergoing antireflux surgery: analysis of a management algorithm. Presented at annual meeting of Society of Laparoscopic Surgery, New York, NY, September 2004.
23. DeMeester TR, Stein HJ. Surgical treatment of gastroesophageal reflux disease. In: Castell D, ed. The Esophagus. Boston: Little, Brown, 1992:579–626.
24. Hunter JG, Smith CD, Branum GD, et al. Laparoscopic fundoplication failures: patterns of failure and response to fundoplication revision. Ann Surg 1999;230: 595–606.
25. Soper NJ, Dunnegan D. Anatomic fundoplication failure after laparoscopic antireflux surgery. Ann Surg 1999;229:669–677.
26. Hunter JG, Swanstrom L, Waring JP. Dysphagia after laparoscopic antireflux surgery. The impact of operative technique. Ann Surg 1996;224:51–57.

27. Watson DI, Pike GK, Baigrie RJ, et al. Prospective double-blind randomized trial of laparoscopic Nissen fundoplication with division and without division of short gastric vessels. Ann Surg 1997;226:642–652.

28. Watson DI, Davies N, Devitt PG, Jamieson GG. Importance of dissection of the hernia sac in laparoscopic surgery for large hiatal hernias. Arch Surg 1999;134:1069–1073.

29. Velanovich V. Medication usage and additional esophageal procedures after antireflux surgery. Surg Laparosc Endosc Perc Tech 2003;13:161–164.

30. Lord RV, Kaminski A, Oberg S, et al. Absence of gastroesophageal reflux disease in a majority of patients taking acid suppression medications after Nissen fundoplication. J Gastrointest Surg 2002;6:3–10.

31. Galvani C, Fisichella PM, Gorodner MV, et al. Symptoms are a poor indicator of reflux status after fundoplication for gastroesophageal reflux disease: role of esophageal functions tests. Arch Surg 2003;138:514–518.

32. Contini S, Scarpignato C. Endoscopic treatment of gastro-esophageal reflux disease: a systemic review. Digest Liver Dis 2003;35:818–838.

33. Utley D. The Stretta procedure: device, technique, and pre-clinical study data. Gastro Endosc Clin N Am 2003;13:135–145.

34. Houston H, Khaitan L, Holzman M, Richards WO. First year experience of patients undergoing the Stretta procedure. Surg Endosc 2003;17:401–404.

35. Triadafilopoulos G. Clinical experience with the Stretta procedure. Gastro Endosc Clin N Am 2003;13:147–155.

36. McClusky D 3rd, et al. Fluoroscopic guided Stretta procedure increases accuracy and reliability. Presented at SAGES annual meeting, Denver, CO, March 2004.

37. McClusky DA 3rd, Khaitan L, Smith CD. Utility of radiofrequency ablation after failed antireflux surgery. Presented at Digestive Disease Week, New Orleans, May 2004.

38. Chadalavada R, Lin E, Swafford V, et al. Comparative results of endoluminal gastroplasty and laparoscopic antireflux surgery for the treatment of GERD. Surg Endosc 2004;18:261–265. Epub 2003;DOI:10.1007/s00464-003-8921-3.

39. Swain P, Park P, Mills T. Bard EndoCinch: the device, the technique, and pre-clinical studies. Gastrointest Endosc Clin N Am 2003;13:75–88.

40. Rothstein R, Filipi C. Endoscopic suturing for gastroesophageal reflux disease: clinical outcome with the Bard EndoCinch. Gastrointest Endosc Clin N Am 2003;13:89–101.

41. Watson D, Jamieson GG, Game PA, et al. Laparoscopic reoperation following failed antireflux surgery. Br J Surg 1999;86:98–101.

42. Pera M, Deschamps C, Taillefer R, Duranceau A. Uncut Collis-Nissen gastroplasty: early functional results. Ann Thorac Surg 1995;60:915–920.

43. Ritter MP, Peters JH, DeMeester TR, et al. Treatment of advanced gastroesophageal reflux disease with Collis gastroplasty and Belsey partial fundoplication. Arch Surg 1998;133:523–528.

44. Johnson AB, Oddsdottir M, Hunter JG. Laparoscopic Collis gastroplasty and Nissen fundoplication: a new technique for the management of esophageal foreshortening. Surg Endosc 1998;12:1055–1060.

45. Donahue PE, Samelson S, Nyhus LM, Bombeck CT. The floppy Nissen fundoplication. Effective long-term control of pathologic reflux. Arch Surg 1985;120:663–668.

46. Jamieson G. The results of anti-reflux surgery and re-operative anti-reflux surgery. Gullet 1993;3:41–45.

47. Hunter JG. Approach and management of patients with recurrent gastro-esophageal reflux disease. J Gastrointest Surg 2001;5:451–457.

48. DePaula A, Hashiba K, Bafutto M, Macado CA. Laparoscopic reoperations after failed and complicated antireflux operations. Surg Endosc 1995;9:681–686.

49. Smith CD, McClusky DA 3rd, Rajad MA, et al. When fundoplication fails: redo? Presented at the 116th annual meeting of the Southern Surgical Association; submitted to Annals of Surgery.

50. Kirk RM, Stoddard CJ. Complications of Surgery of the Upper Gastrointestinal Tract. Bailliere Tindall, 1986:148–159.

51. Hill L, et al. The Esophagus—Medical and Surgical Management. Philadelphia: WB Saunders, 1988:193–197.

52. Patti MG, Pellegrini CA, Horgan S, et al. Minimally invasive surgery for achalasia. Ann Surg 1999;230:587–594.

53. Hunter JG, Trus TL, Branum GD, Waring JP. Laparoscopic Heller myotomy and fundoplication for achalasia. Ann Surg 1997;225:655–665.

54. Sharp KW, Khaitan L, Scholz S, et al. 100 consecutive minimally invasive Heller myotomies: lessons learned. Ann Surg 2002;235:631–639.

55. Patti MG, Molena D, Fisichella PM, et al. Laparoscopic Heller myotomy and Dor fundoplication for achalasia: analysis of successes and failures. Arch Surg 2001;136:870–877.

56. Morino M, Rebecchi F, Festa V, Garrone C. Preoperative pneumatic dilatation represents a risk factor for laparoscopic Heller myotomy. Surg Endosc 1997;11:359–361.

57. Thompkins RB. Reoperative Esophageal Surgery. JB Lippincott, 1988:33–40.

58. Ellis H. Failure after esophagomyotomy for esophageal motor disorders. Causes, prevention, and management. Chest Surg Clin N Am 1997;7:476–488.

59. Raiser F, Perdikis G, Hinder RA, et al. Heller myotomy via minimal-access surgery. An evaluation of antireflux procedures. Arch Surg 1996;131:593–597.

60. Zaninotto G, Costantini M, Portale G, et al. Etiology, diagnosis, and treatment of failures after laparoscopic Heller myotomy for achalasia. Ann Surg 2002;235:186–192.

61. Peters JH, Kauer WK, Crookes PF, et al. Esophageal resection with colon interposition for end-stage achalasia. Arch Surg 1995;130:632–637.

CHAPTER 11

Reoperative Colorectal Surgery

Mark Lane Welton, MD

Précis

Reoperation is common and an integral part of the treatment of patients with complicated colon and rectal diseases. The critical juncture in the management of these patients is often at the initial operation where the surgeon must anticipate the second operation and prepare for the reoperation. We will review the preoperative planning and the intraoperative decision-making that facilitates the surgical management of the colorectal patient.

Introduction

Planned reoperation in colon and rectal surgery is common. Patients with perforated diverticular disease, inflammatory bowel disease, and complicated perianal sepsis often require multiple or staged procedures. The critical point in the management of these patients is preparing for the reoperation, whether it is by creating a loop ileostomy instead of an end ileostomy or placement of a Seton in anticipation of a definitive repair of a fistula in ano. In this article we will review the preoperative planning and the intraoperative decision-making that facilitates the surgical management of the colorectal patient.

Whenever a second operation is planned, the surgeon will benefit by anticipating his/her needs for the second operation during the first. If a proctectomy is planned for a subsequent operation, it is best to avoid dissection in the pelvis. Do not mobilize the rectum. Transect the bowel at the sacral promontory, and leave those planes undisturbed. Similarly, if it is planned to mobilize the splenic flexure at a subsequent operation, it is often better to leave that to the second operation, because adhesions may form between the mobilized colon and surrounding structures that are harder to disrupt than the original attachments. Finally, one must consider reentry into the abdomen. Seprafilm is the only adhesion barrier approved for general abdominal surgery. Although no studies thus far show conclusively that

Seprafilm decreases the incidence of bowel obstruction, we have found that placing the product over a rectal stump, over the small bowel and under the omentum, and under the incision has greatly simplified our planned reoperations. Studies have confirmed the safety and efficacy of Seprafilm with fewer and less dense adhesions at reoperation.[1,2] This has been our experience. When the agent is placed over the rectal stump, the small bowel is less likely to be stuck to the top of the rectal staple line, and the pelvic dissection is less complicated. This has resulted in decreased time spent lysing adhesions and shorter reoperation times. We also routinely wrap stomas with Seprafilm when the stoma is considered temporary.[3] Seprafilm makes the peristomal dissection easier and the operative time is significantly decreased.

Reoperation for Stomas

Creation of temporary and permanent stomas is a frequent practice in colon and rectal surgery. "Protecting" diverting stomas are made proximal to anastomosis created after colonic resections for diverticulitis, low rectal cancer, restorative proctocolectomy, and many other high risk anastomoses. The operative difficulty associated with closure of stomas is greatly underestimated and often relegated to the junior resident. Senior residents and faculty, however, quickly gain appreciation for the difficulties associated with this "minor surgery." We will describe our approach to these operations in some detail.

The loop ileostomy is taken down by disconnecting the mucocutaneous junction with electrocautery. The dissection is carried into the subcutaneous tissue sharply with electrocautery or Metzenbaum scissors. A Scott or Lone Star retractor may help in the larger patients but simple retraction with Army-Navy retractors is satisfactory for most. It is helpful to stay right on the bowel surface during the dissection, as the tissues will separate most easily when this is done. If the surgeon veers too far into the fat to avoid creating an enterotomy, it is generally quite a bit more difficult to define a good dissection plane. The stoma may be kept closed with Allis clamps to avoid spillage as the dissection progresses. Once the fascia are visualized, it is often preferable to sweep around the stoma with a finger to gently break up loose adhesions between the loop of bowel involved in the stoma, and other loops of bowel and the abdominal wall. This may identify a few residual adhesions that may be sharply divided under direct visualization. In large patients, these last few bands may be at the base of a long, narrow, deep hole. A small incision made at the skin level (that can be excised with the elliptical closure) and a small extension of the fascial defect can radically improve exposure and avoid an injury to poorly visualized underlying small bowel that would mandate a large midline incision. Once the stoma has been completely mobilized, the bowel is drawn out of the abdomen and an anastomosis may be created with suture or staples.

A stapled anastomosis is created by passing the arm of a gastrointestinal anastomosis (GIA) stapler down the proximal and distal lumens of the bowel. The stapler is closed while ensuring the mesentery is rotated as far from the staple line as possible. It is not possible to appose the antimesenteric surfaces precisely, because the bowel wall and mesentery are not divided completely when a loop ileostomy is created. After the stapler is fired, the staple line is inspected for hemostasis. Bleeding along the staple may be controlled with interrupted absorbable sutures placed on the staple line from the luminal surface. The enterotomy can then be closed with either a linear stapler or interrupted absorbable sutures.

A sutured anastomosis is generally created by "freshening" the edges and closing the enterotomy with one layer of absorbable suture placed full thickness in an interrupted fashion.

After the bowel is closed, the abdomen is irrigated and the fascia closed with slowly absorbable suture. The skin edges can be excised in an elliptical fashion and the skin closed primarily. The skin may also be closed loosely over Telfa wicks with staples, or left open and packed.

We have attempted to avoid loop colostomies, preferring the loop ileostomy because of stoma size and ease of management. When we create a loop colostomy it is generally a divided loop, which makes the stoma somewhat smaller but allows for the possibility of stoma closure through a peristomal incision. If a loop colostomy is created for a distal rectal obstruction, then the bowel may still be divided and a corner of the distal loop brought up at the same stoma site to allow for decompression of the distal obstruction with a mucus fistula without burdening the patient with an entirely separate stoma site.

Closure of the divided loop colostomy is achieved through the approaches described for the loop ileostomy. An exception is when the loop colostomy is being converted to an end at the time of proctectomy. Here again, the divided loop with a corner mucus fistula, as described above, is preferred, because the majority of stoma may be left untouched while the edge of the mucus fistula is taken down. Repair of the colostomy is completed with a few interrupted absorbable sutures.

We prefer to close an end ileostomy (or end colostomy) by detaching the stoma from the skin at the mucocutaneous junction with electrocautery. As with the loop stomas, the dissection is carried into the abdomen, care taken to stay on the bowel surface. Once the abdomen is entered, the surgeon passes a finger into the abdomen to bluntly dissect the bowel off the midline incision. The abdomen may then be entered sharply with cautery while the surgeon's hand protects the underlying bowel. The abdomen may then be explored and intestinal continuity reestablished.

Reoperation for Stoma Complications

Peristomal complications include obstruction, hernia, prolapse, stricture, ischemia, and fistula. Small bowel obstructions occur in roughly 5% to 14% of patients and may be directly related to the stoma or intra-abdominal adhesions.[4-8] If a patient develops a bowel obstruction at the stoma, and the stoma is temporary as in the case of a stoma created proximal to an ileoanal pouch or a low rectal anastomosis, then the surgeon may wish to treat the obstruction conservatively at first, while the distal bowel is evaluated for integrity radiographically. If the distal anastomosis is intact, then closure of the stoma and reestablishment of intestinal continuity will resolve the obstruction and minimize the number of operations the patient must undergo.

If the stoma is permanent, and the obstruction is felt to be at or near the stoma, then a peristomal incision may be created and local exploration may reveal the site of obstruction in the subcutaneous tissue or just below the fascia. If not, then the peristomal incision may be used to clear the midline incision of adherent bowel and ease reexploration through the old midline incision. If the site of obstruction is localized preoperatively and is thought to be remote to the stoma, then a standard midline incision should be carried out.

All patients who undergo stoma creation have, by definition, a hernia, with bowel passing through the muscular defect. Hernias become problematic if a bowel obstruction develops because of the hernia, if a stoma appliance cannot be fitted because of the hernia, or if skin necrosis develops because of pressure from the intestinal contents within the hernia. Some hernias may become large enough that loss of domain of the abdominal contents becomes a significant issue. Parastomal hernias more commonly occur with colostomies than with ileostomies and may develop in approximately 10% of stomates, with 10% to 20% of these requiring operative interventions.[9]

Bowel obstruction within a peristomal hernia may be easily addressed by a peristomal incision at the mucocutaneous junction. Adhesive bands within the hernia sac may lead to obstruction or the bowel may be twisted upon itself. Once the adhesive bands are lysed and the bowel is returned to the abdominal cavity, the surgeon may try to sweep the bowel free of the abdominal wall and simply clear the peritoneal surface of bowel so that the colostomy or ileostomy may simply be translocated to the other lower quadrant in a mirror fashion, especially if the patient was satisfied with the location of their stoma. A skin defect is created in a matching location in the opposite lower quadrant, and a fascia defect created over the operating surgeon's hand holding a laparotomy sponge. This is the preferred first treatment of a symptomatic peristomal hernia.[10] If the hernia recurs, then a mesh repair is suggested.[10]

A mesh hernia repair may also be achieved with a peristomal incision, where the bowel is mobilized and the mesh in place above the fascia. A defect is created in the mesh and the bowel is passed through it. The stoma is recreated with interrupted sutures between the bowel wall and skin. If a longstanding hernia led to stretching of the skin, it may be necessary to narrow the skin defect somewhat with interrupted sutures. This seems to work well and does not interfere with the fit of the appliance. A laparoscopic repair of parastomal hernias has been described in which mesh is stapled over the abdominal wall defect.[11] However, stoma translocation is often such a minimally invasive procedure that a laparoscopic approach may not realize tremendous benefit when comparisons are made.

Stoma prolapse may occur in 1% to 3% of ileostomies and end colostomies.[12] Transverse loop colostomies are associated with prolapse in up to 25% of the cases and for this reason transverse loop stomas have largely been replaced by diverting loop ileostomies when proximal diversion is necessary. Nonetheless, prolapse may occur with any stoma. Prolapse that does not result in bowel obstruction is not an urgent problem. Some may intermittently prolapse more or less and reduce spontaneously without any obvious clinical sequelae. However, prolapse may result in obstruction, strangulation, erosion of the bowel surface by chronic contact with the stoma appliance. or an unsightly bulge in the patient's clothing. These issues are relatively easily addressed with a peristomal incision that disconnects the bowel wall from the skin. Care is taken to stay right at the mucocutaneous junction so that the stoma skin defect is not significantly enlarged, resulting in a flatter stoma. The prolapsing bowel is delivered and the redundant length transected without entering the abdomen. The stoma is matured with interrupted 3-0 chromic catgut suture. An ileostomy must be matured in a standard "Brooke" fashion, in which the suture is placed full thickness bowel wall, then in a seromuscular fashion 3 to 4 cm proximal on the bowel and then to the dermis of the skin. Only eight sutures are required, and only four need to be placed in this fashion. The intervening sutures may simply be placed full thickness bowel wall to dermis. Colostomies do not need to be "Brooked" in this fashion. A flush colostomy functions well and the skin does not need to be protected from the effluent of a colostomy, as it does from the caustic effluent of an ileostomy.

Ischemia of the bowel used to create a stoma frequently leads to a stricture or stomal stenosis. An ischemic stoma may best be avoided by transecting the bowel that will be used for the stoma early in the conduct of the operation so that it can be observed for adequacy of blood supply throughout the remainder of the case. If the blood supply appears poor, a more proximal segment may be selected. Tension on the bowel at the end of a case can stretch a viable stoma into ischemia. This may be particularly problematic in obese patients whose bowel may not be adequately mobilized to be drawn tension-free through a generous abdominal wall. In this instance, it may be beneficial to create an end loop stoma, where the bowel is divided but the end is not brought up to the abdominal wall; rather, a portion just proximal to the end with less tension on the blood supply is brought up for the stoma.

If during the conduct of the operation it does not appear that there is too much tension on the bowel, and the blood supply seems adequate, but postoperatively the stoma becomes ischemic, close observation is warranted. This may occur in 1% to 10% of colostomies and 1% to 5% of ileostomies.[13–17] It is not necessary to take back a necrotic stoma, as long as the bowel remains viable at the level of the fascia. The level of transition to viability may be visualized directly with a flashlight and glass blood-draw tube. If the bowel is necrotic below the level of the fascia, then intraperitoneal spillage and sepsis will occur and immediate surgery is indicated. A stoma that necroses but stays viable above the fascia will stricture, but can be revised at a later date.

Strictures occur in 2% to 12% of colostomies and only rarely in ileostomies.[4,5,18,19] Isolated strictures at the skin level may be repaired by simply disconnecting a portion of the bowel from the skin at the mucocutaneous junction and incising the skin perpendicular to the stoma defect, disrupting the fibrotic band and creating a larger aperture. The stoma is recreated with a few interrupted absorbable sutures placed between the bowel and abdominal wall.

In more complicated cases, it may be necessary to disconnect the entire stoma and mobilize the bowel circumferentially down through the fascia and into the abdomen to obtain a tension-free anastomosis. The surgeon may even be forced to reenter the abdomen through the midline to gain enough mobility to create a healthy, tension-free stoma.

Fistulas at the stoma site may be secondary to Crohn's disease, a technical error in the creation of the stoma, or perforation from a foreign body. Fistulas may develop in 7% to 10% of patients with Crohn's disease.[5,20] However, a fistula in a patient with Crohn's disease cannot be assumed to be secondary to the disease process, as a technical error with full-thickness placement of an intended seromuscular stitch may result in a fistula. Patients should not suffer through extended courses of steroids for this type of "pseudo-Crohn's" disease. Thus, it is incumbent upon the surgeon to establish that there is disease activity at the stoma site before a fistula is attributed to Crohn's disease. If it is Crohn's disease, it may be possible to manage the fistula locally by expanding the ring of the appliance to capture the effluent and protect the skin while waiting for medical therapy to assist in controlling the disease. In other instances it is valuable to view the peristomal disease as if it were perianal disease and attempt to maintain sepsis control with Setons, Pezzar drains, unroofing abscesses, performing fistulotomies, etc., until the disease remits. If the Crohn's disease is the source of the fistula and it is limited, resection and creation of a new stoma may control the symptoms.

When the source of the fistula is a clear technical error, reoperation and revision of the stoma locally should resolve the situation.

Recurrent Rectal Cancer

If rectal cancer recurs locally, it often presents a significant challenge to the surgeon that is best approached with a multidisciplinary team approach. Prior to embarking on a large operation it is critical to adequately image the patient to exclude extrapelvic disease or distant metastases as well as to assess resectability. The preoperative assessment should include computerized tomography (CT) scans of the chest, abdomen, and pelvis, and may include magnetic resonance imaging (MRI), positron emission tomography (PET), and even PET/CT scan. CT and MRI are limited in their ability to differentiate fibrosis from recurrence, but interval increase in size or enhancement with gadolinium on MRI are suggestive of recurrent disease. Bony and prostatic invasion or involvement of the sciatic nerve are often best visualized with MRI. PET scans detect increased metabolic activity, but cannot distinguish inflammation from recurrence. CT-guided biopsy can generally establish the diagnosis preoperatively.

Once the imaging has excluded extrapelvic disease, the team can focus on how best to approach the pelvic recurrence. If the patient did not receive pelvic radiation therapy as part of their initial treatment, this often helps shrink the tumor away from vital pelvic structures, facilitating the pelvic reoperation. It also allows a time interval for extrapelvic disease to present. The chemoradiation therapy is generally standard low-dose chemotherapy (bolus, infusional, or oral 5-fluorouracil) with roughly 5040 cGy delivered over 6 weeks with a 6-week waiting period. The chest, abdomen, and pelvis should be reimaged with CT. The involved surrounding structures dictate the consultations required.

Curative reoperation for recurrent rectal cancer requires the ability to obtain a negative circumferential margin (anterior, posterior, and lateral). Previously opened planes may harbor tumor, and the surgeon must therefore attempt to stay outside in previously unoperated tissues. Adherent scar, inflammation, and tumor are generally indistinguishable and should be resected with the tumor en bloc when possible. This is true for involved surrounding structures where tumor or inflammation may extend into the uterus, vagina, bladder, or prostate. The sacrum may be resected en bloc as well up to the level of S-2, above which sacral instability becomes problematic. If it appears that the bone cortex is intact but the tumor abuts the sacrum, resection with intraoperative radiation therapy or placement of after-loading catheters reportedly improves local control in the absence of gross disease. Some have found the after-loading catheters difficult to place in a satisfactory fashion and have moved to excluding intra-abdominal contents from the pelvis at the time of surgery, and placing the catheters under radiographic guidance postoperatively.

Lateral pelvic sidewall is often the rate-limiting step, in that these structures cannot be resected. A grossly positive lateral margin subjects the patient to all the morbidity of the procedure with no proven survival benefit.

The patient is placed in the modified lithotomy position. Cystoscopy and ureteral catheter placement is performed by the urologic service to assist in the identification of the ureters intraoperatively. This is a critical step in nearly all reoperative pelvic surgery. It may not prevent injury to the ureters, as the tumor, radiation, or chronic inflammation can obscure the catheters, but if the ureters are injured, the wire within the catheter is generally visible, facilitating identification of the injury and intraoperative repair. The use of intraoperative indigo carmine or methylene blue may also be helpful when there is a question of ureteral injury, but when ureteral catheters are present the dye may pass down the catheters and not extravasate into the abdomen or pelvis, giving a false sense of security. If confusion persists as to where the ureters may be, dissection up out of the irradiated pelvis generally allows identification of the ureters and tracing of the structures into the pelvis.

After placement of ureteral catheters, the abdomen may be reentered through the old midline incision, and the upper abdomen is explored. If an end colostomy exists, there may be no need to address the stoma. If a stoma does not exist, we prefer to create the stoma site before making the midline incision, as this decreases the chances of creating a stoma that traverses the abdominal wall tangentially. Further, it allows the surgeon to enter through "virgin" territory and sweep the bowel off the old midline incision, thereby decreasing the chance of injuring the bowel adherent to the old midline incision.

After entry, careful adhesiolysis should performed to the extent that is necessary to mobilize the small bowel and colon out of the pelvis. Adherent loops of small bowel may be transected proximal and distal to the tumor with a gastrointestinal stapling device to allow en bloc resection. If possible, the ureters are identified in the abdomen and traced into the pelvis. Vessel loops may be used to encircle the ureters so that traction may be placed on them where necessary during the pelvic dissection. When a colorectal anastomosis is anticipated, it is often helpful to transect the bowel early, at a point on the bowel that appears satisfactory for creation of a stoma. This provides the surgeon a good handle for anterior traction on the bowel and improved exposure of the presacral space. It also allows time for the bowel to declare viability while the abdomen is open and the surgeon can choose a more proximal segment of bowel if needed.

Placing anterior traction on the colorectal remnant, dissection is started in the presacral space and carried as far distally as possible. Once tumor is excluded above S-2, the dissection is carried as far distally as possible, and a biopsy is taken of the distal margin. If this is negative, the anterior plane is explored. If the tumor is large, posterior or even adherent to sacrum, it is often preferable to dissect anteriorly, especially if these planes have not been violated previously. In women, this native plane can be developed by performing a hysterectomy and coming through the vagina to identify the rectum distal to the recurrence. In a man, this may be anterior to the bladder and prostate. The lateral dissection is carried down to the levator ani muscles. The dissection can often then be continued in a distal-to-proximal fashion, when it was nearly impossible to find the proper plane by dissecting in a proximal to distal fashion.

At times it may be necessary for the surgeon to proceed with dissection in a proximal-to-distal fashion in the absence of an identifiable plane. In this situation, hydrodissection has been advocated. Saline is injected between the sacrum and the tissue to be resected to develop a space where a potential space exists and promote cautery dissection without entry into the presacral plexus.

In other circumstances, the surgeon may need to proceed cautiously and violate planes that are ordinarily avoided in order to remove the tumor en bloc. In those circumstances, the surgeon should attempt to identify the ureters, iliac vessels, hypogastric vessels, etc., before they pass into the pelvis, tracing them into the pelvis with careful sharp dissection. Before proceeding into the portion of the dissection where the surgeon will pass into planes normally avoided, the anesthesiologists should have large-bore intravenous access, blood should be available in the room, and the surgical team prepared for blood loss. Prolene, 2-0, and 4-0 should be available as well as long needle drivers, long forceps, and side biting Satinsky clamps. The argon beam coagulator (ABC) is an excellent tool for dissection in this circumstance. The ABC may be set at ~150 and used to carve out the tumor with a margin. If bleeding is encountered, "resting" on the source with ABC is often effective at gaining control. Sterile tacks are rarely used but they can be helpful.

They must be applied with enough pressure to crush the boney cortex of the sacrum, thereby controlling the interosseous venous plexus. This venous plexus communicates with a venous plexus on the dorsal aspect of the sacrum, making intra-abdominal control challenging. In these situations it is often best to pack the pelvis with laps and return in 24 to 48 hours after resuscitation is complete.

The abdominal phase of the operation is complete and the patient is turned prone. Through a large perineal incision, the dissection is carried anteriorly and the pelvis is entered. The levator ani muscles are divided. The sacrospinous and sacrotuberous ligaments are divided posteriorly. The gluteal muscles are lifted from the posterior sacrum and the operating surgeon's finger may be passed through the sciatic notch to guide the level of sacral transection. A laminectomy is performed at that level, and the sacral nerves and dural sac are divided and ligated. The anterior sacral cortex and presacral fascia are divided and the specimen retrieved.

At the completion of these operations, a large pelvic cavity and skin defect may be left that is difficult to close. Omental flaps have been recommended to fill the pelvis, but in the reoperative situation this is often not possible. We prefer to work with the plastic surgeons to mobilize a right rectus flap if a cystectomy with an ileal urinary conduit is not performed. This flap may be harvested with a large skin island that is helpful in closing the perineum, where tissue may have lost elasticity from irradiation. When an ileal urinary conduit is necessary then gracilis or gluteal flaps may be chosen.

Abdominal sacral resection for recurrent rectal cancer is associated with significant morbidity (80% to 100%), blood loss of 3 to 12 L, and mortality of 0% to 9%. However, the 5-year survival is 31% to 33%, suggesting that in well-selected patients, local control and cure may be achieved.[21,22]

Recurrent Colon Cancer

As with recurrent rectal cancer, the initial evaluation of the patient with recurrent colon cancer must exclude distant unresectable disease. A complete colonoscopy is preferable, but if the bowel proximal to the lesion will be sacrificed in the planned operation, as in an ileocolectomy for a recurrent cancer at the hepatic flexure, the proximal bowel does not have to be visualized. If the proximal bowel will not be sacrificed, as in a recurrent descending colon cancer, the preoperative evaluation may consist of a complete colonoscopy, a colonoscopy and barium enema when the bowel proximal to the recurrence could not be directly visualized with a colonoscope, or virtual colonoscopy (CT colonography), which is limited in its availability and documented efficacy. If necessary, we prefer intraoperative evaluation of the proximal bowel with colonoscopy after the anastomosis has been performed with the colonoscope passed per anus.

Colon cancer that invades surrounding organs such as the spleen, a kidney, small bowel, stomach, the abdominal wall, etc., may be resected with curative intent. Reexploration in the elective situation is generally achieved through the old midline wound. After the abdomen is entered, carcinomatosis should be excluded prior to initiating a large and potentially morbid procedure. If carcinomatosis is encountered and the patient is relatively asymptomatic, a confirmatory biopsy and abortion of the planned operation may be in the patient's best interest. Advances have been made with chemotherapy for colorectal cancer, and some patients are now experiencing dramatic responses to the newer agents. Tumor that can be monitored with serial CT imaging is necessary for inclusion in trials, and that may be a reason to abort the planned procedure.

If the patient is experiencing obstructive symptoms or requiring frequent transfusions, then resection with primary anastomosis or creation of a stoma may be beneficial. Resection as a palliative procedure has the benefit of removing tumor that may continue to be a source of blood loss, may perforate, or may invade other vital structures. The disadvantages to resection include the possibility of a permanent stoma, anastomotic dehiscence, and need to resect surrounding structures to extirpate the tumor. Patients with carcinomatosis may have extensive studding of the bowel with tumor, making anastomosis hazardous, and in this instance a stoma may be the best option. However, when a clear surface on the bowel proximal and distal to the recurrence can be identified, and the tumor can be removed, then en bloc resection is preferred. Intestinal continuity is reestablished in a standard fashion when possible.

Reoperation for Abscess/Fistulous Disease

One of the most vexing problems that can face the general and colorectal surgeon is recurrent perianal sepsis. Patients have often undergone multiple previous procedures, and compromise of the sphincter mechanism is a concern. Certainly STDs (e.g., gonorrhea, syphilis, herpes, chancroid, granuloma inguinale, lymphogranuloma venereum), tuberculosis, Crohn's disease, malignancy, pelvic disease, pilonidal sinus, hidradenitis suppurativa, and actimomycosis must all be considered. A detailed history will define patients at risk. Cultures of the perianal skin and wound may be confirmatory. When Crohn's is suspected, preoperative evaluation with colonoscopy, upper gastrointestinal series, and CT may be of benefit. However, unless Crohn's disease or another intra-abdominal source, such as a perforated colon cancer or diverticular disease, is suspected then preoperative imaging studies are often of limited benefit. We prefer an initial thorough exam under anesthesia. Occult masses may be palpated with a bidigital exam (one finger in the anus/rectum and one finger palpating the perineum). Particular attention should be paid to the deep postanal space to exclude an occult source for multiple fistulas. This is the most common cause, in our experience, for recurrent disease when the patient has been treated elsewhere. The deep postanal space is best appreciated by pinching the tissue between the rectum and the coccyx in a sweeping massaging fashion with one finger in the anus and another on the perineum. Induration in this region may suggest the occult source of the patient's problems. The surgeon may also pass a crypt hook or lacrimal probe through an external opening, and this may identify the direction of the tract. Methylene blue diluted with saline may be injected through the external opening with an 18-gauge angiocatheter, and the internal opening may be visualized with an anoscope as blue extravasates from the primary or internal opening. Hydrogen peroxide can be used in a similar fashion. Anoscopy with exploration of the crypts with crypt hooks may suggest a primary internal opening. If these maneuvers fail, intraoperative sound with hydrogen peroxide may also reveal an otherwise occult source. It is unusual for a source to not be identified with one of these techniques. If none is, the surgeon may either leave a drainage catheter in place or widen the external opening and curette the tract with the hope of establishing more adequate external drainage of the resolving abscess.

When the source is found at this evaluation, the surgeon may perform a definitive fistulotomy or place a Seton or catheter to control sepsis and allow a more definitive repair as a staged operation. The decision to proceed with a fistulotomy must take into consideration the amount of muscle that would be transected with the planned procedure. If the tract is superficial, then a fistulotomy may be carried out. The edges of tract may be saucerized to decrease the chance the edges will come together and lead to a recurrent fistula. The crypt should be ablated. If the tract is deeper, the edges may be marsupialized by taking the edge of the tract at the skin and sewing it in a running fashion with a rapidly absorbable suture to the smooth, mature tract at the bottom of the fistula wound. This eases wound management for the patient and may also decrease the rate of recurrence.

When it is unclear how much muscle is involved it is appropriate to place a catheter such as a Pezzer drain through the external opening, or a Seton through both the external and internal openings, and return for a definitive repair at a subsequent operation. This allows for resolution of the associated inflammation. At reoperation a fistulotomy is often possible because with the decrease in inflammation it becomes clear that it is safe to divide the tissue overlying the tract. If not, the surgeon may choose to seal the tract with fibrin glue or commercial products that achieve the same result.

Generally, if fibrin glue repair is attempted, the tract is curetted or abraded with a sponge to prepare the surface of the fistula. The glue is injected through the external opening. It is critical to maintain a constant and steady pressure on the syringe with the glue so as to avoid sealing the catheter through which the glue is being injected. The glue should extrude through the internal opening, where a plug of material will accumulate. The catheter is slowly withdrawn, laying down a tract of glue from proximal to distal. After this is complete, some surgeons suture closed the internal or primary opening, but this is not mandatory. The success rate of fibrin glue repair is roughly 50%, but because the risks are minimal many surgeons and patients prefer multiple attempts with this procedure prior to other repairs that have associated risks to the continence mechanism.[23–25]

Mucosal advancement flaps, rectal sleeve advancement, and anal mucosal advancement flaps are all effective means by which complicated perianal fistulas may be repaired. A mucosal advancement flap is an effective option when the rectal mucosa is healthy and pliable.[26,27] This is often the case after cryptoglandular sources of perianal sepsis have been controlled with catheters or Setons. It is also the case when anorectal Crohn's disease has been controlled with maximal medical therapy and surgical drainage. It is of utmost importance that the surgeon assesses the mobility of the rectal mucosa before initiating the dissection to mobilize the rectal mucosal flap. This is most reliably performed by sweeping an anoscope in a proximal-to-distal manner, such that the healthy, supple mucosa can be seen bunching up under the lip of the scope. Diseased mucosa will appear flat and glistening, and will not fold up and appear mobile. Once mobility has been assured, a rectangular flap is mobilized, with the distal aspect of the flap incision, the apex of the flap, below the internal opening of the fistula. A broad-based flap is created with the incisions extending along two parallel lines up into the rectum. The dissection is next carried out under the flap, taking care to mobilize the entire rectal mucosa, submucosa, and a thin layer of the internal sphincter, which becomes the circular muscle of the rectum as the dissection is carried more proximally. Care is taken to avoid injury to the external sphincter during this process. The internal opening of the tract will by necessity be transected as the dissection carries proximally. This is often the most difficult portion of the dissection, as the planes may be obliterated by chronic inflammation. Once the tract is transected, it becomes easier to develop the plane once again, and this mobilization has to be carried proximally enough to allow a tension-free anastomosis between the rectal mucosa and the anus. The flap is sutured to the surrounding tissues by placing the interrupted sutures at the proximal margins of the flaps on either side. The flap is then secured down both sides and the mucocutaneous junction re-created with interrupted absorbable sutures. If a Pezzer drain was initially used through the external or secondary opening to control sepsis preoperatively, it may be left in place to counterdrain the flap. It can be removed in the office at 4 to 6 weeks. Initial success rates of 80% to 85% are reported, but Crohn's disease may lead to recurrent fistulization.[26,27]

If the rectal mucosa has been previously mobilized and is no longer suitable for use as a flap, the surgeon may consider an anal mucosal flap.[28] This mobilizes the relatively more supple anal mucosa proximally into the rectum. The internal opening is excised and the anal mucosa mobilized as a diamond flap, in much the same way as a flap is created for anal stenosis. When the diamond flap is mobilized, care is taken to avoid undermining and devascularizing the tissue. Once enough tissue is mobilized, the flap is sutured in place with interrupted absorbable sutures.

Finally, rectal sleeve advancement can be performed for repair of complicated recurrent perianal fistulous disease secondary to Crohn's disease when a stricture is present, or even after a restorative proctocolectomy with an ileoanal pouch for ulcerative colitis.[29] Although it is possible to perform a rectangular pouch advancement, flap repair of a fistula as described above with a tongue of the pouch brought down over an internal opening, it is often easier to mobilize the entire pouch circumferentially, and this may lead to less tension on the anastomosis. When Crohn's disease has led to circumferential stricturing, it is not possible to visualize the bowel with an anoscope above the stricture. This limits the ability of the surgeon to mobilize a standard rectangular flap, and it is preferable to mobilize the bowel circumferentially. This allows for resection of the stricture, resection of the bowel that is the internal source of the fistula, and repair of the fistula with healthy proximal bowel. The rectal mucosa is divided circumferentially distal to the stricture and fistula. The dissection is carried full thickness on the bowel wall, taking care to avoid injury to the underlying sphincter mechanism. The fistula is transected as the dissection is carried proximally, but once above the stricture and fistula, the tissue tends to become much healthier and the planes easier to follow. The entire circumference of the bowel is mobilized distally, the stricture and fistula are resected, and the anastomosis to the distal rectal mucosa or anus is created with an absorbable suture in an interrupted fashion.

REFERENCES

1. Beck DE, Cohen Z, Fleshman JW, et al. A prospective, randomized, multicenter, controlled study of the safety of Seprafilm adhesion barrier in abdominopelvic surgery of the intestine. Dis Colon Rectum 2003;46:1310–1319.
2. Beck DE. The role of Seprafilm bioresorbable membrane in adhesion prevention. Eur J Surg Suppl 1997;577:49–55.
3. Tang CL, Seow-Choen F, Fook-Chong S, Eu KW. Bioresorbable adhesion barrier facilitates early closure of the defunctioning ileostomy after rectal excision: a prospective, randomized trial. Dis Colon Rectum 2003;46:1200–1207.
4. Porter JA, Salvati EP, Rubin RJ, Eisenstat TE. Complications of colostomies. Dis Colon Rectum 1989;32:299–303.
5. Londono-Schimme EE, Leong AP, Phillips RK. Life table analysis of stomal complications following colostomy. Dis Colon Rectum 1994;37:916–920.
6. Goldblatt MS, Corman ML, Haggit RC, et al. Ileostomy complications requiring revision: Lahey clinic experience, 1964–1973. Dis Colon Rectum 1977;20: 209–214.
7. Senapati A, Nicholls RJ, Ritchie JK, et al. Temporary loop ileostomy for restorative proctocolectomy. Br J Surg 1993;80:628–630.
8. Feinberg SM, McLeod RS, Cohen Z. Complications of loop ileostomy. Am J Surg 1987;153:102–107.
9. Pearl RK. Parastomal hernias. World J Surg 1989;13:569–572.
10. Rubin MS, Schoetz DJ Jr, Matthews JB. Parastomal hernia. Is stoma relocation superior to fascial repair? Arch Surg 1994;129:413–419.
11. Hansson BM, Van Nieuwenhoven EJ, Bleichrodt RP. Promising new technique in the repair of parastomal hernia. Surg Endosc 2003;17:1789–1791.
12. Shellito PC. Complications of abdominal stoma surgery. Dis Colon Rectum 1998;41:1562–1572.
13. Wara P, Sorensen K, Berg V. Proximal fecal diversion: review of ten years' experience. Dis Colon Rectum 1981;24:114–119.
14. Bakker FC, Hoitsma HF, Den Otter G. The Hartmann procedure. Br J Surg 1982;69:580–582.
15. Stothert JC Jr, Brubacher L, Simonowitz DA. Complications of emergency stoma formation. Arch Surg 1982;117:307–309.

16. Wexner SD, Taranow DA, Johansen OB, et al. Loop ileostomy is a safe option for fecal diversion. Dis Colon Rectum 1993;36:349–354.
17. Khoo RE, Cohen MM, Chapman GM, et al. Loop ileostomy for temporary fecal diversion. Am J Surg 1994;167:519–522.
18. Cheung MT. Complications of an abdominal stoma: an analysis of 322 stomas. Aust N Z J Surg 1995;65:808–811.
19. Carlsen E, Bergan A. Technical aspects and complications of end-ileostomies. World J Surg 1995;19:632–636.
20. Greenstein AJ, Dicker A, Meyers S, Aufses AH Jr. Periileostomy fistulae in Crohn's disease. Ann Surg 1983;197:179–182.
21. Wanebo HJ, Antoniuk P, Koness RJ, et al. Pelvic resection of recurrent rectal cancer: technical considerations and outcomes. Dis Colon Rectum 1999;42:1438–1448.
22. Mannaerts GH, Rutten HJ, Martijn H, et al. Abdominosacral resection for primary irresectable and locally recurrent rectal cancer. Dis Colon Rectum 2001;44:806–814.
23. Abel ME, Chiu YS, Russell TR, Volpe PA. Autologous fibrin glue in the treatment of rectovaginal and complex fistulas. Dis Colon Rectum 1993;36:447–449.
24. Aitola P, Hiltunen KM, Matikainen M. Fibrin glue in perianal fistulas—a pilot study. Ann Chir Gynaecol 1999;88:136–138.
25. Lamont JP, Hooker G, Espenschied JR, et al. Closure of proximal colorectal fistulas using fibrin sealant. Am Surg 2002;68:615–618.
26. Shemesh EI, Kodner IJ, Fry RD, Neufeld DM. Endorectal sliding flap repair of complicated anterior anoperineal fistulas. Dis Colon Rectum 1988;31:22–24.
27. Hyman N. Endoanal advancement flap repair for complex anorectal fistulas. Am J Surg 1999;178:337–340.
28. Robertson WG, Mangione JS. Cutaneous advancement flap closure: alternative method for treatment of complicated anal fistulas. Dis Colon Rectum 1998;41:884–887.
29. Simmang CL, Lacey SW, Huber PJ Jr. Rectal sleeve advancement: repair of rectovaginal fistula associated with anorectal stricture in Crohn's disease. Dis Colon Rectum 1998;41:787–789.

CHAPTER 12

Reoperative Vascular Surgery

Michel A. Bartoli, MD; Robert W. Thompson, MD, FACS

Précis

Reoperative procedures are extremely common in vascular surgery. These operations require careful and sound judgment, comprehensive preoperative planning, and consideration of multiple approaches and strategies. The surgeon undertaking reoperative vascular procedures must therefore allow for the unexpected, remain flexible to different intraoperative findings, and employ creative solutions as well as expert technical precision in the conduct of the operation. The purpose of this presentation is to briefly review two examples of common reoperative problems in abdominal vascular surgery, graft limb occlusion following aortofemoral bypass and infection of aortic prostheses.

Introduction

Reoperative procedures are extremely common in vascular surgery, and they comprise a substantial number of the procedures performed by any individual practicing in this field. Reoperative procedures may be indicated either for progression of vascular disease or for direct failure of a previous vascular reconstruction. More recently, reoperative procedures have also come to include open operations performed for failure of previous endovascular procedures.

As in all areas of surgery, the best strategy for arterial reoperations is prevention: select the best operation that can be performed for a given problem the first time around, accomplish the procedure in the most technically precise manner, and ensure optimal postoperative care to avoid complications. However, progression of disease, failure of arterial reconstructions, or infection of prosthetic graft materials seem almost inevitable outcomes in the practice of vascular surgery, making careful, long-term follow-up necessary for all patients having arterial reconstruction. Early recognition of problems requiring reoperation is essential to achieve optimal outcomes. Indeed, patients presenting for reoperations are likely to have had progression of systemic and local cardiovascular disease, and they are inevitably older than at the time of the primary procedure; reoperations thereby represent some of the greatest challenges to surgeons performing vascular procedures, with heightened potential for postoperative complications and procedural failure. Nonetheless, patients presenting for vascular reoperations often harbor life- and/or limb-threatening problems for which an effective solution must be sought.

Successful reoperative vascular surgery requires careful, sound judgment, comprehensive preoperative planning, consideration of multiple approaches and strategies, allowance for the unexpected, and creative intraoperative flexibility as well as expert technical precision in the conduct of the operation. These challenging problems should therefore be referred to a regional center and undertaken by an experienced vascular surgeon, unless precluded by emergent life-threatening complications requiring immediate management (e.g., hemorrhage), when temporizing maneuvers must be employed prior to referral and definitive care.

A comprehensive discussion of reoperative vascular surgery is obviously beyond the scope of this article; thus, the purpose of this presentation is to briefly review several of the more common reoperative problems in abdominal vascular surgery, with an emphasis on general strategic principles and options by which to approach these difficult situations. The chapter is therefore focused on reoperations after two types of abdominal aortic reconstructions: aortobifemoral bypass for aortoiliac occlusive disease (AOD) or graft repair of abdominal aortic aneurysms (AAAs). Reoperations following these procedures are considered for two general conditions: (1) stenosis or occlusion of a previous aortic graft limb, or (2) infection of an aortic prosthesis.

Aortofemoral Graft Limb Occlusion

INCIDENCE

Graft limb occlusion is one of the more common long-term complications developing in patients following aortofemoral bypass grafts for AOD. The overall incidence of this complication is relatively low, however, with 5-year patency rates for aortofemoral bypass reaching 90%.[1]

ETIOLOGY

Acute graft limb occlusion in the early postoperative period is almost always caused by technical complications during construction of the distal anastomoses, such as angling or kinking of the graft, improper suture technique with elevation of an intimal flap, or incomplete evacuation of blood from the graft limb at the time of insertion. These problems are best addressed by prompt return to the operating room and will not be discussed further here. In contrast, graft limb occlusion most frequently appears after several months to years of successful graft function. These complications are typically caused by anastomotic neointimal hyperplasia and/or significant progression of atherosclerotic disease.

CLINICAL PRESENTATION

Graft limb occlusion may present as the acute onset of limb-threatening ischemia, suggesting acute thrombosis or thromboembolism to more distal vessels. This is more common if the original procedure was performed for aortic aneurysm disease, if an end-to-end anastomosis was performed in a graft placed for AOD, or if there is significant occlusive disease in the ipsilateral femoral-popliteal-tibial outflow tract vessels. Chronic graft limb occlusion may also present as the gradual development of pain at rest or the recurrence of short-distance claudication. Some patients may develop graft limb occlusion with minimal symptoms at rest, particularly if the original operation was for AOD, an end-to-side proximal anastomosis was performed, or there is minimal outflow tract disease. Thus, the acuity of symptoms depends on the original indication for the aortofemoral procedure and the manner in which the graft was placed, the adequacy of the collateral circulation, the status of the distal outflow vessels, and the time course over which graft limb occlusion develops.

DIAGNOSIS

The diagnosis of graft limb occlusion is relatively straightforward, indicated by the history and physical findings of a weakened or absent femoral artery pulse on palpation. Assessment of the circulation to the foot and lower leg is necessary to determine the urgency of revascularization, based on evidence of resting tissue perfusion, ischemic pain, and motor or sensory dysfunction. Supplemental evidence is provided by a decrease in leg pressures by noninvasive vascular laboratory studies, but these tests are of most value in assessing the status of the distal circulation by the presence or absence of segmental changes in arterial pressure. To prevent propagation of thrombus, patients presenting with graft limb thrombosis are anticoagulated with intravenous heparin at the time of diagnosis.

PREOPERATIVE PREPARATION

Arteriography is essential in delineating the location and extent of occlusion and the status of the inflow and outflow vessels, which will determine the options for reconstruction. This is especially useful in chronic graft limb occlusions and should include complete visualization of the aortofemoral-popliteal circulation. Although intra-arterial thrombolytic therapy may be considered in some cases of acute graft limb occlusion without an immediately threatened limb, prompt revascularization is necessary for limb-threatening ischemia and surgery should not be delayed; moreover, even successful thrombolysis only provides sufficient restoration of inflow through the graft limb and does not correct the underlying problem.[2,3] Finally, an assessment of the overall cardiopulmonary condition is made that may influence the choice of anesthesia for reoperation and the reasonable range of options that can be considered for revascularization. Revascularization should not be delayed for cardiopulmonary testing if acute limb ischemia is present.

OPERATIVE APPROACH

The patient is positioned supine with the abdomen and both lower extremities prepped into the sterile field. If there is no palpable femoral pulse on either side, the sterile field is extended to the shoulder on one side, in anticipation of possible axillofemoral reconstruction. In unstable or acutely ill patients, local anesthesia is used for procedures limited to one or both groins; in stable patients, general or regional anesthesia is preferred.

The affected groin is explored through a vertical incision, and the previous graft limb is exposed. It is often easier to begin this dissection at the level of the inguinal ligament, where there may be less scarring from the previous procedure, and the anatomical structures may be easier to identify. Scalpel dissection is used to avoid injury to adjacent structures, such as the femoral vein and nerves, which are frequently encased in scar from the previous operation. The previous graft limb is used as a guide to its anastomosis with the femoral artery. One expects to find the prosthetic graft densely adherent to the surrounding tissues; however, if the graft is poorly incorporated or perigraft fluid is encountered, graft limb infection should be suspected and measures appropriate to this finding employed (see later discussion). The common femoral artery, as well as the superficial and deep femoral arteries, are all exposed and circumferentially controlled. It is important to avoid injury to the branches of the common and deep femoral arteries during this exposure, since these may serve as important collaterals to the pelvis and/or lower extremity. The superficial and deep femoral arteries are exposed for several centimeters beyond their origins, since reconstruction of the distal anastomosis usually involves these vessels. The previous graft limb is transected just proximal to the femoral anastomosis.

The preferred approach to restore inflow is retrograde thrombectomy of the graft limb.[2–5] This is performed using No. 5 and 6 Fogarty balloon catheters with the contralateral femoral artery transiently compressed each time the catheter is passed into the occluded graft limb, in order to obliterate flow down the companion graft limb and thereby minimize the chance of having any dislodged thrombus pass to the other side. In chronic graft limb occlusions there is often a layer of thrombus adherent to the graft wall, which may also require use of endarterectomy strippers or other devices to remove. Graft limb thrombectomy is considered complete only when there is return of brisk arterial flow through the graft and no further thrombus is retrieved after 2 or 3 additional passes of the catheter. Intraoperative retrograde arteriography or angioscopy may be used to visualize the lumen of the graft limb, as adjuncts to ensure complete thrombectomy.[6] The patent graft limb is then flushed with saline containing heparin (500 units/mL) and clamped.

If satisfactory inflow cannot be achieved by thrombectomy alone, an alternative source of arterial inflow is required. The preferred approach is to open the contralateral groin and isolate the patent graft limb, which can be used as the inflow source by constructing a femoral-femoral bypass graft.[2,7] If neither femoral artery has sufficient inflow to support lower extremity revascularization, an axillofemoral bypass procedure may be considered to achieve inflow, complemented by a femoral-femoral bypass graft to ensure bilateral femoral revascularization. Alternatively, reexposure of the aorta by laparotomy may be considered for replacement of the entire aortobifemoral bypass graft.

Once satisfactory inflow to the femoral level has been achieved, attention is turned to the previous common femoral artery anastomosis. The remaining graft is cut free from the margins of the femoral artery and all suture material removed, and any thrombus at the anastomotic site is evacuated. Inspection of the common femoral artery lumen usually reveals an underlying occlusive lesion, due either to intimal hyperplasia at the anastomotic margins or to atherosclerotic stenosis at the orifice of one or both outflow vessels. The proximal common femoral artery is inspected to determine if any native inflow through this vessel is present. If no inflow from this vessel is apparent, the proximal common femoral artery is divided and oversewn; if the vessel is patent, the reconstruction is designed to preserve retrograde flow from the anastomosis to the proximal femoral artery. At this stage in the procedure, a short length of new prosthetic graft material may be attached to the free end of the previous graft limb in an end-to-end anastomosis. The distal end of this new graft will then be used to reconstruct the femoral anastomosis.

Endarterectomy of the common femoral artery is performed when severe atherosclerosis is encountered, with particular attention to the presence of disease extending into the origins of the superficial and deep femoral arteries. In some cases, graft limb occlusion may be due to intimal hyperplasia at the margins of the previous femoral anastomosis, in which case the thickened material is cut away with a scalpel until a satisfactory lumen is obtained. In the unusual situation in which the occlusive process is limited to the common femoral artery, the distal end of the new graft may then be attached to the common femoral artery in a long end-to-side anastomosis to complete the procedure.

Perhaps the most common finding is chronic occlusion of the superficial femoral artery, in which case the principal outflow for the graft limb is the profunda femoris artery and its collateral branches. Maintenance of the profunda femoris should therefore be considered the key element in any successful reconstruction. Endarterectomy may be extended into the orifice of the profunda femoris to remove any atherosclerotic disease at this level; however, if there is more extensive disease, a longitudinal arteriotomy should created along the anterior wall of the profunda femoris until a soft, disease-free segment is obtained. It is important to anticipate that, in some patients, particularly those with diabetes or early-onset diffuse forms of accelerated atherosclerosis, the disease process may extend several centimeters into the profunda femoris, requiring more extended exposure and reconstruction.

Reconstruction of the profunda femoris may be achieved by several methods, including extension of the prosthetic graft as a long-tongued anastomosis along the anterior wall of the open vessel.[2,4,8] Although this tactic appears expedient, prosthetic patch repair of a relatively small profunda femoris artery may be more prone to late reocclusion secondary to intimal hyperplasia than repair with autologous material. Thus, a more attractive alternative is to perform reconstruction of the profunda femoris by patch angioplasty with saphenous vein. Another option is to utilize an excised segment of the occluded superficial femoral artery that has been disobliterated by endarterectomy. Once profunda femoris reconstruction has been completed in this manner, the distal end of the graft limb can be attached to the common femoral artery in an end-to-end anastomosis.

Restoration of lower extremity perfusion is assessed by inspection of the feet and detection of Doppler signals over the pedal vessels. Patients with occlusion of the superficial femoral artery and insufficient collateral circulation through the profunda femoris may still have persistent ischemia despite satisfactory aorto-femoral reconstruction, in which case an intraoperative decision must be made regarding the need for further revascularization. Intraoperative arteriography may be informative in this setting, and if distal occlusive disease and ischemia remain a concern, extension of the reconstruction with a femoral-popliteal bypass should be considered. This situation is fortunately unusual, and in most cases revascularization of the profunda femoris artery is sufficient to alleviate acute ischemia. Moreover, revascularization with outflow into the profunda femoris artery is usually sufficient to provide durable aortofemoral graft limb patency and limb salvage over time.[8]

Aortic Graft Infection

INCIDENCE

The overall incidence of aortic graft infections is low, occurring in approximately 1% of patients undergoing prosthetic aortoiliac or aortofemoral reconstructions. Prosthetic graft infection is nonetheless one of the most serious complications that can occur after aortic operations, with a high rate of morbidity and mortality. Aortic graft infections may occur with increased frequency in debilitated patients, those with a coexisting infectious process at the time of the original procedure, those with placement of the distal anastomosis at the femoral level, or in patients suffering postoperative complications.

ETIOLOGY

The cause of prosthetic graft infections is generally considered to be microbial seeding of the graft at the time of the original operation, with the most common organisms responsible including gram-positive cocci such as *Staphylococcus aureus* or certain strains of *S. epidermidis*.[9] These organisms can give rise to slowly developing indolent infections, resulting in difficultly in diagnosis and a protracted clinical course. Graft infections with gram-negative organisms are less common but more virulent, usually resulting in a more acute clinical course. These infections often occur early in the postoperative period in association with wound, gastrointestinal, or other systemic complications. Patients with a previous aortic graft may also develop prosthetic graft infections by hematogenous seeding during systemic infectious illnesses, or after interventions and operations that result in transient bacteremia. Appropriate preventive measures taken at the time of the original aortic operation should include liberal use of perioperative antibiotics and bowel preparation. Antibiotic prophylaxis is also indicated in patients with an aortic graft prior to undergoing invasive dental or endoscopic procedures that might result in bacteremia.

Aortic graft infections with *S. epidermidis* deserve special comment, since they may occur years after the primary operation and their enigmatic clinical presentation may make diagnosis particularly difficult. Substrains of *S. epidermidis* that produce bacterial slimes are thought to be especially important in this regard, since they may be harbored within the interstices of textile prosthetic grafts for a long period before producing clinical infection.[10] It is also difficult to establish laboratory cultures of these organisms unless special techniques are used to disrupt their adherence during isolation from excised graft materials.[11,12] Thus, documented infections with *S. epidermidis* are probably underrepresented in large clinical series.

CLINICAL PRESENTATION

Early aortic graft infections become clinically apparent within several weeks to months of the primary procedure. The typical scenario is in a patient who had overt gastrointestinal tract contamination at the time of primary graft implantation, or in whom postoperative complications involving the gastrointestinal, genitourinary, or lower respiratory tract developed in the immediate postoperative period. These patients may present with persistent systemic sepsis, anastomotic complications related to the graft, or gastrointestinal hemorrhage.

Late aortic graft infections generally come to clinical attention more than 6 months after the primary procedure, and often appear after a period of several years. The clinical presentation of these patients varies, but may include fever of uncertain origin or systemic sepsis, anastomotic pseudoaneurysms or graft limb occlusions, or gastrointestinal hemorrhage.

Upper gastrointestinal hemorrhage may arise by three distinct mechanisms in patients with an infected aortic graft.[13] First, bleeding from the upper gastrointestinal tract may occur as a manifestation of systemic sepsis and physiological stress, resulting in gastritis or peptic ulcer. Second, the infected graft may erode into an adjacent portion of the gastrointestinal tract, resulting in bleeding into the lumen from intramural vessels. This most commonly arises in the fourth portion of the duodenum, which normally lies immediately adjacent to the proximal portion of the infrarenal aorta. The third mechanism is erosion of the gastrointestinal tract by a large anastomotic pseudoaneurysm associated with disruption of an infected graft. This can result in direct communication between the aortic lumen and the bowel, producing exsanguinating hemorrhage. While an initial episode of upper gastrointestinal bleeding may appear to stop due to formation of thrombus at the site of communication (described as a "herald" or "sentinel" bleed), after a delay another episode of bleeding may occur with fatal consequences.

DIAGNOSIS

Once aortic graft infection is suspected, prompt evaluation is necessary to attempt confirmation of the diagnosis and to assess the extent of graft infection. Initial studies include a peripheral white blood cell count to detect leukocytosis and blood cultures drawn from the arm and the lower extremities. The most important imaging study is an abdominal CT scan.[14] This is done with the aim of identifying any dilatation or disruption at the site of the proximal and/or distal graft anastomoses and any fluid or gas adjacent to the graft. Either of these findings is strong evidence of graft infection, but their absence cannot be used to completely exclude graft infection. The presence of proximal anastomotic disruption or a pseudoaneurysm should be considered evidence of graft infection, permitting plans for repair to be conducted with this diagnosis in mind. When perigraft fluid is present on the CT scan, its extent along the length of the graft can suggest whether the infection is limited to just one limb of the prosthesis or the entire prosthesis is involved. These findings are therefore helpful not only in making the correct diagnosis, but in planning the appropriate operative strategy.

In patients with upper gastrointestinal hemorrhage, endoscopy is critical in the early stages of evaluation.[13] While location of a source of bleeding not related to the aortic graft may provide reassurance, it should be reinforced that gastritis or peptic ulceration may still represent a response to graft-related sepsis and systemic stress. These sources of bleeding may also coexist with a graft-enteric fistula; thus, efforts to evaluate the fourth part of the duodenum are necessary to determine whether a graft-enteric erosion or fistula is present. Perhaps the most reassuring finding is the visualization of a mucosal defect with a portion of the textile graft visible in the distal duodenum; this not only proves the presence of an infected graft with graft-enteric erosion, but provides evidence that the cause of bleeding is from intramural vessels within the bowel wall rather than the more fearsome possibility of a graft-enteric fistula. A graft-enteric fistula remains a concern, however, when endoscopy reveals a mucosal defect with fresh clot and no visible graft; in this event, the clot should be left undisturbed and prompt preparations made for operative exploration.

Aortography remains a useful step in the diagnostic evaluation. This is most valuable to delineate the anatomy and patency of the previous aortic graft and its adjacent branch vessels, in order to plan the appropriate operative procedures. In current practice, much of this information can also be obtained by high-resolution spiral CT scanning with contrast, when this is available.

PREOPERATIVE PREPARATION

Operative intervention must be carried out expeditiously in all patients with proven aortic graft infection, especially in the presence of anastomotic disruption or active gastrointestinal bleeding. Appropriate steps to stabilize the patient are undertaken, with operation carried out within 12 to 24 hours of presentation or as soon as the necessary diagnostic studies are completed. In stable patients in whom the diagnosis of aortic graft infection requires a series of studies, or in whom the diagnosis is only presumptive, preoperative evaluation of cardiopulmonary status may also be included prior to surgical exploration. Operative treatment should not be delayed for cardiac interventions or prolonged attempts to improve the condition of the patient, however, as this invites development of emergent complications. Prior to operative treatment, patients should be treated with broad-spectrum intravenous antibiotics that include coverage for methicillin-resistant staphylococcus.

OPERATIVE APPROACH

Emergency operation is necessary for unstable patients with anastomotic disruption and intraperitoneal bleeding or for active gastrointestinal hemorrhage. The approach should be through a midline laparotomy to control the proximal aorta above the origin of the graft. Once proximal aortic control is obtained, the graft can be more deliberately assessed and its relationship to the bowel evaluated. The infected aortic graft must be excised and any defect in the bowel repaired. Given the acute nature of these situations, aortic reconstruction is best carried out by in situ repair at the same setting, by one of three alternatives. The first is to perform in-situ repair with a new prosthetic graft. This should be done with a prosthetic material that has been treated with rifampin, to reduce the chances of subsequent reinfection.[15] Although this approach might be considered just a temporizing solution for an unstable patient, with the recognition that another procedure may be required once the patient's immediate survival has been ensured, in-situ aortic repair with rifampin-impregnated materials may also produce satisfactory long-term results.[16–19] A second alternative is in-situ repair with a cryopreserved aortic allograft.[20–23] The third alternative, if such grafts are not available, is to perform reconstruction by in-situ repair with a deep femoral vein, recognizing that harvesting of this conduit is a painstaking process.[24–27]

In stable patients with known or suspected aortic graft infection, a single-stage operation may be performed with aortic graft excision and in-situ repair using a rifampin-impregnated prosthetic graft, a cryopreserved aortic allograft, or a conduit constructed from the deep femoral veins.[16–27] Another alternative in this setting is a staged approach, favored by some as a means to diminish the duration and perioperative stress associated with a single operation.[28,29] The first procedure consists of extra-anatomic revascularization of the lower extremities. If only one graft limb is involved, this may be performed using an ipsilateral axillobifemoral bypass, in which the graft is brought around the groin through a subcutaneous tunnel along the lateral hip, to reach the superficial or profunda femoral artery in the mid-thigh. This allows the new graft to avoid the potentially involved femoral anastomotic site. In this option, the groin is left unexplored during the first stage. If both graft limbs or the entire aortic prosthesis are known to be involved, bilateral lower extremity revascularization is performed in the first stage operation. This may be accomplished by bilateral axillofemoral bypass grafts in a manner similar to that used for unilateral infection, with both groins to be explored at the second-stage operation. An alternative is to perform unilateral axillofemoral bypass as described, followed by bilateral groin exploration. In this case, the femoral artery anastomoses to the previous graft are dismantled, and the femoral arteries are reconstructed with autologous tissues. A femoral-femoral bypass is necessary in this setting, constructed with either autologous saphenous vein or, if available, a cryopreserved saphenous vein conduit. This approach is generally less satisfactory than bilateral axillofemoral revascularization and is therefore reserved for situations where the infected groin wounds must be explored at the first operation (i.e., when expanding femoral pseudoaneurysms or overt purulent infection exists at these sites).[30]

The second stage of treatment is performed 3 to 7 days after lower extremity revascularization. This operation involves laparotomy and excision of the aortic graft, oversewing of the proximal aortic stump, and reconstruction of the common femoral arteries. The operation is usually started by reopening the groin incisions and dismantling the femoral anastomoses. The margins of the femoral artery are also debrided to ensure complete excision of infected tissue, and any surrounding tissues involved in the infectious process are also debrided. The ends of the prosthetic graft limbs are oversewn and passed into the retroperitoneum. The femoral arteries are reconstructed to ensure flow from the superficial femoral arteries (fed by the previously placed axillofemoral grafts) to the profunda femoris arteries. This can be done by simply closing the common femoral artery directly if sufficient tissue is available, or with a saphenous vein patch placed over the femoral bifurcation. A laparotomy is then performed to complete excision of the aortic graft. The proximal aorta is controlled well above the previous graft, usually requiring mobilization of the left renal vein and juxta- or suprarenal exposure. The aorta is clamped and the previous anastomosis dismantled, making sure to excise all remnants of the graft and suture materials. The end of the aorta is debrided as close to the renal arteries as possible, and the tissue is sent for culture. The aortic stump is closed in two layers with monofilament suture, using a running horizontal mattress suture followed by an over-and-over stitch. The remaining graft is excised, taking care not to injure the ureters during extraction of the graft limbs from their retroperitoneal tunnels. Any obviously infected retroperitoneal tissue is debrided aggressively. The aortic stump is covered with omentum, and one or more closed-suction drains are placed in the adjacent retroperitoneal space.

The key principle of surgical treatment in these situations is the complete excision of all infected prosthetic material and appropriate revascularization. In some cases, infection may be confined to a single graft limb, raising the question of whether the entire aortic graft must be excised. Indeed, exploration of the graft limb at the iliac level, through a low retroperitoneal approach, may reveal dense incorporation of the graft without signs that the infection has spread above the groin. When this is encountered, the graft limb may be oversewn and only the lower part excised, with autologous reconstruction used to restore inflow to the femoral level.

REFERENCES

1. Szilagyi DE, Elliott JP Jr, Smith RF, et al. A thirty-year survey of the reconstructive surgical treatment of aortoiliac occlusive disease. J Vasc Surg 1986;3: 421–436.
2. Brewster DC, Meier GH 3rd, Darling RC, et al. Reoperation for aortofemoral graft limb occlusion: optimal methods and long-term results. J Vasc Surg 1987;5: 363–374.

3. Erdoes LS, Bernhard VM, Berman SS. Aortofemoral graft occlusion: strategy and timing of reoperation. Cardiovasc Surg 1995;3:277–283.
4. Bernhard VM, Ray LI, Towne JB. The reoperation of choice for aortofemoral graft occlusion. Surgery 1977;82:867–874.
5. Hyde GL, McCready RA, Schwartz RW, et al. Durability of thrombectomy of occluded aortofemoral graft limbs. Surgery 1983;94:748–751.
6. LaMuraglia GM, Brewster DC, Moncure AC, et al. Angioscopic evaluation of unilateral aortic graft limb thrombectomy: is it helpful? J Vasc Surg 1993;17:1069–1074.
7. Nolan KD, Benjamin ME, Murphy TJ, et al. Femorofemoral bypass for aortofemoral graft limb occlusion: a ten-year experience. J Vasc Surg 1994;19:851–856.
8. Goldstone J, Malone JM, Moore WS. Importance of the profunda femoris artery in primary and secondary arterial operations for lower extremity ischemia. Am J Surg 1978;136:215–220.
9. Kaebnick HW, Bandyk DF, Bergamini TW, Towne JB. The microbiology of explanted vascular prostheses. Surgery 1987;102:756–762.
10. Bandyk DF. Diagnosis and treatment of biomaterial-associated vascular infections. Infect Dis Clin North Am 1992;6:719–729.
11. Tollefson DF, Bandyk DF, Kaebnick HW, et al. Surface biofilm disruption. Enhanced recovery of microorganisms from vascular prostheses. Arch Surg 1987;122:38–43.
12. Bergamini TM, Bandyk DF, Govostis D, et al. Identification of *Staphylococcus epidermidis* vascular graft infections: a comparison of culture techniques. J Vasc Surg 1989;9:665–670.
13. Reilly LM, Ehrenfeld WK, Goldstone J, Stoney RJ. Gastrointestinal tract involvement by prosthetic graft infection. The significance of gastrointestinal hemorrhage. Ann Surg 1985;202:342–348.
14. Low RN, Wall SD, Jeffrey RB Jr, et al. Aortoenteric fistula and perigraft infection: evaluation with CT. Radiology 1990;175:157–162.
15. Gahtan V, Esses GE, Bandyk DF, et al. Antistaphylococcal activity of rifampin-bonded gelatin-impregnated Dacron grafts. J Surg Res 1995;58:105–110.
16. Young RM, Cherry KJ Jr, Davis PM, et al. The results of in situ prosthetic replacement for infected aortic grafts. Am J Surg 1999;178:136–140.
17. Bandyk DF, Bergamini TM, Kinney EV, et al. In situ replacement of vascular prostheses infected by bacterial biofilms. J Vasc Surg 1991;13:575–583.
18. Towne JB, Seabrook GR, Bandyk D, et al. In situ replacement of arterial prosthesis infected by bacterial biofilms: long-term follow-up. J Vasc Surg 1994;19:226–233.
19. Bandyk DF, Novotney ML, Back MR, et al. Expanded application of in situ replacement for prosthetic graft infection. J Vasc Surg 2001;34:411–419.
20. Kieffer E, Bahnini A, Koskas F, et al. In situ allograft replacement of infected infrarenal aortic prosthetic grafts: results in forty-three patients. J Vasc Surg 1993;17:349–355.

21. Koskas F, Plissonnier D, Bahnini A, et al. In situ arterial allografting for aortoiliac graft infection: a 6-year experience. Cardiovasc Surg 1996;4:495–499.

22. Vogt PR, Brunner-LaRocca HP, Lachat M, et al. Technical details with the use of cryopreserved arterial allografts for aortic infection: influence on early and midterm mortality. J Vasc Surg 2002;35:80–86.

23. Noel AA, Gloviczki P, Cherry KJ Jr, et al. Abdominal aortic reconstruction in infected fields: early results of the United States cryopreserved aortic allograft registry. J Vasc Surg 2002;35:847–852.

24. Clagett GP, Bowers BL, Lopez-Viego MA, et al. Creation of a neo-aortoiliac system from lower extremity deep and superficial veins. Ann Surg 1993;218:239–248.

25. Clagett GP, Valentine RJ, Hagino RT. Autogenous aortoiliac/femoral reconstruction from superficial femoral-popliteal veins: feasibility and durability. J Vasc Surg 1997;25:255–266.

26. Gordon LL, Hagino RT, Jackson MR, et al. Complex aortofemoral prosthetic infections: the role of autogenous superficial femoropopliteal vein reconstruction. Arch Surg 1999;134:615–620.

27. Valentine RJ, Clagett GP. Aortic graft infections: replacement with autogenous vein. Cardiovasc Surg 2001;9:419–425.

28. Reilly LM, Stoney RJ, Goldstone J, Ehrenfeld WK. Improved management of aortic graft infection: the influence of operation sequence and staging. J Vasc Surg 1987;5:421–431.

29. Kuestner LM, Reilly LM, Jicha DL, et al. Secondary aortoenteric fistula: contemporary outcome with use of extraanatomic bypass and infected graft excision. J Vasc Surg 1995;21:184–195.

30. Jicha DL, Reilly LM, Kuestner LM, Stoney RJ. Durability of cross-femoral grafts after aortic graft infection: the fate of autogenous conduits. J Vasc Surg 1995;22:393–405.

CHAPTER 13

Reoperative Breast Surgery

Darren R. Carpizo, MD, PhD; Mai Brooks, MD;
Helena Chang, MD, PhD

Précis

The surgical management of breast cancer has changed substantially over the last 25 years. Reoperation in breast cancer is being performed with considerable frequency as women undergo procedures for diagnosis, treatment, and recurrence. This chapter discusses the management principles that guide the surgeon in his or her attempt to minimize reoperation in the breast cancer patient.

Introduction

Breast cancer develops in approximately 212,000 women per year, with an annual mortality rate of approximately 40,000.[1] The surgical management of breast cancer has changed substantially over the last 25 years, with recent long-term studies validating equal survival outcomes with breast conservation therapy and mastectomy for early breast cancer.[2,3] Diagnosis of breast cancer at an early stage permits breast conservation therapy in the majority of patients. The increased use of lumpectomy, however, lends to an increased need for reoperation, either due to margin involvement or local recurrence.

Indeed, reoperation in breast cancer is being performed with considerable frequency as many women first undergo an operation for diagnosis, then another procedure for treatment to the breast and axilla, followed possibly by others to achieve negative margins. Reoperation is also commonly performed when breast cancer recurs. The increased frequency of reoperation in breast cancer patients imparts considerable psychological hardship to patients and economic duress to the health care system. Equally important is the burden of increased surgical morbidity suffered by patients undergoing multiple operations.[4] Similar to most aspects of surgical oncology, avoiding reoperation is often best accomplished by choosing the appropriate initial operation. This chapter discusses the three main areas in which reoperation is most commonly encountered in breast cancer: diagnosis, primary breast cancer treatment, and the management of local recurrence.

Reoperation in Breast Cancer: Diagnosis

Any attempts to avoid reoperation in the breast cancer patient must begin with the first procedure that the breast surgeon encounters to obtain a tissue diagnosis. Excisional biopsy, with or without wire localization, has been traditionally used to obtain a tissue diagnosis; however in the last decade, the image-guided large core needle biopsy has gained popularity. Numerous studies into the accuracy and cost-effectiveness of core needle biopsy have validated its use in comparison to open excisional biopsy.[5–7] Core needle biopsy obviates the need for an initial operation, with its associated morbidity and cost, and minimizes reoperative surgery by allowing the surgeon to plan for definitive local therapy of the breast and axilla in one operation. For these reasons, core needle biopsy has become the preferred method of tissue diagnosis for most surgeons.

When there is a contraindication to breast conservation, and a mastectomy is chosen, the advantage of core needle biopsy is clear. First, it allows for the possibility of immediate reconstruction with the mastectomy procedure, if the patient so desires. Second, since there is no incision from previous excisional biopsy surgery, the surgeon does not need to consider incorporating the initial scar into the mastectomy incision. Taken together, the knowledge of a cancer diagnosis before any surgery is performed may avoid multiple surgeries and achieve the best possible cosmetic result in these women. Even in the setting of breast conservation, the preoperative knowledge of a cancer diagnosis allows the surgeon to perform a better lumpectomy with secured margins and to perform nodal staging surgery during the same procedure.

The number of studies specifically investigating the effect of core needle biopsy on the number of operations required to complete local therapy are few, and they have not consistently shown a clear advantage over open excisional biopsy to obtaining negative surgical margins.[8,9] Nonetheless, these studies have demonstrated that a core needle biopsy reduces the number of surgical procedures required to complete local therapy.

A proposed theoretical advantage of core needle biopsy is preservation of the ability to perform accurate sentinel lymph node (SLN) biopsy. Some studies have suggested that SLN biopsy for breast cancer may be less accurate after excisional biopsy, because surgical removal of the breast tissue leads to disruption of breast lymphatics, decreasing the likelihood of successful lymphatic mapping.[10,11] However, when this was examined prospectively by Wong et al, there was no advantage found to core needle biopsy over excisional biopsy with respect to the accuracy rates in SLN biopsy.[12]

A theoretical disadvantage of core needle biopsy is the concern of seeding tumor cells in the needle tract, and thus predisposing the patient to local recurrence. King and colleagues recently studied the impact of core needle biopsy on cancers treated with breast conservation, focusing on outcomes in local recurrence rates, and found no difference.[13]

Thus, it appears that image-guided core needle biopsy would be the preferred method of tissue diagnosis for all visible abnormalities, benign or malignant. Because the majority of biopsies are benign, the patient is spared an unnecessary operation that can distort the breast. In the setting of a malignant diagnosis, core needle biopsy minimizes reoperative breast surgery without compromising local recurrence risks.

Reoperation in Primary Breast Cancer: Therapy

As more patients today are opting for breast conservation for early stage breast cancers as well as SLN biopsy to stage the axilla, the chances for reoperation in the primary treatment setting are increasing. More specifically, further breast surgery becomes necessary to obtain local control or to clear the axilla if SLN biopsy is positive.

RE-EXCISION LUMPECTOMY

With respect to breast conservation therapy, reoperation in the form of re-excision lumpectomy is most commonly necessary for positive margin status or residual suspicious microcalcifications on postoperative mammography. The impact of margin status on local recurrence rates has been a subject of some controversy in the past. Some authors suggested that microscopically positive margins do not have an impact on local recurrence and that these patients can be treated effectively with radiation.[14–16] However, most studies have found margin status to be one of the most important predictors of local recurrence for both invasive cancer[17–22] and carcinoma in situ.[23,24] Jobsen et al have recently examined this issue in a prospective study designed to identify subsets of patients most likely to recur with microscopically positive margins, and found that positive margins were associated with increased local recurrence and reduced disease-free survival in women aged 40 years or younger.[25] The overall local recurrence rate for women in this age group was 14.7% (21 of 143), while that for women over age 40 years was 4.1% (66 of 1607). They found the 5-year local recurrence risk for women 40 years or younger to be 8.4% for negative margins and 36.9% for positive margins. The 5-year local recurrence risk for women over 40 years was 2.6% for negative margins and only 6.2% for positive margins. In addition, they found the 5-year disease-free survival for women 40 years or younger to be 74.5% for negative margins and 27.4% for positive margins. In contrast, the 5-year disease-free survival rates for women over 40 years was 87.2% for negative margins and 84.3% for women with positive margins. Thus, these authors recommend re-excision for positive margins be limited to women 40 years or younger, and for those women older than 40 years, radiation may be adequate for microscopically positive margins.

Others found that margin status is an important predictor not only of local recurrence, but also of systemic recurrence and disease-specific survival after breast conservation therapy.[26] In view of the available information, we recommend an aggressive approach to the local surgical therapy in breast conservation therapy to achieve complete pathologically negative surgical margins. This is especially important for women 40 years old or younger. Moreover, breast irradiation, while decreasing the risk of local recurrence, is not a substitute for clear surgical margins, as breast radiation boosts have not been shown to provide adequate local control in patients with positive margins.[27]

The decision to reoperate for positive margin status, although generally supported by the literature, is complicated by the high rates of negative re-excision lumpectomies. The frequency of residual tumor in relumpectomy specimens has been estimated to be between 32% and 63%.[28] Moreover, Papa et al recently studied the margin status in re-excision lumpectomies and found that only 47% of re-excision specimens of true positive excisional biopsies were positive for residual tumor.[29] These findings have served as the basis for numerous studies into which factors associated with positive re-excision lumpectomies may predict which women are most likely to have a positive re-excision.[20,28–34] Theoretically, a subgroup of patients whose risk of a positive re-excision is low could be spared an additional operation, with its associated morbidity and cost. Alternatively, some studies have attempted to identify the women most likely to have positive re-excisions so that a more generous re-excision can be performed. When a selective approach is being considered, this type of analysis may guide us for proper patient selection.

From the numerous studies examining positive re-excision patterns over the last decade, only three have employed a multivariate analysis in their identification of significant corollaries. The results of these three studies are summarized in Table 13-1 below.

An examination of the various factors found in common among these studies in Table 13-1 seems to indicate that tumor size and a close surgical margin are the best clinicopathologic predictive factors for positive re-excision lumpectomies. Prospective outcomes-based research is necessary to validate these observations.

Table 13-1 Factors Associated with Positive Re-excision Lumpectomies: A Summary of Multivariate Analyses

Papa et al[29]	Jardines et al[28]	Anscher et al[20]
Number of margins involved with disease (≤2 mm)	Clinical tumor size	Previous excision margin status
Presence of multifocal disease	Histologic appearance Pathologic status of axillary lymph nodes	Extensive intraductal component
Mode of detection (mammography versus physical examination)	Mode of detection	

Nonetheless, these studies provide some guidelines for risk assessment to help identify which patients whose risk of positive re-excision is low enough that re-excision may be omitted or, alternatively, whose risk is high enough that re-excision or even mastectomy is necessary.

INTRAOPERATIVE TECHNIQUES FOR MINIMIZING POSITIVE SURGICAL MARGINS IN INSITU AND INFILTRATING BREAST CANCER

Reoperation after breast cancer surgery most commonly occurs when the margin is involved. Thus, any attempts at avoiding or minimizing re-excision at the initial operation depend on several factors related to the margin. These factors include the method of defining negative/positive and close margins, and the significance of each to local recurrence. Other factors include how to handle the specimen for proper margin assessment and innovative means of ensuring a negative margin at the time of initial excision.

Margin status is generally defined as negative (no tumor within a fixed distance from the cut edge of the tumor), positive (tumor at the margin), or close (tumor closer than the fixed distance for a negative margin). Although many studies exist supporting the correlation between margin status and local recurrence, no uniform standard distance exists to define the margin.[17,33,35–38] The range of margin width reported in these studies varies from 1 mm to 5 mm, and interestingly, there does not seem to be a direct relationship between width of the negative margin and the rate of local recurrence.[39] Nonetheless, the rate of local recurrence has been found to increase over time when the margin is positive.[39] At our institution, we define a negative margin as no tumor cells within 2 mm of the inked margin, a close margin as tumor cells <2 mm from the inked margin, and a positive margin as tumor cells present at the inked margin.

How the surgical specimen has been handled during pathologic examination has also changed over time, in order better to define which aspects of the margins are positive. Some institutions use India ink to stain the entire cut surface of the specimen. If orientation of the specimen is unknown, however, the finding of a positive margin will require re-excision of the entire lumpectomy cavity. Proponents of multicolored inking, in which each margin (superior, inferior, lateral, medial, anterior, posterior) is stained with a different color, argue that when a positive margin is found, only a limited re-excision of that margin is necessary. Gibson et al compared this limited re-excision technique with the standard India ink system with whole cavity re-excision. They found the local recurrence rates to be the same; however, the limited re-excision technique allowed for substantial tissue conservation, with re-excision specimens on average four times smaller than with whole cavity re-excision.[40]

Due to the importance of tumor margin involvement as a predictor of local recurrence, many have investigated innovative means of assessing the margin status of a lumpectomy specimen intraoperatively in order to maximize the chance for adequate initial excision. These methods range from pathologic specimen analysis to intraoperative imaging.[44–46] Other procedures such as cryo-assisted lumpectomy or operative breast endoscopy during lumpectomy are being tested for their role in minimizing reoperation.[41,42]

Excision of ductal carcinoma in situ (DCIS) has been shown to have a high rate of positive margins, ranging from 40% to 50%.[24,43,44] Chagpar et al studied the "intra-operative margin assessment" to obviate the need for future reoperation.[45] In this study, the lumpectomy specimen was radiographed to identify the targeted mammographic lesion, and then the margins were inked with different colors. The specimen was then sectioned into 3 to 5 mm slices, and each slice was both grossly examined by a pathologist and reradiographed. The authors found the rate of positive margins on intraoperative assessment was 54%. They compared a group of 53 patients who underwent intraoperative margin assessment with further excision (during the initial operation) to another group of 56 patients who did not undergo intraoperative assessment, and found that only 13% of the first group required a second operation, as opposed to 30% of the patients who did not undergo intraoperative margin assessment.

Intraoperative ultrasonography for mass lesions has recently been investigated as an innovative means of assessing tumor margin, and several studies have validated its use for intraoperative localization of nonpalpable tumors and assessment of tumor margins.[46,47] The authors hypothesized that intraoperative ultrasound increased the rate of negative margin compared to the gold standard of wire localization for lumpectomy. This hypothesis was recently tested in a prospective randomized trial in which intraoperative ultrasound-guided lumpectomy was compared to wire-localized lumpectomy for invasive cancer. These authors studied the rate of negative margins, as well as the depth of margin assessed and the weight of each lumpectomy specimen.[48] They found that ultrasound guidance led to significantly more accurate lumpectomies that were equal to or smaller in size than wire-localized lumpectomy specimens. Their results are promising and deserve further investigation by others for confirmation. If successful, it would require the breast surgeon to learn a new skill set, and it may improve the outcome of oncologic surgery.

No data exist analyzing the economic impact of intraoperative margin assessment. Specifically, it has not been studied whether the financial cost saved in the prevention of reoperation for positive margins outweighs the cost of intra-operative assessment.

REOPERATION AFTER SENTINEL LYMPH NODE BIOPSY

SLN biopsy has become the procedure of choice for staging of the axilla in the management of early breast cancers. If the SLN is positive for malignancy, the standard of care has been to proceed with a formal axillary lymph node dissection (ALND), thus necessitating reoperation of the axilla. Because this form of reoperation of the axilla has become so frequent, it has raised questions as to whether the additional axillary surgery imparts a significantly higher rate of morbidity and cost to the completion of primary breast cancer therapy in the setting of invasive breast cancer.

Several groups have begun to study the feasibility of intraoperative SLN diagnosis in an effort to stage, and, if necessary, treat the axilla definitively all in one operation.[49–52] The results of these studies have varied considerably, but overall they suggest that intraoperative SLN assessment is feasible for larger tumors (T1c and T2) and for invasive ductal cancers, but not lobular cancers. For example, Weiser et al examined the relationship between sensitivity of intraoperative frozen section analysis of the SLN to tumor size and found that for T1a tumors the sensitivity was only 40%, whereas for T2 tumors it was 76%.[49] When Leidenius et al compared tumors of 375 breast cancer patients, they reported a sensitivity of 83% for intraoperative frozen section of SLN, the highest yet reported. When they separated the invasive ductal and invasive lobular cancers, they found the false negative rate to be 28% for invasive lobular, as opposed to only 8% for invasive ductal. As expected, they found the false negative rate to be substantially higher in lymph nodes that contained micrometastases (38%), than in lymph nodes that contained larger metastases (6%).[51]

Reoperation in Breast Cancer: Recurrence

LOCAL RECURRENCE IN INVASIVE CARCINOMA

Beyond the reason for achieving a tumor free margin, is also necessary for women with local recurrence of breast cancer. Ipsilateral breast tumor recurrence (IBTR) in the setting of breast conservation therapy (BCT) for invasive carcinoma has been extensively studied with respect to its incidence, risk factors that predict it, and its impact on overall survival. Recent reports of 20-year follow-up of two randomized studies comparing women with early breast cancer treated with either BCT or mastectomy have revealed that BCT imparts a greater risk of IBTR than mastectomy, with an incidence between 8.8% and 20%,[2,3] with no difference in overall survival rate. It has been argued by some that if there is no survival difference between BCT and mastectomy, then the IBTR in BCT should not cause distant disease, but rather it should be considered as an increased risk for metastasis.[53]

Others believe that local recurrence after lumpectomy represents a poor prognosis. Several studies have reported a close correlation between IBTR and systemic recurrence.[54–56] Additional studies indicate that patients who develop IBTR indeed do have a decrease in survival and thus argue for aggressive local control at the initiation of surgical treatment, as well as at the time of detection of a local recurrence.[26,27,57,58]

The understanding of the clinical impact of local breast recurrence after breast conservation treatment reflects our limited understanding of the host-tumor relationship. With our current knowledge, we have accepted that, in suitable patients, BCT is as effective as mastectomy in treating early breast cancer. In addition to the biological properties of each tumor, positive surgical margin predisposes to local recurrence; therefore, adequate local surgery is paramount to minimize the risk of local recurrence. Postoperative radiation is beneficial for those treated with

Table 13-2 Risk Factors for Local Recurrence after Breast Conservation Therapy
Factor
Age younger than 35 to 40 years[58–62]
Positive resection margins[20,60,62–64]
Presence of extensive intraductal component (EIC)[58,61,65,66]
Lymphovascular invasion[58,66–69]
Tumor multicentricity[62,70–72]

lumpectomy or mastectomy, in whom the tumor biology dictates a high rate of local recurrence.

Many studies have attempted to identify clinicopathologic risk factors of local recurrence in patients treated with BCT. Information from these studies may guide the selection of initial surgery in patients with early breast cancer. These factors are summarized in Table 13-2.

Factors that correlate with local recurrence after mastectomy have not been as extensively studied as with BCT. Recently Voogd et al used the database of two large randomized clinical trials comparing BCT to mastectomy for stage I and II breast cancers to identify the risk factors that correlated best with local recurrence after both BCT and mastectomy. These authors found that age 35 years and younger and presence of extensive intraductal component (EIC) were associated with an increased risk of local recurrence after BCT, while lobular carcinoma was associated with an increased risk with mastectomy.[58] Lymphovascular invasion and high histologic grade were found to be associated with an increased risk of local recurrence in both treatment groups. The fact that some factors are predictive of recurrence both after BCT and mastectomy suggests that in certain patients, local recurrence is independent of local therapy.

In addition, higher stage breast cancer correlates with local recurrence after mastectomy. This includes T3 and T4 primary breast cancer with positive nodal metastasis. Studies have demonstrated an increased risk of local recurrence after mastectomy for patients with four or more positive lymph nodes.[73–75] These findings have led to the study of postmastectomy radiation (PMR) for patients with four or more lymph nodes involved. These studies were recently reviewed by an NIH consensus conference on the utility of PMR and concluded that patients with four or more positive lymph nodes do benefit from PMR.[76]

LOCAL RECURRENCE IN DUCTAL CARCINOMA IN SITU

Concomitant with the increased use of BCT in treating early invasive carcinomas has been an increase in its use for DCIS. Over the last decade there has been considerable controversy surrounding therapy for patients with DCIS. The application of BCT for DCIS has yielded high local recurrence rates. The result of the National Surgical Adjuvant Breast Project (NSABP) Protocol B-17 attempted to address the question of whether postoperative radiation therapy had a beneficial effect on local recurrence after BCT for DCIS. This study revealed a local recurrence rate of 10% for patients treated with BCT and radiation versus 21% for patients treated with tumor excision alone. Further, the incidence of invasive disease present in the local recurrence was significantly reduced by BCT with radiation.[77,78]

Subsequent to the NSABP B-17, several 8-year follow-up analyses of the patients in this study have been performed. One purpose of these follow-up analyses is to determine which clinicopathologic factors best correlate with local recurrence after BCT, possibly identifying subsets of patients whose risk of local recurrence is so low that they can be spared radiation. In a multivariate analysis, Fisher et al identified moderate/marked comedo necrosis and uncertain/involved tumor margin status as independent predictors of local recurrence[79]; however, in their analysis, patients identified as having low risk of recurrence still benefited from radiation therapy. In our own institution, we found that both positive surgical margin (2 mm or less) and the absence of postoperative radiation were associated with local recurrence.[80] We are, therefore, in favor of postoperative radiation in all patients undergoing BCT for DICS, with the exception of those with minimal DCIS or a generous surgical margin.

Alternatively, Silverstein et al devised a scoring system, based on a retrospective database analysis, to separate DCIS patients into three groups according to three independent predictors of local recurrence: pathology, margin, and size.[81] This system, known as the Van Nuys Prognostic Index (VPNI), attempts to identify patients that can be treated with BCT alone, BCT with radiation, or mastectomy. The pathologic score was based on the presence or absence of high nuclear grade and comedo necrosis. The margin width was categorized based upon widely free margins (10 mm or larger), intermediate margins (1 to 9 mm), and close margins (less than 1 mm). The size of the tumors were stratified into tumors smaller than 15 mm, 16 to 40 mm, and larger than 40 mm. The VPNI gives equal weighting to each of the three factors in their predictive value.

Boland et al have recently applied the VPNI to a group of patients in the UK.[82] In their analysis, they categorized their patient population into low, intermediate, and high risk groups based on their VPNI criteria. They found that the most important predictor of local recurrence was the margin width. Tumor grade (either by the Van Nuys pathologic classification or one of their own) also held predictive value; however, the tumor size was of no significance. Whereas Boland et al found the margin width to outweigh the pathologic grade in its predictive value by a factor of 3:1, they found that a disproportionate group of patients fell into the intermediate group (78%) and argued that the VPNI lacks the ability to effectively discriminate patients' tumors and thus cannot be used to stratify patients for adjuvant local therapy.

At this time there is still no consensus on the criteria that identify those patients in whom the risk of local recurrence after BCT for DCIS is low enough to safely omit adjuvant radiotherapy. For a small lesion, in the absence of a high nuclear grade, an excision margin of 10 mm or more may be adequate.[83] Conversely, for large DCIS tumors (larger than 50 mm), of high nuclear grade with comedo necrosis and marginal surgical margins, a mastectomy may be indicated. In-between patients with DCIS in whom a negative margin is accomplished should receive postoperative radiation. A postlumpectomy mammogram is required in all patients with DICS associated with microcalcifications to ensure the absence of residual microcalcifications.

REOPERATION FOR LOCAL RECURRENCE AFTER BREAST CONSERVATION THERAPY: RE-EXCISION VERSUS MASTECTOMY

The management of IBTR following breast conservation therapy is controversial. The limited reports on the recurrence rates for IBTR treated with re-excision vary from 25% to 36% versus 12% when mastectomy is employed for IBTR.[84,85] In a retrospective study, however, Salvadori et al found there to be no statistically significant difference between re-excision versus mastectomy for the treatment of IBTR.[86] After a median follow-up of 73 months following treatment for local recurrence, the relapse rate was 13% (8 of 57) after re-excision of the IBTR, versus 3% (4 of 133) in patients treated with mastectomy. The currently accepted surgery after a failed breast conservation treatment is mastectomy.

REOPERATION FOR LOCAL RECURRENCE FOLLOWING MASTECTOMY: CHEST WALL RECURRENCE

As stated earlier, breast cancer patients are highly heterogeneous and it is no surprise that local recurrence following mastectomy is also heterogeneous in terms of its incidence and biologic behavior. Thus, treatment recommendations for this type of recurrence are not standardized, and there is considerable controversy regarding the use of surgery, chemotherapy, and radiation. The incidence of chest wall recurrence (CWR) has been reported to range by as much as 5% to 40% of breast cancer patients.[87] CWR after mastectomy is frequently associated with distant metastases. Recent studies examining the relationship of clinicopathologic variables to outcomes have been able to stratify patients into several groups that serve to identify patients in whom aggressive therapy, including both systemic and local treatment, for the isolated CWR is indicated.

Features such as primary nodal status, tumor grade, estrogen receptor status, length of disease-free interval, positive margins, and lymphovascular invasion have been reported as having significant prognostic impact on disease-free survival.[88,89] Chagpar et al in a multivariate analysis found that disease-free interval greater than 24 months, initial node-negative disease, and the use of postmastectomy radiation were associated with a low risk for local rerecurrence and development of distant metastases. The authors suggested that those patients with one or two of these factors belong to an intermediate risk group, and those patients with none of these favorable prognosticators were at high risk for subsequent relapse. They found that positive initial node status was the only significant factor predictive of distant metastases and overall survival.[87]

In contrast, variations in the characteristics of CWR, including number of nodules, size of CWR, and location of CWR, were found to be of no significance in predicting survival.[90,91] These studies were important in that they demonstrated that long-term survival after CWR is possible. Further, they have identified the subset of patients with the best prognosis who would benefit most from aggressive therapy of the recurrence.

In the absence of prospective randomized trials comparing various treatment modalities, the optimal treatment for CWR remains unclear. Most CWRs are soft tissue recurrences in the skin and subcutaneous tissues, with other sites including the deeper tissues such as the muscle bone (rib/sternum) and pleura. Surgical options range from local excision, to local excision with radiation, to radical extirpation with possible chest wall resection. For soft tissue recurrences, local excision to achieve negative margins is the procedure of choice. For deeper tissue recurrences, muscle resection with or without chest wall resection should be considered. Radiation is frequently added if it has not previously been used in the initial treatment.

Downey et al recently reported on 5-year outcomes in a series of 38 breast cancer patients with CWR that were treated with full thickness chest wall resection. This study found that 1-, 3-, and 5-year survival rates after chest wall resection were 74%, 41%, and 18%, respectively. The operative mortality was 0%.[92] In this study, the majority of patients (33 of 38) has chest wall reconstruction using a rigid prosthesis made of a sandwich of Marlex mesh-methyl methacrylate. Thus, chest wall resection, though a radical procedure, is not only safe, but also seems to provide some survival benefit in patients with full thickness chest wall involvement.

From retrospective analyses it seems clear that there is a survival advantage to the use of radiation for CWR that has made it a standard of care at some major centers.[87,93] Recent data regarding outcomes in patients with isolated CWR treated with radiation found that the survival outcomes varied depending on the initial stage of the disease. More specifically, they divided patients into three groups: one group, T1-2 and N0, had an overall survival of 79.9%, whereas two other groups, T1-2 with one to three positive lymph nodes, and T3-4 with four or more positive lymph nodes, had survival rates of 41.9% and 29.1%, respectively.[94] In summary, patients with CWR are most likely to be treated with local resection to obtain a cancer-free margin. Postoperative radiation is recommended for those who did not already receive radiation, and systemic treatment is mandatory in all patients with CWR.

CHEST WALL RECURRENCE FOLLOWING IMMEDIATE BREAST RECONSTRUCTION

Recent data from the plastic surgical literature studying local recurrence following mastectomy with immediate reconstruction suggested that not all CWRs are the same in terms of their location. With the increased use of immediate breast reconstruction with either autologous tissue or implants following mastectomy, questions have been raised as to whether immediate reconstruction negatively impacts the potential for disease control. Recently Langstein et al examined a large series of patients (1694) who had undergone immediate reconstruction and found their local recurrence rate to be 2.3% (69 patients). These authors reported the survival outcomes based on skin/subcutaneous recurrences versus "chest wall" recurrences. They found that 72% of recurrences were skin/subcutaneous recurrences (28 of 39), as opposed to only 28% (11 of 39) representing chest wall recurrences. At follow-up of 80 months, these authors found that the overall survival rates for the skin/subcutaneous group was 61% versus 45% for the chest wall recurrence group. They also found that the skin/subcutaneous group had a greater chance of remaining disease free after treatment of the recurrence over the chest wall recurrence group (32% versus 9%).[95]

Based upon these data, they argue that breast reconstruction does not negatively impact the incidence of CWR. Patients with skin/subcutaneous recurrences seem to fare better than those with deeper tissue chest wall recurrences. Patients with disease involving the deep chest wall tissues have a higher likelihood of distant disease, a higher rate of relapse, and a lower overall survival.

For the management of local recurrence in the mastectomy patient with immediate breast reconstruction, once again there are no prospective studies to guide therapeutic decisions. As for postmastectomy recurrence in the absence of reconstruction, a multimodality approach consisting of surgery, radiation, and/or chemotherapy is recommended for the best disease control in the reconstructed breast. For skin/subcutaneous tissue recurrence, a simple re-excision with removal of as much reconstructed tissue as necessary to achieve negative margins is recommended. Postoperative radiotherapy after re-excision is now being frequently employed in patients who did not already receive it. Chest wall resection should be considered in selected patient populations.

REOPERATION OF THE AXILLA FOR REGIONAL LYMPH NODE RECURRENCE

Regional lymph node recurrence generally refers to recurrence in the previously treated axilla. It can occur as an isolated event or in conjunction with IBTR or distant metastatic disease. The management of local regional lymph node recurrence is controversial and there are no prospective randomized trials that compare treatment modalities (surgery, radiation, and chemotherapy).

The overall incidence of regional lymph node recurrence, including axillary, supraclavicular, infraclavicular, and internal mammary lymph nodes, is rather low. In several series of patients having undergone treatment for early stage breast cancer, the figure has been reported at approximately 2% to 3%.[59,96,97] These series have all examined this small group of patients with respect to patterns of lymph node recurrence, factors associated with lymph node recurrence, and outcomes, and have highlighted a number of important aspects in the management of regional lymph node recurrence.

It appears from these studies that there are survival differences among patients with regional nodal recurrence. Harris et al recently reported 5- and 10-year overall survival statistics on a group of 39 patients with lymph node recurrences and found that patients with lymph node alone or lymph node plus local breast recurrence had similar 5- and 10-year survival rates (67% and 44% for regional lymph node alone versus 69% and 26% for regional with local recurrence).[98] As expected, patients found to have both lymph node recurrence and distant metastases had 5- and 10-year overall survival rates similar to those in stage IV disease, both only 12%. The factors identified by multivariate analysis of this study that predicted regional lymph node recurrence in patients with early breast cancer were: age over 50 years, T2 breast cancers, and stage II disease.

Thus, it appears from the most recent literature that regional lymph node recurrence after treatment for initial early breast cancer is relatively infrequent. The role of surgery in this type of recurrence is limited to axillary recurrences that are either isolated or are found in conjunction with IBTR, in which ALND or modified radical mastectomy, in conjunction with systemic treatment and radiation, would be indicated. These are the patients who clearly benefit from aggressive therapy. There does not appear to be a role for the surgical management of regional lymph node recurrence in basins other than the axilla, as radiation would be the treatment of choice, nor is surgery indicated for asymptomatic regional lymph node recurrences in the presence of distant disease.

REOPERATIVE SENTINEL LYMPH NODE BIOPSY

The role of SLN biopsy is being extended beyond early stage breast cancer. For example, it is becoming increasingly applied in the setting of large DCIS, as it has been reported that 10% to 15% of these patients have invasive cancer in the surgical specimen.[98] More relevant to this discussion has been its increasing use to stage the axilla in the setting of local recurrence after BCT, following the observation that a number of local recurrences occur simultaneously with regional lymph node recurrence.[96,99]

Port et al recently reported on the feasibility of the technique of SLN biopsy in patients who have previously undergone an operation of the axilla. They examined 32 patients, 22 (69%) of whom had undergone previous SLN biopsy or ALND, 7 (22%) of whom had undergone SLN biopsy after a recent failed SLN biopsy or inadequate ALND, and 3 (9%) of who had previous axillary surgery for an unrelated condition. These authors had previously reported successful identification of the SLN in 97% to 98% of patients undergoing SLN biopsy for initial breast cancer therapy, with a false negative rate of 4% to 5%. In the reoperative setting, they were able to identify the SLN in 87% of patients in whom fewer than 10 nodes had been previously removed. In patients with 10 or more nodes previously removed, however, their success rate was limited to 44%.[100] Thus, it seems that for patients with 10 or fewer nodes previously removed, SLN biopsy is feasible to restage the axilla in the setting of local recurrence.

REFERENCES

1. Jemal A, Murray T, Samuels A, et al. Cancer statistics, 2003. CA Cancer J Clin 2003;53:5–26.
2. Veronesi U, Cascinelli N, Mariani L, et al. Twenty-year follow-up of a randomized study comparing breast-conserving surgery with radical mastectomy for early breast cancer. N Engl J Med 2002;347:1227–1232.
3. Fisher B, Anderson S, Bryant J, et al. Twenty-year follow-up of a randomized trial comparing total mastectomy, lumpectomy, and lumpectomy plus irradiation for the treatment of invasive breast cancer. N Engl J Med 2002;347: 1233–1241.
4. Tran CL, Langer S, Broderick-Villa G, DiFronzo LA. Does reoperation predispose to postoperative wound infection in women undergoing operation for breast cancer? Am Surg 2003;69:852–856.
5. Liberman L, Fahs MC, Dershaw DD, et al. Impact of stereotaxic core breast biopsy on cost of diagnosis. Radiology 1995;195:633–637.
6. Howisey RL, Acheson MB, Rowbotham RK, Morgan A. A comparison of Medicare reimbursement and results for various imaging-guided breast biopsy techniques. Am J Surg 1997;173:395–398.
7. Pettine S, Place R, Babu S, et al. Stereotactic breast biopsy is accurate, minimally invasive, and cost effective. Am J Surg 1996;171:474–476.
8. Morrow M, Venta L, Stinson T, Bennett C. Prospective comparison of stereotactic core biopsy and surgical excision as diagnostic procedures for breast cancer patients. Ann Surg 2001;233:537–541.
9. Liberman L, La Trenta LR, Dershaw DD. Impact of core biopsy on the surgical management of impalpable breast cancer: another look at margins. AJR Am J Roentgenol 1997;169:1464–1465.
10. Borgstein PJ, Pijpers R, Comans EF, et al. Sentinel lymph node biopsy in breast cancer: guidelines and pitfalls of lymphoscintigraphy and gamma probe detection. J Am Coll Surg 1998;186:275–283.
11. Feldman SM, Krag DN, McNally RK, et al. Limitation in gamma probe localization of the sentinel node in breast cancer patients with large excisional biopsy. J Am Coll Surg 1999;188:248–254.
12. Wong SL, Edwards MJ, Chao C, et al. The effect of prior breast biopsy method and concurrent definitive breast procedure on success and accuracy of sentinel lymph node biopsy. Ann Surg Oncol 2002;9:272–277.
13. King TA, Hayes DH, Cederbom GJ, et al. Biopsy technique has no impact on local recurrence after breast-conserving therapy. Breast J 2001;7:19–24.
14. Solin LJ, Fowble BL, Schultz DJ, Goodman RL. The significance of the pathology margins of the tumor excision on the outcome of patients treated with definitive irradiation for early stage breast cancer. Int J Radiat Oncol Biol Phys 1991; 21:279–287.
15. Tartter PI, Kaplan J, Bleiweiss I, et al. Lumpectomy margins, reexcision, and local recurrence of breast cancer. Am J Surg 2000;179:81–85.

16. Touboul E, Buffat L, Belkacemi Y, et al. Local recurrences and distant metastases after breast-conserving surgery and radiation therapy for early breast cancer. Int J Radiat Oncol Biol Phys 1999;43:25–38.

17. Park CC, Mitsumori M, Nixon A, et al. Outcome at 8 years after breast-conserving surgery and radiation therapy for invasive breast cancer: influence of margin status and systemic therapy on local recurrence. J Clin Oncol 2000; 18:1668–1675.

18. Smitt MC, Nowels KW, Zdeblick MJ, et al. The importance of the lumpectomy surgical margin status in long-term results of breast conservation. Cancer 1995; 76:259–267.

19. Smitt MC, Nowels K, Carlson RW, Jeffrey SS. Predictors of reexcision findings and recurrence after breast conservation. Int J Radiat Oncol Biol Phys 2003;57: 979–985.

20. Anscher MS, Jones P, Prosnitz LR, et al. Local failure and margin status in early-stage breast carcinoma treated with conservation surgery and radiation therapy. Ann Surg 1993;218:22–28.

21. Fourquet A, Campana F, Zafrani B, et al. Prognostic factors of breast recurrence in the conservative management of early breast cancer: a 25-year follow-up. Int J Radiat Oncol Biol Phys 1989;17:719–725.

22. Renton SC, Gazet JC, Ford HT, et al. The importance of the resection margin in conservative surgery for breast cancer. Eur J Surg Oncol 1996;22:17–22.

23. Bijker N, Peterse JL, Duchateau L, et al. Risk factors for recurrence and metastasis after breast-conserving therapy for ductal carcinoma-in-situ: analysis of European Organization for Research and Treatment of Cancer Trial 10853. J Clin Oncol 2001;19:2263–2271.

24. Neuschatz AC, DiPetrillo T, Steinhoff M, et al. The value of breast lumpectomy margin assessment as a predictor of residual tumor burden in ductal carcinoma in situ of the breast. Cancer 2002;94:1917–1924.

25. Jobsen JJ, van der Palen J, Ong F, Meerwaldt JH. The value of a positive margin for invasive carcinoma in breast-conservative treatment in relation to local recurrence is limited to young women only. Int J Radiat Oncol Biol Phys 2003;57:724–731.

26. Meric F, Mirza NQ, Vlastos G, et al. Positive surgical margins and ipsilateral breast tumor recurrence predict disease-specific survival after breast-conserving therapy. Cancer 2003;97:926–933.

27. DiBiase SJ, Komarnicky LT, Heron DE, et al. Influence of radiation dose on positive surgical margins in women undergoing breast conservation therapy. Int J Radiat Oncol Biol Phys 2002;53:680–686.

28. Jardines L, Fowble B, Schultz D, et al. Factors associated with a positive reexcision after excisional biopsy for invasive breast cancer. Surgery 1995;118: 803–809.

29. Papa MZ, Zippel D, Kolle M, et al. Positive margins of breast biopsy: is reexcision always necessary? J Surg Oncol 1999;70:167–171.

30. Acosta JA, Greenlee JA, Gubler KD, et al. Surgical margins after needle-localization breast biopsy. Am J Surg 1995;170:643–646.

31. Gwin JL, Eisenberg BL, Hoffman JP, et al. Incidence of gross and microscopic carcinoma in specimens from patients with breast cancer after re-excision lumpectomy. Ann Surg 1993;218:729–734.

32. Kearney TJ, Morrow M. Effect of reexcision on the success of breast-conserving surgery. Ann Surg Oncol 1995;2:303–307.

33. Schmidt-Ullrich R, Wazer DE, Tercilla O, et al. Tumor margin assessment as a guide to optimal conservation surgery and irradiation in early stage breast carcinoma. Int J Radiat Oncol Biol Phys 1989;17:733–738.

34. Schnitt SJ, Connolly JL, Khettry U, et al. Pathologic findings on re-excision of the primary site in breast cancer patients considered for treatment by primary radiation therapy. Cancer 1987;59:675–681.

35. Peterson ME, Schultz DJ, Reynolds C, Solin LJ. Outcomes in breast cancer patients relative to margin status after treatment with breast-conserving surgery and radiation therapy: the University of Pennsylvania experience. Int J Radiat Oncol Biol Phys 1999;43:1029–1035.

36. Freedman G, Fowble B, Hanlon A, et al. Patients with early stage invasive cancer with close or positive margins treated with conservative surgery and radiation have an increased risk of breast recurrence that is delayed by adjuvant systemic therapy. Int J Radiat Oncol Biol Phys 1999;44:1005–1015.

37. Wazer DE, Jabro G, Ruthazer R, et al. Extent of margin positivity as a predictor for local recurrence after breast conserving irradiation. Radiat Oncol Investig 1999;7:111–117.

38. Pittinger TP, Maronian NC, Poulter CA, Peacock JL. Importance of margin status in outcome of breast-conserving surgery for carcinoma. Surgery 1994;116:605–609.

39. Singletary SE. Surgical margins in patients with early-stage breast cancer treated with breast conservation therapy. Am J Surg 2002;184:383–393.

40. Gibson GR, Lesnikoski BA, Yoo J, et al. A comparison of ink-directed and traditional whole-cavity re-excision for breast lumpectomy specimens with positive margins. Ann Surg Oncol 2001;8:693–704.

41. Tafra L, Smith SJ, Woodward JE, et al. Pilot trial of cryoprobe-assisted breast-conserving surgery for small ultrasound-visible cancers. Ann Surg Oncol 2003;10:1018–1024.

42. Dooley WC. Routine operative breast endoscopy during lumpectomy. Ann Surg Oncol 2003;10:38–42.

43. Solin LJ, Fourquet A, Vicini FA, et al. Mammographically detected ductal carcinoma in situ of the breast treated with breast-conserving surgery and definitive breast irradiation: long-term outcome and prognostic significance of patient age and margin status. Int J Radiat Oncol Biol Phys 2001;50:991–1002.

44. Cheng L, Al-Kaisi NK, Gordon NH, et al. Relationship between the size and margin status of ductal carcinoma in situ of the breast and residual disease. J Natl Cancer Inst 1997;89:1356–1360.

45. Chagpar A, Yen T, Sahin A, et al. Intraoperative margin assessment reduces reexcision rates in patients with ductal carcinoma in situ treated with breast-conserving surgery. Am J Surg 2003;186:371–377.

46. Kaufman CS, Jacobson L, Bachman B, Kaufman LB. Intraoperative ultrasonography guidance is accurate and efficient according to results in 100 breast cancer patients. Am J Surg 2003;186:378–382.

47. Smith LF, Rubio IT, Henry-Tillman R, et al. Intraoperative ultrasound-guided breast biopsy. Am J Surg 2000;180:419–423.

48. Rahusen FD, Bremers AJ, Fabry HF, et al. Ultrasound-guided lumpectomy of nonpalpable breast cancer versus wire-guided resection: a randomized clinical trial. Ann Surg Oncol 2002;9:994–998.

49. Weiser MR, Montgomery LL, Susnik B, et al. Is routine intraoperative frozen-section examination of sentinel lymph nodes in breast cancer worthwhile? Ann Surg Oncol 2000;7:651–655.

50. Zervos EE, Badgwell BD, Abdessalam SF, et al. Selective analysis of the sentinel node in breast cancer. Am J Surg 2001;182:372–376.

51. Leidenius MH, Krogerus LA, Toivonen TS, Von Smitten KJ. The feasibility of intraoperative diagnosis of sentinel lymph node metastases in breast cancer. J Surg Oncol 2003;84:68–73.

52. Menes TS, Tartter PI, Mizrachi H, et al. Touch preparation or frozen section for intraoperative detection of sentinel lymph node metastases from breast cancer. Ann Surg Oncol 2003;10:1166–1170.

53. della Rovere GQ, Benson JR. Ipsilateral local recurrence of breast cancer: determinant or indicator of poor prognosis? Lancet Oncol 2002;3:183–187.

54. Haffty BG, Reiss M, Beinfield M, et al. Ipsilateral breast tumor recurrence as a predictor of distant disease: implications for systemic therapy at the time of local relapse. J Clin Oncol 1996;14:52–57.

55. Elkhuizen PH, van de Vijver MJ, Hermans JZ, et al. Local recurrence after breast-conserving therapy for invasive breast cancer: high incidence in young patients and association with poor survival. Int J Radiat Oncol Biol Phys 1998;40:859–867.

56. Rouzier R, Extra JM, Carton M, et al. Primary chemotherapy for operable breast cancer: incidence and prognostic significance of ipsilateral breast tumor recurrence after breast-conserving surgery. J Clin Oncol 2001;19:3828–3835.

57. Hayward J, Caleffi M. The significance of local control in the primary treatment of breast cancer. Lucy Wortham James clinical research award. Arch Surg 1987;122:1244–1247.

58. Voogd AC, Nielsen M, Peterse JL, et al. Differences in risk factors for local and distant recurrence after breast-conserving therapy or mastectomy for stage I and II breast cancer: pooled results of two large European randomized trials. J Clin Oncol 2001;19:1688–1697.

59. Fowble BL, Schultz DJ, Overmoyer B, et al. The influence of young age on outcome in early stage breast cancer. Int J Radiat Oncol Biol Phys 1994;30:23–33.

60. Kini VR, White JR, Horwitz EM, et al. Long term results with breast-conserving therapy for patients with early stage breast carcinoma in a community hospital setting. Cancer 1998;82:127–133.

61. Voogd AC, Peterse JL, Crommelin MA, et al. Histological determinants for different types of local recurrence after breast-conserving therapy of invasive breast cancer. Dutch Study Group on local Recurrence after Breast Conservation (BORST). Eur J Cancer 1999;35:1828–1837.

62. Fredriksson I, Liljegren G, Palm-Sjovall M, et al. Risk factors for local recurrence after breast-conserving surgery. Br J Surg 2003;90:1093–1102.

63. Macmillan RD, Purushotham AD, Mallon E, et al. Tumour bed positivity predicts outcome after breast-conserving surgery. Br J Surg 1997;84:1559–1562.

64. Schnitt SJ, Abner A, Gelman R, et al. The relationship between microscopic margins of resection and the risk of local recurrence in patients with breast cancer treated with breast-conserving surgery and radiation therapy. Cancer 1994;74:1746–1751.

65. Kurtz JM, Jacquemier J, Amalric R, et al. Risk factors for breast recurrence in premenopausal and postmenopausal patients with ductal cancers treated by conservation therapy. Cancer 1990;65:1867–1878.

66. Sinn HP, Anton HW, Magener A, et al. Extensive and predominant in situ component in breast carcinoma: their influence on treatment results after breast-conserving therapy. Eur J Cancer 1998;34:646–653.

67. Borger J, Kemperman H, Hart A, et al. Risk factors in breast-conservation therapy. J Clin Oncol 1994;12:653–660.

68. Locker AP, Ellis IO, Morgan DA, et al. Factors influencing local recurrence after excision and radiotherapy for primary breast cancer. Br J Surg 1989;76: 890–894.

69. Cowen D, Houvenaeghel G, Bardou V, et al. Local and distant failures after limited surgery with positive margins and radiotherapy for node-negative breast cancer. Int J Radiat Oncol Biol Phys 2000;47:305–312.

70. Cowen D, Jacquemier J, Houvenaeghel G, et al. Local and distant recurrence after conservative management of "very low-risk" breast cancer are dependent events: a 10-year follow-up. Int J Radiat Oncol Biol Phys 1998;41:801–807.

71. Leopold KA, Recht A, Schnitt SJ, et al. Results of conservative surgery and radiation therapy for multiple synchronous cancers of one breast. Int J Radiat Oncol Biol Phys 1989;16:11–16.

72. Kurtz JM, Jacquemier J, Amalric R, et al. Breast-conserving therapy for macroscopically multiple cancers. Ann Surg 1990;212:38–44.

73. Beenken SW, Urist MM, Zhang Y, et al. Axillary lymph node status, but not tumor size, predicts locoregional recurrence and overall survival after mastectomy for breast cancer. Ann Surg 2003;237:732–739.

74. Overgaard M, Hansen PS, Overgaard J, et al. Postoperative radiotherapy in high-risk premenopausal women with breast cancer who receive adjuvant chemotherapy. Danish Breast Cancer Cooperative Group 82b Trial. N Engl J Med 1997;337:949–955.

75. Ragaz J, Jackson SM, Le N, et al. Adjuvant radiotherapy and chemotherapy in node-positive premenopausal women with breast cancer. N Engl J Med 1997;337:956–962.

76. Eifel P, Axelson JA, Costa J, et al. National Institutes of Health Consensus Development Conference Statement: adjuvant therapy for breast cancer, November 1–3, 2000. J Natl Cancer Inst 2000;93:979–989.

77. Fisher B, Costantino J, Redmond C, et al. Lumpectomy compared with lumpectomy and radiation therapy for the treatment of intraductal breast cancer. N Engl J Med 1993;328:1581–1586.

78. Weng EY, Juillard GJ, Parker RG, et al. Outcomes and factors impacting local recurrence of ductal carcinoma in situ. Cancer 2000;88:1643–1649.

79. Fisher B, Dignam J, Wolmark N, et al. Lumpectomy and radiation therapy for the treatment of intraductal breast cancer: findings from National Surgical Adjuvant Breast and Bowel Project B-17. J Clin Oncol 1998;16:441–452.

80. Wong E, Julliard G, Parker R, et al. Outcomes and factors impacting local recurrences of ductal carcinoma in situ (DCIS). Cancer 2000;88:1643–1649.

81. Silverstein MJ, Lagios MD, Craig PH, et al. A prognostic index for ductal carcinoma in situ of the breast. Cancer 1996;77:2267–2274.

82. Boland GP, Chan KC, Knox WF, et al. Value of the Van Nuys Prognostic Index in prediction of recurrence of ductal carcinoma in situ after breast-conserving surgery. Br J Surg 2003;90:426–432.

83. Silverstein MJ, Lagios MD, Groshen S, et al. The influence of margin width on local control of ductal carcinoma in situ of the breast. N Engl J Med 1999;340: 1455–1461.

84. Dalberg K, Liedberg A, Johansson U, Rutqvist LE. Uncontrolled local disease after salvage treatment for ipsilateral breast tumour recurrence. Eur J Surg Oncol 2003;29:143–154.

85. Kurtz JM, Spitalier JM, Amalric R, et al. The prognostic significance of late local recurrence after breast-conserving therapy. Int J Radiat Oncol Biol Phys 1990; 18:87–93.

86. Salvadori B, Marubini E, Miceli R, et al. Reoperation for locally recurrent breast cancer in patients previously treated with conservative surgery. Br J Surg 1999;86:84–87.

87. Chagpar A, Meric-Bernstam F, Hunt KK, et al. Chest wall recurrence after mastectomy does not always portend a dismal outcome. Ann Surg Oncol 2003;10: 628–634.

88. Schmoor C, Sauerbrei W, Bastert G, Schumacher M. Role of isolated locoregional recurrence of breast cancer: results of four prospective studies. J Clin Oncol 2000;18:1696–1708.

89. Freedman GM, Fowble BL. Local recurrence after mastectomy or breast-conserving surgery and radiation. Oncology (Huntingt) 2000;14:1561–1581; discussion 1581–1582, 1582–1584.

90. Schwaibold F, Fowble BL, Solin LJ, et al. The results of radiation therapy for isolated local regional recurrence after mastectomy. Int J Radiat Oncol Biol Phys 1991;21:299–310.

91. Halverson KJ, Perez CA, Kuske RR, et al. Survival following locoregional recurrence of breast cancer: univariate and multivariate analysis. Int J Radiat Oncol Biol Phys 1992;23:285–291.

92. Downey RJ, Rusch V, Hsu FI, et al. Chest wall resection for locally recurrent breast cancer: is it worthwhile? J Thorac Cardiovasc Surg 2000;119:420–428.

93. Deutsch M. Radiotherapy for postmastectomy local-regional recurrent breast cancer. Am J Clin Oncol 2000;23:494–498.

94. Chagpar A, Kuerer HM, Hunt KK, et al. Outcome of treatment for breast cancer patients with chest wall recurrence according to initial stage: implications for post-mastectomy radiation therapy. Int J Radiat Oncol Biol Phys 2003;57: 128–135.

95. Langstein HN, Cheng MH, Singletary SE, et al. Breast cancer recurrence after immediate reconstruction: patterns and significance. Plast Reconstr Surg 2003; 111:712–722.

96. Harris EE, Hwang WT, Seyednejad F, Solin LJ. Prognosis after regional lymph node recurrence in patients with stage I-II breast carcinoma treated with breast conservation therapy. Cancer 2003;98:2144–2151.

97. Recht A, Pierce SM, Abner A, et al. Regional nodal failure after conservative surgery and radiotherapy for early-stage breast carcinoma. J Clin Oncol 1991;9: 988–996.

98. Cox CE, Nguyen K, Gray RJ, et al. Importance of lymphatic mapping in ductal carcinoma in situ (DCIS): why map DCIS? Am Surg 2001;67:513–519, 519–521.

99. Moran MS, Haffty BG. Local-regional breast cancer recurrence: prognostic groups based on patterns of failure. Breast J 2002;8:81–87.

100. Port ER, Fey J, Gemignani ML, et al. Reoperative sentinel lymph node biopsy: a new option for patients with primary or locally recurrent breast carcinoma. J Am Coll Surg 2002;195:167–172.

CHAPTER 14

Reoperative Surgery for Intestinal Fistulas

David R. Fischer, MD; Michael S. Nussbaum, MD, FACS

Précis

The critical points to the successful management of gastrointestinal fistulas are recognition of the fistula, control of infection and further contamination, restoration of fluid and electrolyte losses, and the reestablishment of a positive nutritional balance prior to undertaking major, definitive, corrective procedures.

Introduction

The word fistula comes from the Latin meaning a pipe or a flute and is defined as an abnormal communication between two epithelialized surfaces. Gastrointestinal fistulas continue to cause significant morbidity and mortality, even though many factors important to their management are known. Over the past 35 to 40 years, mortality for gastrointestinal fistulas has diminished from approximately 40% to 60% down to 15% to 20%. This improvement in prognosis is attributable to general advances in fluid and electrolyte/acid-base therapy, blood administration, critical care advances, ventilatory management, antibiotic regimens, and nutritional management. Formerly, malnutrition and electrolyte imbalance were the causes of death in the majority of these patients. In the present era of fistula treatment, mortality is largely attributable to uncontrolled sepsis and sepsis-associated malnutrition.

The mechanism of fistula formation is varied. Congenital fistulas are caused by errors in development. Acquired fistulas may occur as a result of inflammatory disease, abdominal trauma, surgical complications, radiation, and benign or malignant neoplasms. Spontaneous causes of gastrointestinal fistula account for 15% to 25% of these fistulas. These include radiation, inflammatory bowel disease, diverticular disease, appendicitis, ischemic bowel, indwelling tubes, perforation of duodenal ulcer, pancreatic and gynecologic malignancies, and intestinal actinomycosis or tuberculosis.[1–4] The remaining 75% to 85% of gastrointestinal fistulas are of iatrogenic origin occurring as the result of technical complications of surgical procedures. These include dehiscence of anastomoses, mechanical injury to the bowel during dissection, or the accidental suture of the bowel during abdominal closure. Other technical complications resulting in fistulas are those that occur at delayed periods following operations such as intraperitoneal bleeding and abscess formation with or without suture line dehiscence.

Treatment of patients with gastrointestinal fistulas requires an understanding of metabolic and anatomic derangements. In order for patient mortality to be minimized, nutrition, volume, and electrolyte derangements must be promptly corrected. Additionally, ongoing losses must be anticipated and prevented. Malnutrition is easier to prevent than correct. Once established, malnutrition is difficult to correct, especially in the face of concomitant sepsis. Following the initial stabilization period and the establishment of nutrition support, management can be divided into phases involving determination of the anatomy of the fistula and the likelihood of spontaneous closure, which may then be followed by definitive surgical therapy, and, finally, the healing process.

Clinical Findings

Postoperative fistula formation is heralded by fever and abdominal pain until bowel contents discharge through the abdominal incision. Spontaneous fistulas from neoplasm or inflammatory disease usually develop in a more indolent manner. The loss of gastrointestinal contents either prematurely by diversion to the body surface or by "short circuiting" within the gastrointestinal tract may result in profound fluid and electrolyte losses, the specific nature depending upon the portion of the gastrointestinal tract whose contents are lost. Malabsorption with severe nutritional and vitamin deficiencies may also ensue. Fistulas commonly are associated with one or more abscesses, which often drain incompletely with fistulization. Therefore, persistent sepsis may occur, the result of contamination of a normally sterile space or organ system by gastrointestinal flora traversing the fistula. Gastrointestinal hemorrhage, intestinal obstruction, and excoriation and erosion of the skin by gastrointestinal secretions may also complicate the course of the fistula patient. These problems may be superimposed on other abnormalities inherent to the underlying disease that produced the fistula.

The present approach and understanding of fistula management has developed significantly over the past 40 years. In their classic 1960 paper, Edmunds, Williams, and Welch called attention to the serious nature and the high mortality of patients with such fistulas and pointed out the relationship between infection, malnutrition, fistula output, and mortality.[5] In addition, they advocated earlier surgical intervention in all high-output fistulas and recommended total resection of the fistula with end-to-end anastomosis, or complete bypass of the fistula when resection was not possible. With early correction of the fistulas, malnutrition and its attendant complications were thereby less likely to develop. The overall mortality in their series was 44%.[5]

The signal study in 1964 by Chapman et al emphasized that the key to successful management was to "get control of fistula," combat sepsis, and from the very beginning maintain adequate nutritional support.[6] They stressed the vital role of nutrition and reported a decreased mortality of 14% in those patients treated with an excess of 3000 calories per day using a combination of intravenous (peripheral administration of protein hydrolysates) and tube feedings. They also emphasized that supportive and surgical treatment go hand in hand; the two are not mutually exclusive. Their indications for operative closure of the fistula included the presence of distal intestinal obstruction, continued massive loss of fluid from the fistula despite control of the infection and an adequate nutritional regimen, and persistence of the fistula even without high losses over a prolonged period. In a follow-up report in 1971, Sheldon et al documented the success of such a treatment regimen, noting that most patients could be given adequate nutrition by standard methods such as tube and enterostomy feedings. At the time of their report, total parenteral nutrition was a new technique that had been used in only a few select patients.[7]

With the widespread advent of parenteral nutrition in the 1970s, the overall reduction in mortality to the range of 15% to 20% was achieved consistently in a variety of reports. In their reviews of large series of patients, Reber et al in 1978 (786 patients) and Soeters and associates in 1979 (404 patients) reported that the addition of parenteral nutrition in large scale to the treatment of gastrointestinal fistulas improved the spontaneous closure rate.[8,9] Parenteral nutrition, however, had no impact on fistula mortality, and maintenance of adequate nutrition using more conventional methods was equally effective.[8,9] Nevertheless, parenteral nutrition has greatly simplified the nutritional management of patients with gastrointestinal fistulas. Once a patient is both malnourished and septic, it becomes quite difficult to replete such a patient. Although these patients often have abdominal abscesses and bacteremia, parenteral nutrition is safe, and the overall incidence of septic complications due to the central line or parenteral nutrition are no greater than in other clinical situations.

It is much better to begin to provide nutritional support as soon as the patient is stabilized. Full caloric and nitrogen replacement can be provided within a few days of instituting nutrition support.[10] Utilizing a combination of enteral nutrition techniques along with parenteral nutrition, adequate caloric and nitrogen intake should be achieved rapidly. It is advantageous to provide at least a portion of the calories through the enteral route, since the gastrointestinal tract is a much more efficacious way of providing nutrition, maintaining the intestinal mucosal barrier and immunologic integrity, as well as stimulating hepatic protein synthesis, which has been found to be of critical value in the determination of the outcome in fistula patients.[11] As little as 20% to 25% of nutrition supplied enterally is usually sufficient to provide the advantages of enteral nutrition, and the remainder can be supplied via parenteral nutrition. Conversely, the decreased fistula output that usually accompanies the institution of parenteral nutrition can greatly simplify the management of high-output fistulas. In addition to this adjunctive role in combination with parenteral nutrition, tube feeding continues to be an important measure in the complete nutritional management of some fistula patients with distal and low-output fistulas, when the fistulas are nearly healed, or when parenteral nutrition is difficult or impossible to institute.

Advances in patient monitoring, correction of fluid, electrolyte, and acid/base imbalances, and parenteral nutrition have largely alleviated electrolyte disturbances secondary to high-output fistulas and malnutrition. In the present era, mortality is mostly determined by uncontrolled sepsis and sepsis-associated malnutrition. Malnutrition in the presence of uncontrolled sepsis cannot be treated without effective surgical drainage of the septic source. As long as uncontrolled sepsis persists, the patient's condition will continue to deteriorate. The therapeutic use of appropriate antibiotics for intra-abdominal abscess and intra-abdominal sepsis should be carefully reserved for septicemia and cholangitis as well as in preparation for operation. Once signs of intra-abdominal sepsis have occurred, the use of antibiotics does not obviate the necessity to treat the process surgically or via percutaneous drainage. Abdominal exploration may be required in septic patients who are losing ground, even if diagnostic studies have not pinpointed an abscess. Once sepsis is controlled or when no sepsis is present, parenteral/enteral nutrition should result in improved nutritional status, allowing skin lesions to heal and the future operative field to become quiescent. Early operative intervention in the presence of malnutrition is not necessary and may be detrimental. Even if the regimen of bowel rest in conjunction with intravenous and enteral nutrition does not lead to successful spontaneous fistula closure, the patient is generally in better nutritional and metabolic condition to withstand an operation to correct the fistula.

Staging or Classification

Gastrointestinal fistulas can be classified by their anatomic characteristics, being either internal or external (enterocutaneous) fistulas. The actual anatomic course of the fistula should be defined. In general, the anatomy of a fistula will suggest the etiology and help to prognosticate spontaneous closure.[12,13] Fistulas can be classified physiologically in terms of the output over a 24-hour period. These can be classified as low (less than 200 mL per day), moderate (200 to 500 mL per day), and high (greater than 500 mL per day).[9,12] An accurate measure of fistula output as well as the chemical make-up of the effluent can provide assistance in the prevention and treatment of metabolic deficits and correcting ongoing fluid, electrolyte, and protein losses. The anatomic and etiologic factors are much more important in predicting spontaneous closure than the actual output of the fistula. The underlying disease process will prognosticate both closure rate and mortality.

Management

Management of an intestinal fistula is a difficult and complex process. However, if one uses a systematic approach in dealing with these difficult problems the treatment becomes manageable and potentially rewarding. In general, management can be compartmentalized into five stages: stabilization, investigation, decision, definitive therapy, and healing.[14]

As outlined above, the first step in the management of any intestinal fistula is stabilization of the patient. This is usually accomplished within the first 24 to 48 hours of management. These patients are typically in a vulnerable state of health. They may be febrile and septic from what was thought to be a wound infection treated by opening the wound, and now the wound drainage contains succus entericus and the patient is deteriorating. Alternatively, they may be immunocompromised secondary to ongoing therapy (e.g., cancer radiation treatment, chemotherapy, etc.) or additional infectious processes. Therefore, the most important priority is to stabilize the patient. Patients will typically require rehydration from third-spacing of fluid, emesis, fistula output, or a combination of these and other causes. Rehydration usually will require isotonic fluid until the patient is euvolemic again. Depending on the site of the fistula, replacement of fistula output varies. Small bowel, pancreatic, and biliary losses are isotonic. Colonic losses may be hypotonic, and gastric fistulas may present with the classic hypokalemic, hypochloremic metabolic alkalosis. Although certain patterns can be predicted, electrolyte levels in an aliquot of the fistula output as well as in the patient's serum should be measured and corrected appropriately, according to the particular electrolyte profile. In order to optimize the patient's hemodynamic status, blood transfusion may be required. There is no specific hemoglobin or hematocrit level that requires transfusion; rather, transfusion should be based on the patient's overall hemodynamic status, oxygen-carrying capacity, and oxygen delivery.

Often, these patients will be in a severe catabolic state and have extremely low protein and albumin levels. This is important for several reasons. First, the patients will have a low capillary oncotic pressure, which may contribute to profound edema especially after resuscitation has begun. To minimize this, the patient may be given albumin for a limited period of time to help increase oncotic pressure and minimize edema. More importantly, however, the patient is in a state of nutritional emergency. Before these patients can be stabilized and potentially heal the fistula, positive nitrogen balance must be obtained. If nutritional therapy is not started early, these patients are at great risk for developing multisystem organ failure, infection, and other complications of severe malnutrition that could lead to death.

Nutrition can be given by several routes. Typically, these patients are too ill to eat or certainly cannot take in enough calories even if they can take some oral nutrition. Usually either enteral tube feeding or parenteral nutrition will be required.[8–10,12] The choice of which to use depends on the fistula anatomy. In general, enteral nutrition is preferable to parenteral nutrition, and probably decreases the incidence of multisystem organ failure and sepsis if administered appropriately. Enteral nutrition is not without complication, however, and the process should be closely monitored. Complications such as diarrhea, aspiration, and ischemic bowel are not uncommon without careful clinical monitoring. Enteral nutrition can be given for upper gastrointestinal fistulas, especially when the feeding tube can be placed beyond the fistula (for instance, a feeding tube placed beyond the ligament of Treitz for a gastric or pancreatic fistula). In general, feeding tubes should be placed when possible beyond the ligament of Treitz to decrease potential aspiration risk. Enteral feeding should also be used for distal fistulas (e.g., colonic fistulas), as long as the feeds do not significantly increase the fistula output. On the other hand, parenteral nutrition can be a valuable tool in the treatment of fistulas as well. Patients with small-bowel fistulas may not be able to tolerate enteral nutrition without increasing the fistula output. In these cases, and in others in which patients cannot tolerate enteral feeds, parenteral nutrition is indicated.

Importantly, the stabilization phase often requires control of a septic source. Typically, this will require drainage of an intra-abdominal abscess, and drainage is ideally accomplished in an image-guided, percutaneous fashion. Also, fistula drainage must be controlled and the skin of the abdominal wall protected. Specialized nursing assistance by an enterostomal therapist is frequently necessary and can be quite helpful in the management of these often complex wounds. A sump suction catheter works very well to control fistula drainage (this can be constructed by placing a soft rubber catheter in the wound with an angiocath placed in the side of the catheter to create a sump system by applying low continuous wall suction through the catheter. An ostomy appliance can then be placed around the tube to collect any excess drainage). Alternatively, a wound vacuum drainage system works very well to control the fistula drainage and protect the skin.

The next phase of management is investigation. After stabilization is accomplished in the first 24 to 48 hours, investigation takes place usually over the next 7 to 10 days. Investigation implies a thorough evaluation of the gastrointestinal tract, defining the anatomy of the fistula and identifying any complicating features such as abscess, stricture, or distal obstruction.[12,13] This can be accomplished by several investigational methods. Probably the most important first test is a fistulogram. This will define the length and width of the fistula as well as its anatomic location. This is best performed by the responsible surgeon in collaboration with the radiologist. Another useful test is a computed tomography (CT) scan and/or ultrasonography. This can further define the anatomy of the vicinity of the fistula and evaluate for any ongoing or unrecognized intra-abdominal processes or abscesses, as well as distal obstruction. A CT scan will be required in almost all patients for these reasons, especially to rule out any undrained collections. Other tests such as upper GI series with small bowel follow-through and barium enema are occasionally helpful in further elucidating the exact anatomy and location of the fistula. Endoscopic evaluation, including, colonoscopy, esophagogastroduodenoscopy, and endoscopic retrograde cholangiopancreatography (ERCP), may be helpful in certain specific clinical situations.

Prognosis and Treatment

The next step in fistula management is decision on management and the timing of such management. When one is making these decisions, the likelihood of spontaneous closure must be determined. The likelihood of closure depends on several factors. The first is anatomic location. In general, anatomic locations that are favorable for closure are the oropharynx, esophagus, duodenal stump, pancreas, biliary tree, and jejunum. Unfavorable locations include the stomach, lateral duodenum, ligament of Treitz, and ileum. As mentioned previously, nutritional status is very important. Patients with poor nutritional status, as measured by overall assessment, albumin, short-turnover proteins (serum transferrin, thyroxin-binding prealbumin, retinol-binding protein), injected skin antigens, etc, are much less likely to close a fistula no matter what the anatomic location.[11] More importantly, if a patient's nutritional status is poor, the mortality rate is higher. Another important factor is the presence or absence of sepsis. The absence of sepsis has positive predictive value for closure, whereas the converse is true in the presence of sepsis. Etiology of the fistula also is predictive of closure. Postoperative fistulas and fistulas secondary to appendicitis or diverticulitis are likely to close. Fistulas associated with active Crohn's disease are unlikely to close until the Crohn's disease is quiescent. Fistulas associated with cancer will usually require excision of the tumor along with the fistula. In addition, the presence of a foreign body will prevent closure of the fistula without operative intervention.

The condition of the bowel or other organ involved in the fistula is also important. Healthy adjacent tissue is a favorable factor. Other favorable factors include a small fistula, quiescent disease, and the absence of an abscess. On the other hand, total disruption of the bowel negates closure as do distal obstruction, abscess, malignancy and/or irradiation, epithelialization of the fistula tract, and active disease. Typically a long fistula tract (longer than 2 cm) is more likely to close than a short fistula tract. Similarly, a thin, narrow tract is a favorable prognostic indicator (i.e., less than 1 cm^2). Therefore, short, wide tracts are unlikely to close spontaneously.[12,13] Nutrition has been mentioned as an important factor in stabilization and spontaneous closure. The short-turnover proteins can provide prognostic information. Specifically, a serum transferrin level of less than 200 mg/dL predicts a low likelihood of spontaneous closure.[11] Considering all of the above factors, one determines whether to observe the fistula for spontaneous closure or plan early operation after stabilization. When one determines that the fistula is likely to close and does not operate, if the fistula has not closed after 4 to 5 weeks without sepsis, an operation will likely be required.

The next important decision is to determine if definitive operative therapy is necessary and the timing of such therapy. In situations which are favorable, between 80% and 90% of fistulas that are going to close spontaneously will close within 4 to 5 weeks. When spontaneous closure is unlikely or spontaneous closure has not occurred within that time frame, an operation will be required. When operative therapy has been decided upon, the operation must be carefully planned. Whenever possible the operation should not occur until the patient is stable, not septic, and in an adequate nutritional state. The most favorable time to reoperate on patients is either within ten days of diagnosis or after four months.[13] Unfortunately, reoperation for intestinal fistula usually occurs during an unfavorable time, within 2 to 3 months of the original operation.

When planning the operation for these patients, the surgeon should allow adequate time for a difficult and prolonged procedure. Depending on the complexity of the abdominal wound, component release and other reconstructive maneuvers may be required to achieve closure of the abdominal wall. It is frequently helpful to enlist the expertise of a plastic surgeon in the abdominal wound closure. Thus, preoperative consultation and evaluation by the plastic and reconstructive surgery team should be considered. Preoperative preparation should include a mechanical bowel preparation whenever feasible, preoperative abdominal wall preparation with antiseptic (e.g., chlorhexidine) scrubs beginning at least 24 hours in advance, and perioperative antibiotics directed toward bowel and skin flora as well as any specific organisms identified by recent culture and sensitivity information.

Whenever possible, a new incision or extension of the prior incision over "virgin" abdominal wall will make reentry into the abdominal cavity easier and safer. Once the peritoneal cavity is entered, the entire intestinal tract should be mobilized and a complete enterolysis should be performed whenever possible, especially if there is any question of distal obstruction. A useful adjunct during this portion of the operation is to use laparotomy pads that are soaked in saline solution to "rehydrate" the adhesions before attempting adhesiolysis. Utilizing a combination of gentle compression and palpation with one hand and sharp dissection with either scissors or a scalpel in conjunction with the use of copious amounts of saline-soaked sponges, one can usually carry out a complete mobilization of the involved intestine. In general, if an intestinal fistula cannot be repaired primarily, it will recur. Fistulas require complete resection back to healthy tissue with enteroenterostomy. If the anastomosis is performed on healthy bowel, the choice between a stapled or hand-sewn anastomosis does not matter. More importantly, the anastomosis should be under no tension, there must be adequate blood supply, and there can be no distal obstruction. A feeding jejunostomy or nasoenteric tube should be placed. Ongoing nutritional repletion is an extremely important part of a successful outcome and most patients will not be able to take enough calories by mouth during the postoperative recovery period. A gastrostomy tube may also be a useful adjunct in the postoperative period. Depending on the state of the intestinal tract, the extent of enterolysis required, and the underlying process that led to fistula formation, a prolonged postoperative ileus will commonly occur, and decompression via a gastrostomy while downstream enteral nutrition is given, may be very beneficial. Because of the usual extensive nature of the dissection during such operations, formation of intra-abdominal adhesions is likely. Any methods for decreasing such adhesions utilizing materials such as hyaluronic acid-carboxymethylcellulose membrane (Seprafilm) may be beneficial in preventing postoperative complications.[15] Finally, abdominal wall closure is extremely important to allow for the best chance of success and to prevent recurrent fistulization. The assistance by surgeons with specific skills in abdominal reconstruction (plastic and reconstructive surgery) is often quite helpful in these situations, and their advice and consultation should be readily sought.

Follow-Up

Most postoperative fistula patients are in a profoundly catabolic state in the early postoperative period and are at risk for nutritional complications. Again, optimal nutrition is as important postoperatively as preoperatively. Supplemental nutrition via enteral, parenteral, or a combination is frequently required, and, with time, the patient can be transitioned to complete intake by mouth—even when the patient cannot tolerate full caloric intake via the enteral route, providing a portion of their needs enterally remains an important objective. It may be useful to cycle tube feeds at night once the patient is eating to attempt to stimulate appetite. Meals from home also occasionally help with appetite stimulation. A dietitian consult can be very helpful as well. A period of home tube feeds or (less commonly) home parenteral nutrition is not unreasonable in these patients, as reestablishing normal eating habits may be a long process. The final phase of the treatment of fistulas, then, is healing, and this phase is highly dependent on good nutrition after a well-performed operation. If the patient cannot tolerate at least 1500 kcal enterally, parenteral nutrition should be continued until this goal is achieved. Once the enteral intake approaches this range, the parenteral nutrition can be weaned.

Prognosis

The overall mortality rate if one includes all fistulas is approximately 20%. The prognosis with a postoperative fistula is not as high. Postoperative fistulas have a less than 2% mortality and approximately a 12% morbidity. Delayed complications may include short bowel syndrome, depending upon the extent of the intestinal resection, prior resections, and underlying disease state (e.g., Crohn's disease). In patients with a marginal amount of bowel remaining, some intestinal adaptation may occur, and, with time, weaning of parenteral nutrition may be possible. The surgeon must be vigilant for recurrent fistulas postoperatively. These patients are also highly susceptible to adhesive small bowel obstruction. It is probably wise to treat a postoperative small bowel obstruction in these patients with long-tube decompression, rather than risk further complications with another operation in the early postoperative period.

Summary

The reoperative management of intestinal fistulas provides a surgeon with multiple challenges. Careful attention must be paid to the physiologic, metabolic, and immunologic derangements in these patients. An organized and tolerant approach to the stabilization, investigation, planning, and implementation of medical and surgical therapy, and the healing phase should allow for a successful outcome in the majority of patients.

REFERENCES

1. Patrick CH, Goodin J, Fogarty J. Complication of prolonged transpyloric feeding: Formation of an enterocutaneous fistula. J Pediatr Surg 1988;23: 1023–1024.
2. Galland RB, Spencer J. Radiation-induced gastrointestinal fistulae. Ann Coll Surg Engl 1986;68:5–7.

3. Rubin SC, Benjamin I, Hoskins WJ, et al. Intestinal surgery in gynecologic oncology. Gynecol Oncol 1989;34:30–33.
4. Schein M. Free perforation of benign gastrojejunocolic and gastrocolic fistula: report of two cases. Dis Colon Rectum 1987;30:705–706.
5. Edmunds LH, Williams GH, Welch CE. External fistulas arising from the gastrointestinal tract. Ann Surg 1960;152:445–471.
6. Chapman R, Foran R, Dunphy JE. Management of intestinal fistulas. Am J Surg 1964;108:157–164.
7. Sheldon GF, Gardiner BN, Way LW, Dunphy JE. Management of gastrointestinal fistulas. Surg Gynecol Obstet 1971;133:385–389.
8. Reber HA, Roberts C, Way LW, Dunphy JE. Management of external gastro-intestinal fistulas. Ann Surg. 1978;188:460–467.
9. Soeters PB, Ebeid AM, Fischer JE. Review of 404 patients with gastrointestinal fistulas: impact of parenteral nutrition. Ann Surg 1979;180:393–401.
10. Dudrick SJ, Maharaj AR, McKelvey AA. Artificial nutritional support in patients with gastrointestinal fistulas. World J Surg 1999;23:570–576.
11. Kuvshinoff BW, Brodish RJ, McFadden DW, Fischer JE. Serum transferrin as a prognostic indicator of spontaneous closure and mortality in gastrointestinal cutaneous fistulas. Ann Surg 1993;217:615–623.
12. Fischer JE. The pathophysiology of enterocutaneous fistulas. World J Surg 1983;7:446–450.
13. Fazio VW, Coutsoftides T, Steiger E. Factors influencing the outcome of treatment of small bowel cutaneous fistula. World J Surg 1983;7:481–488.
14. Pritts TA, Fischer DR, Fischer JE. Postoperative enterocutaneous fistula. In: Holzheimer RG, Mannick JA, eds. Surgical Treatment-Evidence-Based and Problem-Oriented, 2001:134–139.
15. Vrijland WW, Tseng LN, Eijkman HJ, et al. Fewer intraperitoneal adhesions with use of hyaluronic acid-carboxymethylcellulose membrane: a randomized clinical trial. Ann Surg 2002;235:193–199.

Index